Healing
Fixers
Mixers
& Elixirs

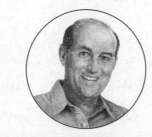

www.jerrybaker.com

Other Jerry Baker Books:

Jerry Baker's Grow Younger, Live Longer!
Healing Remedies Hiding in Your Kitchen
Jerry Baker's Cure Your Lethal Lifestyle
Jerry Baker's Top 25 Homemade Healers
Jerry Baker's Supermarket Super Remedies
Jerry Baker's The New Healing Foods
Jerry Baker's Anti-Pain Plan
Jerry Baker's Oddball Ointments and Powerful Potions
Jerry Baker's Giant Book of Kitchen Counter Cures

Grandma Putt's Green Thumb Magic
Jerry Baker's The New Impatient Gardener
Jerry Baker's Supermarket Super Gardens
Jerry Baker's Bug Off!
Jerry Baker's Terrific Garden Tonics!
Jerry Baker's Giant Book of Garden Solutions
Jerry Baker's Backyard Problem Solver
Jerry Baker's Green Grass Magic
Jerry Baker's Great Green Book of Garden Secrets
Jerry Baker's Old-Time Gardening Wisdom

Jerry Baker's Backyard Birdscaping Bonanza
Jerry Baker's Backyard Bird Feeding Bonanza
Jerry Baker's Year-Round Bloomers
Jerry Baker's Flower Garden Problem Solver
Jerry Baker's Perfect Perennials!

Jerry Baker's Vital Vinegar Cookbook "Cures"
Jerry Baker's Live Rich, Spend Smart, and Enjoy Your Retirement
Jerry Baker's Vinegar: The King of All Cures!
Jerry Baker's Fix It Fast and Make It Last
Jerry Baker's Solve It with Vinegar!
America's Best Practical Problem Solvers
Jerry Baker's Homespun Magic
Grandma Putt's Old-Time Vinegar, Garlic, and 101 More Problem Solvers
Jerry Baker's Supermarket Super Products
Jerry Baker's It Pays to be Cheap

To order any of the above, or for more information on Jerry Baker's amazing home,
health, and garden tips, tricks, and tonics, please write to:

Jerry Baker, P.O. Box 1001, Wixom, MI 48393

Or, visit Jerry Baker online at: **jerrybaker.com**

Healing
Fixers
Mixers
& Elixirs

352 Do-It-Yourself Natural Formulas for a Healthier and More Beautiful You!

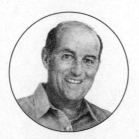

by Jerry Baker

Published by American Master Products, Inc.

NOTICE—All efforts have been made to ensure accuracy. This is a reference volume only, not a medical manual. Although the information presented may help you make informed decisions about your health, it is not intended as a substitute for prescribed medical treatment. If you have a medical problem, please seek competent medical help immediately. Jerry Baker assumes no responsibility or liability for any injuries, damages, or losses incurred during the use of or as a result of following this information.

Herbal research is still in its infancy, and the interaction between herbs and pharmaceutical products remains largely unknown. Herbal remedies and nutraceuticals can have effects similar to those of pharmaceutical products. As a result, they are not without risk. They can interact with each other or with conventional medications, and some people may experience an allergic reaction or other adverse effects when starting an herbal or nutraceutical regimen. That's why you should always check with your doctor before you use them.

Women who are pregnant or breastfeeding and children under age 18 should not use herbal or nutraceutical products without their doctor's specific recommendation.

IMPORTANT—Study all directions carefully before taking any action based on the information and advice presented in this book. When using any commercial product, always read and follow label directions. When reference is made to any trade or brand name, no endorsement by Jerry Baker is implied, nor is any discrimination intended.

Executive Editor: Kim Adam Gasior
Managing Editor: Cheryl Winters-Tetreau
Research and Writer: Zach Gasior
Copy Editor: Nanette Bendyna
Production Editor: Debby Duvall
Interior Design and Layout: Sandy Freeman
Indexer: Nan Badgett

Publisher's Cataloging-in-Publication
(Provided by Quality Books, Inc.)

Baker, Jerry.
    Healing fixers, mixers, & elixirs : 352
do-it-yourself natural formulas for a healthier and more
beautiful you! / Jerry Baker.
      p. cm.
      Includes index.
      ISBN-13: 978-0-922433-01-8
      ISBN-10: 0-922433-01-1

    1. Health. 2. Beauty, Personal. I. Title.
II. Title: Healing fixers, mixers, and elixirs.

RA776.B35 2011   613
       QBI11-600017

Printed in the United States of America
14 16 15 13 hardcover

CONTENTS

PART TWO
A More Beautiful You!

INTRODUCTION

Have you ever shelled out big bucks for an over-the-counter drug that delivered side effects you hadn't bargained for—and maybe didn't help your condition at all? Have you ever fallen for an ad that promised a certain pricey cosmetic would shave years off your appearance—only to find that it didn't make you look even five minutes younger, and furthermore, it irritated your skin? If you're like most folks I know, the answer to both of those questions is "You bet—and way too often!"

Well, friends, it's time to stop spending your hard-earned money on health and beauty aids that frequently do little more than clutter up your bathroom. In this book, I've gathered scads of my favorite remedies, routines, tonics, and toddies that'll cure whatever ails you and yours—with no unpleasant side effects. Plus, I've included scores of grooming aids and beauty treatments that will keep your whole family looking great—with none of the harsh chemicals you find in many commercial products.

This book is chock-full of miraculous methods, timely tricks, and potent potions that will help you solve problems ranging from acne to anemia, earaches to eye bags, and tired feet to toothaches. Many of these sensational solutions are as old as the hills. (For instance, you'll learn a centuries-old secret for easing arthritis pain using—believe it or not—a cabbage leaf.) Others are more recent "discoveries" by scientists who are finding more proof every day that Mother Nature's cure-alls really *do* work. Just one example: Studies show that you can actually improve your memory by eating plenty of foods that are rich in antioxidants, such as oranges, broccoli, carrots, and blueberries.

But wait—that's not all! You'll also find fantastic features like *What Would Grandma Do?*, where you'll learn some of this amazing lady's tried-and-true techniques for stopping nosebleeds, soothing painful hangnails, removing stubborn splinters, curing the common cold—and much, much more.

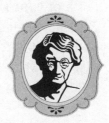

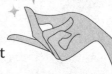

In *Eureka!*, I'll clue you in on a whole bunch of brainstorms that will make you sit up and say, "Why didn't I think of that?!" Sneak preview: One of the easiest ways in the world to prevent wrinkles is simply to wear great big sunglasses every single time you go outdoors—thereby avoiding both radiation damage, which occurs even when the sun's not shining, and the constant muscle contractions that form those crinkles around your eyes.

Snappy Solutions and *Nifty, Thrifty Tips* include fast, fun, and foolproof ideas for improving your health and good looks while conserving two resources that, for most of us, are in mighty short

supply these days: time and money. Just to whet your appetite, you'll learn how to relieve asthma symptoms, beat the blahs, whiten your teeth, soothe chapped lips, and soften your skin using common foods that you probably have in your kitchen right now.

And in *Take My Advice*, readers ask for help and I give my take on solving their various vexing predicaments, ranging from itchy skin to muscle cramps, and a whole lot in between.

Finally, *Dial a Doc* tells you when you need to set home remedies aside and get professional medical help—fast. Even Grandma Putt didn't have all the answers, so don't hesitate to seek your doctor's advice.

Before we get started, though, there's a little fine print (isn't there usually?). Even though all the formulas in this book contain only pure, natural ingredients, it's not possible to predict an individual person's reactions to a particular recipe or treatment. And there is always a chance you could be allergic or sensitive to one or more of them. So if you're the least bit uncertain about the ingredients in an oral remedy, check with your doctor. And always test any topical mixer on a small patch of your skin before you proceed with a full-scale treatment.

Also, remember that this book is not intended to replace your doctor's expert advice. What it will do is show you how to put my all-natural fixers, mixers, and elixirs to work solving common health and beauty problems—and gain a lifetime of good health and good looks in the process!

Part One

Here's to Good Health!

I think it's safe to say that we all agree with the old saying, "When you've got your health, you've got everything." Unfortunately, it's probably also safe to say that few of us even think about how well our bodies are working until something goes wrong—you reach out to pick a flower and get stung by a bee (ouch!); you bend over to pick up a box and wrench your back (yikes!); you help yourself to an extra slice or two of pepperoni pizza (urp!) and wind up with a nasty case of heartburn.

Of course, it's not only our bodies that can get out of kilter. Our minds and spirits are prone to their own kinds of trouble and woe. For example, we all lose track of our car keys or reading glasses every now and then, but when "Where did I put those . . . ?" becomes a daily mantra, it could be a sign that the old gray cells are not exactly cookin' on high, as my Grandma Putt used to say. Then there are times when, for no apparent reason, you catch a case of the blues that just won't quit. Or maybe work pressure (or the lack of work) has sent your stress level soaring higher than a kite.

In this section, I'll share some of my favorite natural fixers, mixers, and elixirs for dozens of aches, pains, burdens, and bothers—physical as well as mental. Plus, because we all know (or *should* know!) that prevention is the best cure for any ailment, I'll let you in on scads of super secrets for heading off those same ills before they put a damper on your day.

A Seedy Solution

There are scads of remedies for acid reflux disease, but for my money, this quick fixer is one of the most effective. It's provided relief to generations of sufferers, and it can help you, too!

Coriander seeds
Cumin seeds
Sugar

➡ Combine equal parts of the coriander, cumin, and sugar. Twice a day, after breakfast and dinner, put 2 teaspoons of the mixture into a glass of cool water, and sip slowly. You'll feel better fast!

Vim and Vinegar

■ As strange as it may seem to drink an acid to get rid of an acidic problem, for some people apple cider vinegar is one of the most effective cures for reflux disease. It's a simple recipe—just add 2 teaspoons of apple cider vinegar to an 8-ounce glass of water, and drink one glass of the water three times a day. Increase the vinegar to 3 teaspoons or so if you're taking the elixir immediately following a heavy meal. **Note:** For this treatment to work, you need to use unprocessed apple cider vinegar from a health-food store, not the filtered kind from the supermarket.

Nifty, Thrifty Tips

Turmeric, the spice that gives curry its distinctive flavor, can help support fat digestion and ease acid reflux. You can buy turmeric capsules at health-food stores, but it's easy (and a whole lot cheaper) to make your own. Just get some gel capsules at the drugstore and fill them with turmeric powder. Make sure you buy the powder in bulk, at either a health-food store or your local supermarket. It'll cost you a fraction of the price you'd pay for the fancy bottled brands—and it'll be much fresher to boot.

Papaya Acid Reflux Reducer

Millions of Americans have heartburn, but taking antacids and other drugs may not be effective and can often cause side effects. A natural way to reduce acid reflux and soothe indigestion and gassiness is to drink a cup of this exotic elixir.

1 cup of papaya juice
1 tsp. of organic sugar
2 pinches of ground
    cardamom

➡ Pour yourself a glass of papaya juice and add the organic sugar and cardamom. Stir the mixture, and sip it slowly to calm your rumbling stomach. Like papaya, cardamom aids digestion and reduces gas and cramping. Your stomach (and peace of mind) will thank you.

Grandma's Marshmallow Tea

■ Marshmallow tea, a reflux remedy that must be used by half the world's grandmothers, soothes the gastrointestinal tract all the way through, from beginning to end. To make the mixture, soak 1 heaping tablespoon of marshmallow root in 1 quart of cold water overnight. Strain, and drink throughout the day to soothe your aching gut.

Forget the Fat

■ High-fat meals stay in the stomach longer than low-fat meals do, and as a result, they cause more acid to accumulate, which slows down the digestive process. If you follow a sensible diet that's low in fats, moderate in proteins, and high in complex carbohydrates (which are easily digested), you won't have problems.

Snappy Solutions

Instead of buying antacids for your acid reflux, try this little sleep remedy. Elevate the head of your bed on 6-inch blocks, or sleep on a special foam rubber wedge to allow gravity to minimize the reflux of your stomach contents into your esophagus. You can find a variety of wedges at drugstores and medical-supply shops.

Anti-Allergy Juice

A lot of allergy sufferers I know swear by this jewel-toned sipper as an effective—and delicious—treatment for their seasonal woes. What's more, besides helping to relieve your runny nose, weepy eyes, and other allergy symptoms, it's chock-full of vitamins that will fine-tune your whole internal system.

3 carrots
½ beet with greens
½ cucumber

➡ Wash the vegetables thoroughly, cut them into sections about 1 inch by ½ inch, and process them in your juicer (either all together or separately, depending on the size of the container). Drink two to three 8-ounce glasses of the combo a day.

Travel with Life Support

■ Anaphylaxis (which causes swelling of the airways and other symptoms) occurs when the body is overwhelmed by its immune response to an allergen—typically fish, peanuts, bee or wasp venom, contact with latex (gloves or balloons), or drugs such as penicillin and aspirin. It goes without saying (I hope!) that if you know you're allergic to any of these substances, you'll do your level best to avoid them. But don't take chances: Always carry Benadryl® and ask your doctor about self-injectable epinephrine (such as an EpiPen®), which can stave off the allergic response until you can get to the hospital for further treatment.

✚ If you have throat tightening; tingling or swelling of the lips or mouth; shortness of breath, wheezing, or light-headedness, dial 911 immediately. You may be having an anaphylactic reaction—a potentially fatal, whole-body allergic response in which histamines flood your mucous membranes with fluid that can swell your throat and airways, shut off your breathing, and even stop your heart.

Dial a Doc

Ragweed Reliever

It's not surprising that Mother Nature provides her own springtime solutions just as allergy season rolls around. Try these spring greens and flowers to make the best remedy for allergy relief.

➡ Pick the herbs, and before they wilt, steep ¼ cup of them in the water overnight. Strain and then drink the tea throughout the day. **Caution:** Use gloves when handling fresh nettles to avoid being stung. Steeping them will remove their sting.

Cleavers
Elderflowers
Eyebright
Nettles
1 qt. of water

Seal the Perimeter

■ During pollen season, keep the windows of your car and house closed, and stay in air-conditioned spaces whenever possible. Be cautious during early-morning hours because pollen counts are at their highest between 5 a.m. and 10 a.m. Never hang your clothes outside to dry, where they can collect pollen, and wash your hair every night to keep from contaminating your pillowcase.

Mask Your Mug

■ Don't leave home without it . . . a face mask, that is! There was a time when seeing masked people jogging, dusting, or mowing the lawn would make us think that aliens had landed, but not anymore. These inexpensive masks (available at any drugstore) are a great way to protect airways from allergy overload.

Q: *I have a runny nose and sore throat. Is it allergies or just a cold?*

A: Check the color of the mucus that you are sneezing and coughing up. If it's on the thick side with a yellow or greenish color, you've probably got a cold. With allergies, your mucus is usually thin and colorless.

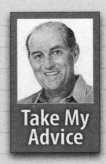

Take My Advice

Sniff Away Sniffles Solution

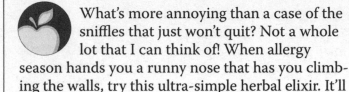

What's more annoying than a case of the sniffles that just won't quit? Not a whole lot that I can think of! When allergy season hands you a runny nose that has you climbing the walls, try this ultra-simple herbal elixir. It'll have you breathing easier in no time at all.

Eucalyptus
Rosemary
1 cup of boiling water

➡ Put 1 tablespoon each of the fresh herbs into the water, place a towel over your head to make a tent, and sniff the fumes for five minutes. (Be careful not to scald your face—lower it slowly over the steam.)

Move Mites Out

■ Dust mites are major allergens, and since they love to sleep in your bed, wash your bedding often. They live in feather as well as synthetic pillows, but you can wash the synthetic versions frequently to drown the little buggers.

Honey, Please Pass the Pollen

■ Bee pollen and locally made honey have long been touted as allergy preventives. By eating them before allergy season hits, you ingest minute amounts of the plants, grasses, and trees that may be the cause of your allergies. This stimulates your immune system and may increase your resistance to pollen, thereby lessening the severity of your allergies when the season is in full swing. A typical dose is 1 teaspoon of honey per day. **Caution:** Never give honey to children under 1 year of age.

What Would Grandma Do?

🦋 GRANDMA PUTT's *favorite hay fever treatment still works wonders for me. Soak a washcloth in the hottest water you can stand, wring it out, and lay it across your nose and sinuses. If you keep the cloth as hot as you can, it seems to work on the same principle as hot soup or spicy food: It loosens and liquefies mucus.*

Dandy Dandelion Tea

Lawn lovers may curse pesky dandelions, but these weeds are super sources of iron and they're gentle on the liver. This tasty tea is a fine way to fend off anemia— or just about anything else that ails you.

2 tsp. of fresh dandelion roots and leaves
½ cup of spring water

➡ Put the roots and leaves into the water. Bring the water to a boil, then remove the pan from the heat and let the mixture steep for 15 minutes. Make a cup three times a day and drink to your good health! **Caution:** Use only dandelion plants that you know have not been treated with pesticides or other chemicals.

Try a New Wrinkle

■ Dried fruits, including figs, dates, prunes, and raisins, but especially peaches and apricots, are rich in iron. And it's easy to work them into your daily diet. Grab a handful at snack time, bake them into breads, muffins, and cookies, or use them in entrees (chicken, turkey, and fish recipes lend themselves especially well to fruity ingredients).

Q: *A friend of mine insists that you can get all the iron you need just by eating food that's cooked in old-fashioned cast-iron pots. Isn't that just an old wives' tale?*

Take My Advice

A: Yes and no. You probably won't get *all* the iron you need that way. But it is true that if you cook tomatoes and other acidic foods in iron pots, you more than double the iron you take in. The iron may discolor some foods, but it won't affect the taste. Experts, however, say the iron from cast-iron cookware doesn't get absorbed into your body quite as well as iron that comes directly from foods.

Start at the Root

When a doctor diagnoses iron-deficiency anemia, it means that you're not getting enough iron in your diet or that your body isn't absorbing iron well. Mineral-rich herbs can boost your iron levels, so use one or more of these herbs in a tea.

Dried alfalfa leaf
Dried dandelion root
Dried yellow dock root
1 cup of boiling water

➡ Steep 1 heaping teaspoon of a mixture of the herbs in the water for 20 minutes. Drink 1 cup two or three times per day to boost your iron intake.

Strawberry Tea

■ Strawberry leaves are berry, berry good for treating anemia. Pick a bunch of fresh leaves and crush about 3 teaspoons of them, or use 1 teaspoon of dried leaves. Place them in 1 cup of boiling water. Let steep for five minutes, scoop out the leaves, and enjoy the tea!

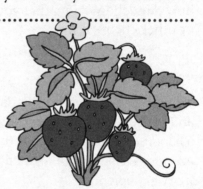

Lemon Lifter

■ Try spicing up leafy greens with vinegar. Acidic condiments like vinegar and lemon juice help liberate minerals when sprinkled on greens, making the iron they're loaded with more easily absorbed by your body.

Nifty, Thrifty Tips

Blackstrap for breakfast! The syrupy substance that remains after sugarcane is processed—blackstrap molasses—is a rich source of iron. Slather blackstrap on whole-grain bread for breakfast, or stir it into oatmeal. If you don't mind the taste, you can simply swallow 2 tablespoons of blackstrap molasses a day, or stir it into a cup of hot water for iron-rich tea. This amount contains about 10 milligrams of iron—nearly 40 percent of the daily requirement—and just 85 calories.

A Treat for Your Feet

Warm footbaths help erase your cares and pamper your soul. So the next time you feel your anxiety level rising, mix up a basin of this soothing soak.

½ cup of Epsom salts
Fresh lavender or lemon balm

➡ Add the Epsom salts and a sprig or two of the lavender or lemon balm to a basin of warm water. Then sit back in a comfortable chair, ease your feet into the relaxing elixir, and soak your troubles away. **Caution:** If you have diabetes, check with your doctor before soaking your feet in anything.

Lose the Lattes

■ Drinking more than five caffeinated beverages a day boosts lactate, a substance that can induce anxiety in people who are panic-prone. Caffeine also influences noradrenaline, a chemical messenger that induces arousal. Here's a simple fix: Switch to decaf. By the way, sugar also tends to increase anxiety levels, so if your daily beverage of choice is a sugary soft drink, trade it in for water or natural fruit juice.

Pray

■ When your panic level is soaring off the charts, close your eyes, take a deep breath, and admit that it's all just too much. Then ask that all the anxiety and fear be lifted from your shoulders. Believe it or not, it will be.

EUREKA!

PASSIONFLOWER IS TAILOR-MADE for hyped-up people with thumping hearts. But don't bother buying the passionflower soda you see in the stores these days. It doesn't contain enough of the active ingredients to relieve your anxiety. Instead, pick up some passionflower extract at a health-food store. Add 20 to 40 drops to a glass of water, and drink two to three glasses a day. **Caution:** Don't use passionflower if you're pregnant or think you might be.

Gratitude Tea

When worries start a-brewin', sip some chamomile tea. Studies show that this feel-good fixer blocks anxiety-boosting brain chemicals that are triggered by worry.

1 tsp. of dried
    chamomile flowers
1 cup of spring water
Honey

➡ Place the chamomile in a cup and fill it with just-boiled water. Cover the mixture and let it steep for 15 minutes or so. Add honey to taste. As you sip the cooled beverage, allow your worries to slip away. **Caution:** If you're allergic to ragweed or other members of the daisy family, don't take chamomile.

Shift Your Focus

◼ When panic rises in the midst of a crowd, cast your thoughts on something else—*anything* else! Wiggle your toes in your shoes. Read a nearby sign. Fumble for your keys. Ask someone for directions (even if you're not going anywhere). Focusing on concrete, familiar objects and activities keeps your anxiety from commandeering your thoughts—and building up to an all-out panic attack.

Fish for Serenity

◼ Salmon, tuna, and sardines are filled with omega-3 fatty acids, which can improve your mood. There's just one catch: For these essential fatty acids to have any effect, you need to eat fish three times a week. If you can't find a fish that suits your fancy, get the same results by taking 1 gram of fish oil in capsules. Look for fish oil that's been certified free of pesticides and heavy metals.

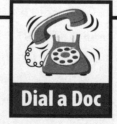

Dial a Doc

✚ If chronic anxiety is seriously limiting the way you live your life, seek help from a mental health professional. You may need cognitive therapy to give you a different way to think about things that happen, talk therapy to address why you're panicking in the first place, or a prescription, such as alprazolam (Xanax), to block the fight-or-flight response and calm your body and mind.

Minty Syrup Sweetener

I must admit that some herbal potions, as life-enhancing as they may be for body and soul, taste absolutely awful—or at best, not exactly what you want when you're already feeling in less than tip-top form, either physically or emotionally. Well, this sweet fixer will take care of that!

1 cup of sugar (or honey)
2 cups of water
6 sprigs of fresh peppermint or spearmint leaves (or mix 'em!)
Zest from 1 small lemon or orange

➡ Heat the sugar and water in a pan, stirring until the sugar is dissolved. Add the mint leaves and citrus zest. Remove the pan from the heat and let the syrup steep for about 30 minutes. Strain out the herbs and pour the liquid into a container with a lid. Stir a teaspoon of the syrup into your next healing elixir; it'll satisfy even the sweetest tooth. Store leftover syrup in the fridge for up to a week.

Confront Your Fears

■ Each time you leave an event in panic or avoid a situation because you're anxious about it, it becomes that much easier to let your fears run your life. But the opposite is also true: Each time you confront your fears, it becomes easier to strip them of their power. The next time you feel anxious, assure yourself, "I may be frightened, but I'm not in danger. I'm not having a heart attack; my heart is simply beating fast."

Snappy Solutions

If the thought of making cup after cup of tea tries your patience to the limit, make your herbal elixirs by the quart instead. Then put the container into the refrigerator, where the brew will keep for three to four days, or freeze it in ice cube trays or plastic cups. Unless the recipe instructions specifically say to reheat the potion, it'll work the same magic whether you warm it up, drink it cold, or eat it like an ice pop. Whatever you do, though, don't let herbal tea sit at room temperature for any length of time—within a few hours, it'll start to go sour.

Pleasing Poppy Potion

This excellent elixir will chill you out without stressing your system. In fact, it's so gentle, you can give it to infants and children at bedtime to soothe away the cares of the day.

1 part fresh California poppy flowers
1 part fresh chamomile flowers
1 part oat straw (the milky green tops)
½ part fresh marshmallow root flowers

➡ Combine the herbs in a heat-proof bowl or teapot. Boil 1 cup of water per tablespoon of herbs (or 1 quart of water per ounce of herbs if you want to make the potion in quantity). Pour the water over the herbs, and let the mixture steep for 30 to 60 minutes. Strain out the solids, and drink as much of the brew as often as you feel the need.

Ix-Nay the What-Ifs

■ Are you a worrywart, constantly mulling over a long list of "what-ifs" for every situation? For instance, let's say you worry, "What if the bus crashes?" To nip your anxiety in the bud, simply counteract your concern with hard facts. Ask yourself, "What's the probability of being in a bus crash?" Then answer, "Unless I'm an extra in the next *Speed* sequel, it has to be pretty low." In other words, talk yourself free of your spiraling emotions—talking back to the negative chatter inside your head can, in some cases, be every bit as effective as taking anti-anxiety drugs.

Nifty, Thrifty Tips

When you're feeling anxious, the last thing you need is some brainless chucklehead droning on about healthcare, socialism, Middle East politics, etc. So no matter what radio or TV talk shows you listen to, or what the subject is, turn off that non-stop chatter, and either slip a Mozart disc into your CD player, or turn your radio dial to a classical music station. According to at least one study, listening to 30 minutes of classical music can be as calming as 10 milligrams of diazepam (Valium)—and it won't cost you a dime.

Skullcap Soother

 Skullcap is a fabulous anti-anxiety herb. Combine equal parts of these herbs to soothe your stress away.

Dried lemon balm
Dried oat straw
Dried skullcap
1 cup of boiling water

➡ Add 1 heaping teaspoon of the herb mixture to the water. Steep for 10 minutes, strain, and drink twice a day.

Get Regular Exercise

■ Exercise will work off pounds. But it'll also chip away at stress and anxiety. That's because when you exercise, your brain releases endorphins that have a calming effect. So take a walk or a run, hop on your bike, or dance the night away. Anything that gets you moving will help. And increasing your heart rate because of exercise rather than anxiety will make you feel more in control.

Lovely Lavender

■ A few drops of lavender oil added to your body lotion can be a source of anxiety-preventing aromatherapy all day long. For a more dramatic effect, add a drop of lavender oil to a dab of your favorite salve, and rub it into your temples or solar plexus (stomach) for a reminder to relax and breathe deeply.

EUREKA!

AS ANXIETY SETS IN, you tend to breathe more shallowly, and this makes you even more anxious. So the next time you're feeling panicky, try breathing with your diaphragm the way singers and yoga practitioners do—with long, slow, deep breaths. Put your hand on your stomach. If it expands like a balloon, you're breathing properly. Now breathe in deeply to the count of 4, hold your breath to the count of 8, and exhale to the count of 7. Repeat the exercise four times, and you should feel much calmer.

Anti-Arthritis Clover Tea

Now, please understand that clover won't cure arthritis, but if you start the day with a cup of clover tea, it'll go a long way toward easing some of your aches and pains.

1 tsp. of dried alfalfa leaves
1 tsp. of dried
    red clover blossoms
1 cup of boiling water

➡ Add the herbs to the water, steep for five minutes, strain out the herbs, and sip away. Add a teaspoon of honey if you want to sweeten it up a bit. **Caution:** Alfalfa and red clover should be avoided when taking warfarin (Coumadin).

Dust Off the Old Schwinn

■ One of the best ways to control arthritis is to strengthen the thigh muscles that support the knee. The best kind of exercises for this are non-weight-bearing ones, like riding a bicycle. So roll your old bike out of the garage, and pedal around the neighborhood for as long as your legs feel comfortable.

Warm Up with a Walk

■ When you sit still, the synovial fluid between your joints can become as stiff as molasses in a Wyoming winter. Although you may not feel like walking when your joints are stiff, it's actually the ideal way to keep the synovial fluid warm and flowing—and your weight in check so you don't overload your joints.

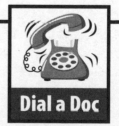

Dial a Doc

✚ The U.S. Food and Drug Administration estimates that anywhere from 10,000 to 20,000 Americans with arthritis accidentally kill themselves with nonsteroidal anti-inflammatory drugs (NSAIDs) every year in an attempt to ease their pain. Believe it or not, this is more than the number of people who overdose on heroin! So if your pain doesn't ease with your regular dosage of an NSAID, *don't take any more!* Ask your doctor for a more effective pain medication instead.

Arthritis Hand Pain Remedy

 When arthritis in your hands flares up, sip a glass of cider vinegar tea for fast, soothing relief. You'll be back to business in no time.

➡ Pour the ingredients into a glass, mix well, and then sip and enjoy.

**2 parts honey
1 part apple cider
vinegar
Warm water**

Flatten Pain with Fruit

■ Raisins, pears, apples, and other fruits, as well as nuts and beans, all contain the trace element boron, which can relieve pain and joint stiffness and actually appears to protect against arthritis. If you don't eat fruit on a regular basis or don't live in a particularly arid area (where concentrations of boron in the soil and water are highest), consider taking a daily multivitamin supplement that provides 1 to 3 milligrams of boron. **Caution:** Higher than indicated doses of boron can cause nausea, vomiting, and skin rashes.

Turn the Pain Around

■ Sometimes, you can help counteract the crippling effect of rheumatoid arthritis simply by turning a doorknob differently. Why? Because arthritis causes more damage to the outside of your wrist joint (the side with the pinkie finger), making it difficult to turn a doorknob to the left with your left hand, for example. So switch hands and open doors by turning the knob the opposite way with your right hand, and vice versa with your left.

What Would Grandma Do?

🦋 WHENEVER MY GRANDMA PUTT'S *arthritic knee started acting up, she went to the garden and cut a head of cabbage. Cabbage leaves have been used for centuries to soothe inflammation, and a sturdy outer leaf is just the right shape to place over a bent knee or elbow. Blanch a leaf or two, then apply it, either warm or cool, to inflamed joints. Wrap it in gauze or an elastic bandage to hold it in place.*

Healing Ginger Tea

 Ginger is a powerful anti-inflammatory—just what you need to take the edge off arthritis pain.

1 cup of water
1 tsp. of grated fresh ginger
Honey, to taste

➡ Boil the water, pour it into a mug, and stir in the ginger. Steep for 10 to 15 minutes, then strain. Sweeten the tea with honey. Drink 2 cups a day, and your knees may soon begin to feel as nimble as that other famous Ginger's.

Echinacea Antidote

◼ If you start to feel the old aches and pains of your arthritis creeping in during the day, try making this excellent echinacea antidote. In a stainless steel saucepan, mix 3 teaspoons of fresh echinacea root and 1 cup of water. Bring the mixture to a boil, and let it simmer for 10 minutes. Strain, then sip. **Caution:** If you have an autoimmune disease, such as rheumatoid arthritis, lupus, or multiple sclerosis, consult your doctor before taking echinacea.

Add Some Arnica

◼ To soothe aching joints, add a few drops of arnica oil to your favorite healing salve. Try using a warming wintergreen, lavender, or rosemary salve as a base, since all three can help increase circulation to the painful area. Just add 3 or 4 drops of arnica oil to every ½ teaspoon of salve. Rub it into your joints three or four times each day. But be careful: Arnica is for external use only and shouldn't be used on broken skin.

Nifty, Thrifty Tips

Some research has found that if you drink five or more cups of coffee a day, you increase your risk of developing rheumatoid arthritis. Other research disputes this claim. Either way, if you have arthritis and you are a heavy coffee drinker, try cutting back and see how you feel. You'll save the money you normally spend on your a.m. java jolt, and you just might save your joints.

Herbal Aspirin

 Doctors usually recommend aspirin or other anti-inflammatory drugs to ease the pain of common osteoarthritis. But here's a homemade elixir that may give you the same soothing relief. **Caution:** If you've been diagnosed with rheumatoid arthritis or any other autoimmune condition, substitute devil's claw for the echinacea, and follow the same instructions.

1 cup of water
3 tsp. of powdered chamomile flowers
2 tsp. of powdered echinacea root
2 tsp. of ground ginger
1 tsp. of powdered meadowsweet leaves and flower tops
Honey and/or lemon (optional)

➡ Boil the water and pour it into a mug. Add the herbs and stir well. Let steep for 10 to 20 minutes. Add honey and/or lemon as desired. Drink up to 3 cups a day, or if you're over 65, 2 cups. **Caution:** Don't take chamomile if you're allergic to ragweed.

Egg It On

■ This vintage mixer has brought quick relief to generations of arthritis sufferers: Just blend 2 egg whites, ½ cup of apple cider vinegar, and ¼ cup of olive oil in a bowl, and massage the lotion into your painful parts. (Don't get the lotion on clothing, sheets, or furniture!) Wipe off the excess with a soft cotton cloth.

Shed the Excess Baggage

■ Arthritis pain is more intense and gets worse more rapidly in people who are overweight. By simply losing 5 to 10 pounds you'll lighten the load considerably on all your weight-bearing joints—hips, knees, ankles, and feet.

What Would Grandma Do?

🦋 *If* ARTHRITIC FINGERS *make it hard for you to grip a pen, this trick from Grandma Putt will make it easier: Find a tube-shaped, foam hair curler, shove the pen through the opening, and scribble to your heart's content (or at least until you've finished your shopping list).*

Marvelous Mustard Rub

Whenever painful arthritic joints prevent you from falling asleep at night, call on this oh-so-warming mixer at bedtime.

½ tsp. of ground ginger
¼ tsp. of dry mustard
1 tbsp. of olive oil or sesame oil

➥ Mix the ginger and mustard with the oil, and dab a drop on the bend of your arm to test for irritation. Wait 10 minutes, and if your skin shows no reaction, rub the mixture into your afflicted body parts until you feel a warm, tingling sensation. Wrap strips of clean, soft cotton fabric (such as pieces cut from an old T-shirt or flannel sheet) around the oiled area to protect your sheets, and go to bed. Before you know it, you'll be drifting off to dreamland. Come morning, wash the rub off, lathering well to make sure you get rid of all the residue.

Sassy Sassafras

■ A whole lot of folks I know swear by this old-time fixer for arthritis—and rheumatism, too: Steep 3 tablespoons of sassafras root in a fifth of whiskey (any kind will do) for two weeks. Take 1 tablespoon three times a day before meals. (You can find sassafras root in health-food stores.)

Give Pain Relief the Green Light

■ Fend off arthritis pain by drinking plenty of green tea. Medical studies show that it contains the strongest known form of antioxidants and that consuming 4 to 6 cups a day seems to reduce the incidence of rheumatoid arthritis and all kinds of other nasty conditions, including heart disease and cancer.

Nifty, Thrifty Tips

You can spend a lot of time, money, and energy trying different ways to relieve arthritis pain and stiffness. But you may be able to solve the problem quickly (and deliciously) with this old-time remedy: Just eat 15 to 20 sweet bing cherries every day. Before you know it, you could be moving smoothly again.

Power-Packed Pain Reliever

When you've got a full day of activities planned and not a whole lot of time to complete them, the last thing you need is arthritis pain putting a crimp in your schedule. For a quick fix, combine equal parts of these herbs to make a mellow mixer. Then sip it to ease the aches during painful flare-ups.

Dried black cohosh
Dried devil's claw
Ground ginger
Dried passionflower
1 cup of boiling water

➡ Add 1 teaspoon of the herb mixture to the water. Steep, covered, for 20 minutes, and then strain. Drink a cup two or three times a day.

Put Cold on Heat

■ When an arthritic joint is inflamed, it may be painful, swollen, or even feel hot. If so, then put out the fire with ice. Place an ice pack on the sore joint for no more than 20 minutes at a time. Repeat the treatment once an hour, continuing for as long as it seems to help.

Warm the Stiffness

■ When your joints are stiff and achy, but there's no swelling, heat may work better than cold. For one thing, it feels good, and for another, it promotes the flow of healing nutrients into sore joints. Moist heat seems to work best, so you may want to use a warm compress instead of a heating pad. Simply soak a small towel in hot water, wring it out, and drape it over your painful joint. When the towel cools, soak it again, and reapply it as necessary.

EUREKA!

IF YOU'RE LIKE MOST PEOPLE, you probably don't drink enough water. And not drinking enough water may actually make arthritis symptoms worse. So be sure everyone in the family drinks at least eight glasses every day, whether they're actually thirsty or not! Research has proven that by the time you feel thirsty, your body's water levels have already dropped too low.

Raisin Relief

When arthritis pain racks your body, try this remarkable recipe that's safe, natural, and has been around for ages. Lots of folks swear by it, including the late, great radio commentator Paul Harvey.

1 box of yellow raisins
1 pint of gin

➡ Put the raisins in a bowl, add enough gin to cover them completely, and let 'em sit—uncovered—until the liquid is all gone. Transfer the gin-soaked raisins to a closed container, and eat nine a day for blessed relief.

Magnetic Magic

■ Although scientists aren't sure why, studies show that wearing knee wraps embedded with magnets may help you get out of a chair more easily and walk faster and less stiffly. Look for wraps with "unipolar" magnets, then place the positive end of the magnet directly over your sore knee. (Unipolar magnets have only one pole and it's usually negative.) You should feel relief within 30 minutes.

Measure Those High Heels

■ Skinny stilettos are murder on your knees—but they're not the only culprits. In fact, high, wide-heeled pumps or boots may predispose you to osteoarthritis (OA) of the knees, too. The problem, it seems, isn't the stability of the platform but the height of the heel. Women who regularly wear heels higher than 2 inches are twice as likely to develop OA as those who don't. Heels shift your body weight away from your ankles and onto your hips and the inner part of the knee joints, and arthritis of the knee is often the result.

Snappy Solutions

If you're taking a pain reliever for arthritis, down your dose before noon. The pain and inflammation tend to be worse in the late afternoon and evening, so starting your treatment early will help head off trouble.

Wild Yam Arthritis Tamer

The little things you do during your day can put a lot of wear and tear on your joints. A warm cup of this tea works wonders on the aches, pains, and swelling associated with arthritis.

1 oz. of dried wild yam root
1 oz. of dried willow bark
3 pints of water

➡ Place the ingredients in a saucepan on the stove, and allow the mixture to simmer for 20 to 25 minutes. Then strain out the solids, and pour the tea into a pitcher with a lid on it. You can drink this tasty tea hot or cold, up to 3 cups a day. It can also be stored in the refrigerator for up to three days.

Bring On the Heat

■ Capsaicin, the component that makes red peppers hot, helps stop the production of substance P, an inflammatory prostaglandin that's present in arthritic joints. To ease arthritis pain, check your local drugstore for capsaicin cream and apply it directly to inflamed joints three or four times a day for a week. Just be careful not to get it in your eyes or on any areas of broken skin, and wash your hands thoroughly after using it.

Q: *I have arthritis in my hip, but I hate to keep popping pain relievers all day long. What else can I do to relieve the discomfort?*

A: The next time arthritis in your hip flares up, sit comfortably, close your eyes, and slow your breathing. Then imagine that you're running a marathon or doing the rumba with pain-free, swaying hips. Fully conjure this vision and pay attention to all of the details as it runs through your mind. Do it again the next day, and the next. When you repeatedly visualize pain-free scenarios like this, you can reduce discomfort and even improve mobility.

Take My Advice

Cinnamon Stick Tea

This potent tea treats asthma by relaxing your bronchial muscles so you can breathe more freely. (Look for the herbs in health-food stores.)

➥ Mix equal parts of the first four ingredients with a half part of ginger. Add 1 heaping teaspoon of the blend to the water. Bring it to a boil, and simmer, covered, for 15 minutes. Strain, and drink. **Caution:** If you have high blood pressure, eliminate the licorice.

Cinnamon stick
Dates
Licorice root
White peony root
Grated fresh ginger
1 cup of cold water

Say Ohm

■ Yoga is a perfect form of exercise for those with asthma. You'll become stronger and more limber, but more importantly, you'll learn deeper and more efficient breathing techniques. Find a local class led by an experienced teacher.

Kick Butt

■ It turns out that karate isn't just an excellent way to ward off bad guys—it's also a solid defense against asthma attacks. That's because the exclamation that accompanies the powerful kicks forces you to exhale quickly and deeply, so you draw in a deep breath before you continue. And deep, full-lunged breathing (also required when you're walking, running, or swimming) opens airways.

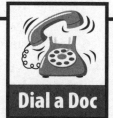

Dial a Doc

✚ Whether you typically have mild, moderate, or severe asthma, if you have wheezing, shortness of breath, or tightness in your chest that doesn't respond to inhaled or oral medications, call 911 and seek medical attention immediately. Other danger signs include difficulty talking, rapid or shallow breathing, flaring nostrils, tightly stretched skin on your neck and/or around your rib cage with each breath, and gray or bluish skin around your mouth or under your fingernails.

Relief from the Vegetable Garden

Believe it or not, one of the simplest and most effective—not to mention healthiest—asthma-relief remedies comes straight from your vegetable garden, or from the produce section of your local supermarket. **Note:** For the ultimate in nutrition and flavor, use veggies that have been grown organically.

4 to 5 carrots
   (greens removed)
2 celery stalks
2 curly endive leaves

➡ Wash the vegetables thoroughly. Cut the carrots and celery into 1-inch-long pieces, and tear the endive leaves into strips. Process the pieces in your juicer, pour the potion into a glass, and drink up. For maximum benefits, drink this and all fresh juices immediately.

Muffle the Cold

■ Asthma is often triggered by very cold air. So when the temps fall below freezing, wear a scarf or mask over your mouth to warm and moisturize the air you breathe. And always carry your quick-relief inhaler with you.

Don't Touch That Vacuum

■ Vacuum cleaners can kick up 2 to 10 times the number of allergens that normally float around your house. The extra onslaught can persist for up to a full hour after you turn off the vac. If you have chronic asthma, look into the special vacuum cleaners that eliminate this dusty "exhaust." (They're expensive but worth it to relieve your lungs.) Or wear a dust mask when you vacuum. Better yet, hire a cleaning service and get out of the house while they work.

Snappy Solutions

Scientific studies have shown that the limonene in citrus peels seems to neutralize inhaled ozone, which often triggers asthma symptoms. So if you feel the early warning signs of an attack, grab the skin of a citrus fruit—any kind will do—and take a sniff.

Triple Your Fun Juice

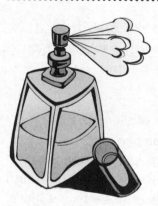 Put a little more punch in your anti-asthma juice arsenal with this variation on the theme. Celery, carrots, and apples all contain important nutrients—especially vitamin A, potassium, and magnesium—that help ease asthma symptoms. That makes this elixir a must in your recipe collection.

4 stalks of celery
2 large carrots, with
　　green tops removed
1 large apple, cored

➡ Wash the vegetables and fruit, and cut them into pieces that fit your juicer. Whirl them into a juice, pour it into a glass, and drink up. **Note**: If you have a sweet tooth, or you're making this juice for a child, use just 3 stalks of celery. For maximum benefits, drink fresh juices immediately.

There's Something in the Air . . .

■ Be aware that some seemingly beneficial aromas may be harmful to a person with asthma. The chemical "perfumes" in room deodorizers, carpet cleaners, and even some cat litters, for example, can set off an attack. To play it safe, always read package labels carefully, and opt for brands that are free of perfumes and dyes. And steer clear of scented candles, incense, and aromatherapy oils.

EUREKA!

THE SON OF a friend of mine had chronic asthma when he was young. His mom believed that if she learned to strengthen his breathing, it would relieve his asthma. So she sent him for clarinet lessons. Not only did all that tooting relieve his asthma, but he's now a talented professional musician! So, if you suffer from asthma, maybe it's time to go blow your horn.

Athlete's Foot Fighter

The best defense against athlete's foot is to keep your feet dry. But since that can't always happen, you can use this fungus-fightin' formula to dry out your feet and fight off the loathsome condition.

20 to 30 garlic cloves, minced
2 to 4 tsp. of ground cinnamon
2 to 4 tsp. of ground cloves
5 oz. of 100-proof vodka
Baking soda

➤ Put the garlic, cinnamon, and cloves in a jar. Add the vodka, seal the jar up tight, and let it sit at room temperature. Keep it out of the sunlight, and shake up the mixture every few days. After two weeks, it'll be ready for use. Apply it to your feet twice a day with cotton balls, then dust your feet with baking soda after they've dried.

Powder Up

■ Wash and thoroughly dry your feet twice daily, then slip 'em into a fresh pair of all-cotton socks sprinkled with baking soda or anti-fungal powder. Wearing cotton right next to your skin allows your feet to breathe and lets any residual moisture evaporate. Dust the insides of your shoes, too, for extra protection.

Expose Yourself

■ Let those tootsies hang out in the fresh air and sunshine if you're not going anywhere. Just don't walk barefoot around the house. Not only will you track powder all over, but you'll also plant contagious fungus seedlings where you go. And you don't want to be known as Johnny Fungusseed, do you?

What Would Grandma Do?

WHEN I CAME DOWN with a bad case of athlete's foot, my Grandma Putt turned to one of her favorite cooking ingredients to kill that nasty fungus—apple cider vinegar! She knew how much fungi hate acids like vinegar, so she would fill a tub with equal parts of apple cider vinegar and warm water and have me soak my feet for 10 minutes every day. You can try the same foot soak for your own problem.

Athlete's Foot Remedy

Anyone can get athlete's foot, even armchair quarterbacks. And the fungus can leave your feet feeling like they're stuck in a raging fire. But you can kick it with a mixer made with these herbs that boost the immune system and fight the fungus from the inside out.

Dried calendula
Dried cleavers
Dried echinacea
Dried oregano
1 cup of boiling water

➡ Combine equal parts of these herbs, and add 1 heaping teaspoon of the mixture to the water. Steep, covered, for 15 minutes. Strain and drink up to 3 cups a day. For mild cases of athlete's foot, you can make an external wash with the same herbs, using ½ cup of the mixture per 1 quart of water. Let the mixture cool to a comfortable temperature, then soak your feet for 15 to 20 minutes, and dry them well.

Take Time for Thyme

■ Soak your itchy feet in hot water to which you've added a few drops of oil of thyme to relieve the itching and burning. Soak until the water cools, pull your feet out, and dust 'em with a mixture of equal parts of myrrh and goldenseal root powder. Then pull on a pair of heavy cotton socks. Repeat this every day until you've ditched the itch. **Caution:** Do not use on sensitive or cracked skin.

Soak Those Piggies

■ To soothe the itch of athlete's foot and start the healing process, place your feet in a basin of warm water spiked with 2 to 3 teaspoons of tea tree oil, and soak for about 15 minutes twice daily. If you have sensitive skin, start with a gentler herb, such as goldenseal, chamomile, or calendula, and go from there.

Nifty, Thrifty Tips

If athlete's foot is making your feet cracked and scaly, skip the expensive healing ointments and invest in an aloe vera plant. This desert native is simply miraculous for healing damaged skin. Just break off a big leaf, squeeze out the gel, and rub it all over your feet.

Toes-ty Garlic Soak

Are your tired old dogs feelin' kind of funky, fungusy, or just plain foul? Well, put your foot down—in a tub of garlic water! Garlic has been scientifically proven to stop fungal infections dead in their tracks.

5 to 6 garlic cloves
Rubbing alcohol
Warm water

➡ Crush the garlic cloves, and drop them in a tub filled with a mixture of warm water and a little rubbing alcohol. Gently place both feet in the tub, and let them soak for about 10 minutes a day. Of course, the garlic footbath may cause your loved ones—and even the family dog—to temporarily steer clear of you! **Caution:** If you have diabetes, you should check with your doctor before trying this garlicky cure.

Season Your Feet

◼ Mamma mia! Try applying a generous film of olive oil to your feet, then placing a clove of raw, peeled garlic between each of your toes every night for a week. Don't bruise or break open the clove because garlic juice can burn your skin. Wear a pair of all-cotton socks to bed, then wash and dry your feet in the morning. Although the smell might force you to sleep alone, this treatment should stop the itch in a hurry. **Caution:** Do not use if you have broken or cracked skin.

Snappy Solutions

Foot soaks are definitely relaxing, and their healing properties are spot-on. But often we just don't have the time during the day to sit down and soak our feet. Instead, work in this quick fix right after something that's already part of your daily routine. If you're prone to athlete's foot, dry each toe separately after you shower. Then use a paper towel between them to absorb every drop of moisture. Or you can use a blow-dryer (set on low) to make sure your tootsies are totally dry. It may sound silly, but it'll feel oh-so-good.

Bad Back Easer

Back pain can be so crippling that it'll spoil your entire day—not to mention a good night's sleep. Relieve the pain with this herbal mixer that's tailor-made to help keep your schedule running smoothly.

Dried chamomile
Dried peppermint
Fresh ginger
1 cup of boiling water

➡ Mix equal parts of chamomile and peppermint together. Add 1 teaspoon of the herb mixture and a ¼-inch slice of ginger to the water. Steep, covered, for 10 minutes. Strain and drink a cup three or four times a day. **Caution:** Do not take chamomile if you have a ragweed allergy.

Don't Sit on Your Wallet

■ That lump of a wallet in your back pocket can damage the nerves in your buttocks, leading to lower back pain and even sciatica. Folks who regularly drive with their wallet in their back pocket seem to be most at risk, so put your wallet in a cup holder or the glove compartment before you hit the road.

Choose Comfortable Shoes

■ If your feet aren't comfortable, your back will suffer. So wear shoes that are suitable for whatever it is you're doing. If you're walking through the countryside or strolling along cobblestone streets, choose an excellent walking shoe that offers good support and flexible soles. Oh, and ladies? Remember that high heels throw your center of gravity out of whack, which wreaks havoc on your back.

When back pain persists without abating for more than three days, it's time to see a doctor. If the pain is accompanied by a fever, pain at night or when resting, or bowel or bladder changes, get to your doctor pronto. You should also see a doctor at the first sign of back pain if you have a history of cancer or diabetes, since it may indicate a tumor or nerve damage.

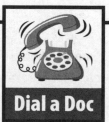

Dial a Doc

Hot Herbal-Tea Toddy

A bad back is not just painful, it can put you out of commission for hours—or even days—at a time. To relieve the agony, combine these herbs to create a great pain-pulverizing elixir.

Fresh ginger
Dried Jamaican dogwood
Dried passionflower
1 cup of boiling water

➡ Combine these herbs in equal parts. For muscle spasms, add skullcap or valerian to the herb mixture. Add 1 teaspoon of the mixture to the water. Steep, covered, for 10 minutes. Drink a cup three to four times a day, and your pain will be gone before you know it

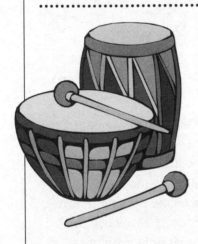

Get Rhythm

■ In some nations, day laborers chant or sing while they do backbreaking work, such as carrying loads of goods on their heads. They've been doing it for centuries, so why not give it a try? Hum if it helps make your movements slow and regular, instead of quick and jerky. And take a lesson from people who carry baskets on their heads by walking in a balanced, undulating rhythm. Remember: Their baskets don't fall—and their backs don't wrench, either.

Snappy Solutions

You'll do your body a lot of good in the long run if you avoid nighttime neck cricks. While your back is usually injured during the day, your neck (the uppermost part of your back) is more often hurt during sleep, when you toss and turn. If you frequently wake up with a stiff neck, discuss it with your doctor—a crick can signal the onset of a cervical disk herniation. Make sure your pillow keeps your neck and back in alignment, and if it doesn't, then buy a new one!

The Ultimate Back Bath

When your back is causing you so much pain that you don't even want to think about standing at the stove simmering herbal concoctions, this tried-and-true muscle-relaxing mixer has your name written all over it. I've used it for years, and take my word for it: Sore-back remedies don't come any simpler—or more effective—than this one. I like to think of it as a liquid mustard plaster.

1 scant handful of dry mustard
1 handful of sea salt

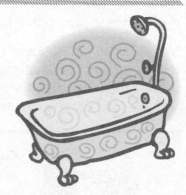

➡ Mix the mustard and sea salt into a tub of water that's as hot as you can stand it. Then ease in, relax, and say "Aaahhh."

Try Herbal Aspirin

■ Willow bark is a natural source of aspirin-like salicylates, which ease pain. But unlike aspirin or ibuprofen, it won't irritate your stomach while it's easing your backache. To make a pain-relieving elixir, pick up some willow bark from a health-food store and steep 2 teaspoons in 1 cup of boiling water, then strain and sip. You can also take willow bark capsules or apply willow bark ointment directly to your back (both are available at health-food stores). Don't use the stuff in any form, however, if you already take aspirin; the double dose of salicylates may be too much for your system.

EUREKA!

SWEEP YOUR BACK SPASMS away with a plain old broomstick. Here's how: First, remove the handle from the head. Next, roll the handle in a towel to pad it, then lie on your back on top of it, lining up your spine along the broomstick. Stay there for five minutes. Gravity will pull your shoulders down and stretch out the muscles around your spine.

Tub Time Tonic

A tub full of warm water is just about the best friend a sore back ever had. When you add this combo of healing herbs, you've got a muscle-soothing fixer that can't be beat.

1 large handful of dried chamomile
1 large handful of dried comfrey root
1 large handful of dried eucalyptus
1 large handful of dried sage
1 qt. of water

➡ Pour the water into a pan, toss in the herbs, and simmer for 15 minutes. Strain out the solids, and add the liquid to a warm bath. Then soak for half an hour or so, and let the aromatic oils in the herbs take your aches and pains down the drain.

Don't Move!
■ After any injury to your back, rest it for one or two days (complete immobility has been shown to worsen back pain, even with acute injury). Put an ice pack on your back for 15 or 20 minutes—or lie on the ice pack if that's easier—then repeat every one to two hours. Don't go beyond 20 minutes, or you may risk frostbite. And don't use a heating pad or hot-water bottle because heat may actually make the pain worse in the early stages after an injury.

Face the Fat Facts
■ Excess weight causes a severe strain on your spine. As your abdomen balloons outward, you pull your spine out of alignment. In other words, a big gut pulls your back out of whack, because you've changed your center of gravity. So let your back pain prompt you to take responsibility for the underlying conditions that caused the problem, such as overeating and avoiding exercise.

✚ Call your doctor instantly if back pain is causing any numbness in your groin or legs, or if you lose control of your bowels or bladder. You could have a serious spinal injury that needs immediate attention.

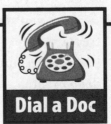

Dial a Doc

Gladder Bladder Tonic

When you've got to go a lot, or you can't go at all, the culprit may be your bladder. If you've got minor bladder and urinary problems, try this herbal elixir to take the edge off of the going.

1 tsp. of dried bearberry (also known as uva ursi) leaves
1 tsp. of dried corn silk
1 tsp. of dried marshmallow root
1 cup of boiling water

➤ Combine the bearberry, corn silk, and marshmallow root, and scoop a teaspoon of the mixture into the water. Let it steep for 15 minutes, strain out the solids, and your tea is ready for sippin'! If your bladder difficulties don't go away within a couple of days, talk to your doctor to make sure they aren't a symptom of a much larger problem.

Make Sure You Can Go

■ Chronic constipation can place pressure on the bladder or pelvic-floor muscles, causing incontinence. If you clear up your constipation, your bladder may stop leaking. So eat more whole-grain cereals and breads and at least two servings of fruit (like prunes) daily. Then help your digestive tract get things moving by heading out for a brisk walk every day.

Q: *No matter what I try, if I feel like I have to go, I go. Is there anything I can do to stop myself from going to the bathroom once an hour?*

A: If you go on your bladder's command, then you're training it to need emptying more frequently. So retrain it! When you have to go, relax the muscles outside your pelvis (like your belly), take deep breaths, and count to 3. Do this every time you have to go, and slowly increase the count to 5, then 15, then 50. Gradually lengthen the interval between bathroom visits to three to four hours.

Take My Advice

Sleepy-Time Bladder Beverage

Getting a good night's sleep can be all but impossible when you have an overactive bladder. One solution to that problem is to consume plenty of foods that are high in tryptophan—like all three of the ingredients in this delicious (and nutritious) smoothie.

1 cup of chopped mango (fresh or frozen)
1 cup of frozen unsweetened tart cherries
1 cup of skim milk

➡ Put all of the ingredients in a blender and puree until smooth. Pour the libation into a glass and drink to good sleep! **Note:** Drinking this tonic at bedtime, however, isn't necessary. Simply getting a good supply of tryptophan throughout the day will help you fall asleep faster and sleep more soundly through the night.

Sleep with Valerian

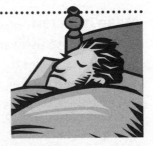

■ This common American plant has a soothing effect on the smooth muscles of the body—and your bladder is actually just one big smooth muscle. So if you find yourself hopping out of bed for bathroom trips every few hours during the night, take one or two valerian capsules before you hit the hay. The herb will gently relax your bladder so you can get a good night's sleep. Look for valerian at your local health-food store, then follow the label directions. **Caution:** Don't take this herb if you're taking antidepressants.

EUREKA!

STUDIES SHOW THAT women who lose 5 percent of their excess body weight—especially if it's bunched around their middles—can reduce their bladder-leaking episodes by more than half. Kick-start your metabolism and shore up your bladder by doing at least 30 minutes of continuous aerobic exercise, such as brisk walking, at least three times a week.

Anti-Retention Wrap

Fluid retention can make your legs feel—and look—like sausages. But this soothing fixer will ease the discomfort and restore your legs' good looks in no time at all.

1 tbsp. of dried peppermint
1 tbsp. of dried yarrow
1 pint of boiling water
Several lengths of gauze,
    muslin, or cheesecloth

➤ Steep the herbs in the water for 15 to 20 minutes. Strain out the solids, and put the liquid in the refrigerator to cool. When the infusion is thoroughly chilled, saturate the cloths with it, then wring them out well and wrap them around your lower legs. Relax with your legs elevated for 20 minutes or so. This will leave your legs refreshed and help discourage fluid retention.

Make It Melon

■ The Chinese use watermelons, cucumbers, and other members of the squash and melon families to reduce fluid retention. These foods—known in botanical circles as members of the cucurbit family—contain cucurbocitrin, which is said to increase the natural leakiness of tiny blood vessels, or capillaries, in the kidneys. This means that more water escapes into the kidneys for elimination.

Make Like Miss Peggy Lee

■ One of the jazz singer's most famous songs is called "Black Coffee." If you don't drink coffee often and have trouble with fluid retention now and then, try a cup—but make sure it's black. Black coffee is a natural diuretic.

EUREKA!

BELIEVE IT OR NOT, the leaf of the lowly dandelion is one of the most potent diuretics you can find (which is why the French call it *pissenlit*, or "urinate in bed"). What's more, it's delicious. Serve the fresh, young leaves in salads, and steam the older ones. **Caution:** Use only dandelion plants that you know have not been treated with pesticides or other chemicals.

Bloat-Busting Tonic

Some days—particularly hot, humid ones—you can retain so much fluid that your body feels as bloated as the Goodyear Blimp. Bloating is a common premenstrual symptom, but can also stem from too much salt in our diets, food allergies, and side effects of medications. To enhance your lymphatic flow, try this herbal mixer.

Dried cleavers
Dried dandelion leaf
Dried ginkgo
Dried hawthorn
Dried horse chestnut leaf
1 qt. of hot water

➥ Combine equal parts of these herbs, and steep 2 tablespoons of the mixture in the water for 15 minutes or so. Let the mixture cool, and drink it throughout the day to chill out. **Caution:** Dandelion is rich in potassium and should not be taken with potassium tablets. And people on blood-thinning medications or aspirin therapy should talk to their doctors before using ginkgo. Do not take this tonic if you are pregnant.

Chug Asparagus Juice

■ When you steam asparagus, save the water, let it cool—then gulp it down. It's one of the best diuretics you can find. (Yes, the taste will have a hint of asparagus, but mostly it'll taste like water.) Other excellent diuretic foods include artichokes, watercresses, and watermelons.

Dial a Doc

✚ If you have an underlying liver, heart, or kidney condition, you need to consult your doctor if you begin to retain fluid. Likewise, talk to your physician if simply pressing on your skin leaves a dent (you may have edema, or very serious fluid retention, which can block blood flow); if you're pregnant and have sudden swelling in your face and hands (which could signal the beginning of preeclampsia—a life-threatening, pregnancy-induced condition); or if you suspect that a food allergy may be the cause of your bloating.

Ear-Clearin' "Sushi" Solution

When congestion is backing up into your ears, try this sweet and spicy tea that'll set your tongue on fire and blow all the congestion right out of your head.

½ tsp. of wasabi or horseradish
3 or 4 thin slices of fresh ginger or garlic
1 cup of peppermint tea

➡ Spread the wasabi or horseradish on the slices of ginger or garlic and pop them in your mouth. The spicy hot spread will clear your sinuses faster than you can take it all in. Then follow with the peppermint tea to cool your mouth down and keep your sinuses wide open.

Onion Power

■ The next time you have an earache, reach for an ordinary onion. Cut it in half, microwave it until it's soft, and let it cool to a comfortable temperature. Then hold the cut end against your ear for 10 to 15 minutes. The heat is very soothing, and the sulfur in the onion may help draw excess fluid from inside your ear.

Snort Some Salt Water

■ Dissolve as much table salt as you can in a glass of warm water without the water becoming cloudy (it should taste like tears), then pour a little of the salt water into the cup of your hand. Sniff the mixture into one nostril, then the other. Repeat several times. This nasal wash acts as a natural decongestant.

What Would Grandma Do?

🦋 ANYTIME I'D TAKE A DIP at the local swimming hole, I'd come back with a lake full of water in my ears. But Grandma Putt knew exactly how to get it out: She'd drop a mixture of vinegar and rubbing alcohol in my ears. The alcohol is a drying agent that helps excess water evaporate. This trick can be used anytime you take a swim in an unchlorinated body of water like a lake or river. Make a 50/50 mixture of the alcohol and vinegar, using white vinegar only; apple cider vinegar may promote fungal growth.

Great Garlic Earache Reliever

Just when you least expect it, an earache can come out of nowhere and deal you a blow that makes you feel like you've gone three rounds in a boxing ring. When that happens, fight back with one of nature's most potent antibiotics.

1 garlic clove
Olive oil

➤ Mash the garlic clove with a fork and saturate it with several drops of olive oil. Let the mash absorb the oil overnight, strain out the garlic, and warm the oil so it's pleasantly tepid, not hot. Tilt your head with your sore ear facing up, and plop 2 or 3 drops of the garlic oil into your ear. Lie down—again with your sore ear up—and let the oil settle for two or three minutes before raising your head. Repeat two to three times a day, and your discomfort should disappear within a day or two.

Bet on Boric Acid

■ Are you prone to ear infections? Then ask your pharmacist to mix up a 3 percent boric acid/70 percent alcohol solution. The boric acid will acidify the ear canal, discouraging any bacterial or fungal invaders from venturing down that path, while the alcohol will dry it up. Squeeze a few drops into your ears each day to keep yourself infection-free. And while you're at the pharmacy, ask your pharmacist for other ear-saving tips.

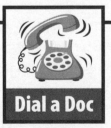

Dial a Doc

✚ If your ear pain is severe, your hearing is diminished, you have blood or pus oozing from your ear, or you had severe pain that stopped abruptly and was followed by hearing loss, call your doctor immediately. Your eardrum may have burst. While a ruptured eardrum usually heals on its own within two months and hearing spontaneously returns to normal, your physician needs to watch closely to stave off infection and prevent permanent hearing loss. And never, ever put anything into your ear if you suspect you have a ruptured eardrum.

Anti-Fog Formula

Stress and poor nutrition can lead to memory loss and poor concentration. Fortunately, stress-relieving techniques and better eating habits can improve brain function. So can potent brain-strengthening mixers like this one.

2 parts fresh or dried ginkgo
2 parts fresh or dried gotu kola
4 parts dried blueberries or bilberries, chopped
1 part fresh or dried reishi mushrooms, chopped
¼ part rosemary
Vodka, gin, or brandy (80 to 100 proof)*
Glass jar with a tight-fitting lid

➡ Chop the ginkgo and gotu kola finely, and put them in the jar along with the berries, mushrooms, and rosemary. Pour in the alcohol until it reaches 3 inches above the top of the solids. Cover the jar with a tight-fitting lid, and put it in a warm, dark place. Let the mixture sit for four to six weeks—the longer, the better. Shake the bottle now and then to keep the solids from packing down. Strain, and pour the liquid into clean, fresh bottles. Label them, and store in a cool, dark place out of reach of children. Take 1 to 2 teaspoons three times a day. **Caution:** If you are on blood-thinning medications or take aspirin regularly, consult your doctor before taking ginkgo.

*If you're sensitive to alcohol, substitute warmed (not boiled!) apple cider vinegar.

Break It Up

■ As we get older, marathon work sessions become more difficult. So when tackling a long project, keep your mind focused by taking a 5-minute rest every 30 minutes.

What Would Grandma Do?

🦋 GRANDMA PUTT *knew that trying to do several things at once would put you on the path to distraction and forgetfulness. "First things first" was her philosophy, and she always finished one task before she started another. It worked, too—and it still does.*

Blueberry Breeze

Blueberries—one of nature's most delicious treats—can help reverse short-term memory loss. So eat 'em by the handful, bake 'em into muffins, cobblers, and pies, stuff 'em into waffles and pancakes—or whirl 'em into this invigorating drink. (This recipe makes 2 servings.)

1 cup of frozen blueberries
1 cup of milk
6 oz. of lemon yogurt
2 tsp. of honey or sugar (optional)
1 tsp. of lemon extract

➡ Pour the ingredients into a blender, and blend until smooth. Then drink up and say, "Thanks for the memory!"

Hey, Coach!

■ Just as athletes can hire coaches to hone their focus on the field, people with attention deficit disorder (ADD) can now hire coaches to hone their own focus in life. To find a coach in your area, contact ADD Resources at www.addresources.org.

Q: *I've just been diagnosed with attention deficit disorder, and my doctor has prescribed drugs that I don't feel comfortable taking. Do you think ADD is a real medical condition? And if so, are there any natural treatments that will help?*

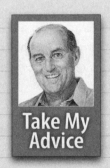

Take My Advice

A: I do think ADD is a real medical condition, but I also think it's overdiagnosed (and many natural-health professionals agree with me). It's definitely worth your while to give alternative remedies a chance before you start popping pills. The most common and frequently effective natural strategy is a change in diet. Before you try anything else, eliminate all processed foods, refined sugars, and food additives, and see if that doesn't do the trick.

Brain Booster

I can't promise that you will suddenly remember everything about Einstein's theory of relativity, or be able to help your kid with his algebra homework. But you can certainly give your brain a healthy workout by drinking this mind-expanding ginkgo mixer every day.

1 tsp. of dried peppermint
½ tsp. of dried ginkgo leaves
½ tsp. of dried gotu kola leaves
½ tsp. of dried rosemary
1 cup of boiling water

➤ Mix all of the herbs together, then scoop 1 teaspoon of the blend into the water. Let it steep for about 10 minutes, strain out the herbs, and sip 1 cup daily to get your brain juices flowing. **Caution:** If you are taking blood-thinning medications or aspirin, consult your doctor before taking ginkgo.

Build Up Your Brain

■ In many cases, forgetfulness can be reversed nonmedically by keeping your blood sugar levels stable. One way to do this is by eating several small meals featuring complex carbohydrates and protein throughout the day, rather than three large meals. Smaller meals could include apple slices smeared with peanut butter; a bagel with banana and low-fat cream cheese; cut-up raw vegetables with low-fat cottage cheese; a small salad and a handful of nuts; a glass of low-fat milk and half a turkey sandwich.

Nifty, Thrifty Tips

Don't get dazzled by all of those pricey newfangled gizmos that are supposed to help train your brain, and instead try snacking on ½ cup of antioxidant-rich blueberries every day to help sharpen your memory. Of course, if the market is fresh out of blueberries, you can munch on other antioxidant-rich fruits and veggies, such as oranges, grapefruit, broccoli, carrots, strawberries, and spinach, which have nearly the same memory-restoring effects.

Brain Brew

There's plenty of talk nowadays about working on puzzles and playing games to keep your mind sharp. But there's not always time to sit down and think your way through a Sudoku grid. So give your brain a healthy workout with this lovely elixir.

2 parts dried ginkgo
1 part dried hawthorn
1 part dried rosemary
1 part dried yarrow
1 cup of hot water

➡ Combine the herbs and add 1 heaping teaspoon of the mixture to the water. Steep, covered, for 15 minutes. Drink 1 or 2 cups per day. **Caution:** If you take aspirin or blood-thinning medication, consult your doctor before taking ginkgo.

Double Your Memory, Double Your Fun

■ Chew on some Doublemint®—or any other kind of gum—and you may ace that exam! Researchers have found that chewing gum improves memory, possibly because it raises the heart rate. This boosts the delivery of oxygen to the brain, which may be the key to recalling facts.

Exercise à Deux

■ While any physical exercise enhances blood circulation and therefore memory, studies show that activities such as tennis that require moving in sync with another person and responding to each other's movements are the best way to keep your brain on its toes. Regular dancing with a partner lowered the risk of Alzheimer's disease among older people by a whopping 75 percent in one study.

EUREKA!

ARE YOU TENSE, distracted . . . and can't remember where you parked the car? Take several deep breaths, then give yourself a foot massage. The soles of your feet correspond to the area of the brain that activates memory. In fact, using a massage oil that contains brahmi is recommended if you tend to freeze up and have trouble recalling things.

Brain-Power Balls

Not a big fan of herbal teas and other "health-foody" concoctions? Then make these delicious brain-function fixers. You *will* remember to down your daily dose—guaranteed!

➡ Mix together equal parts of the nut butter and honey. Combine the powdered herbs, and add just enough of the mixture to the butter-honey combo to make a thick batter. Stir in whatever goodies you prefer from the options listed here. Add enough carob powder to form a breadlike dough, and roll it into small balls. Store them in an airtight container in the fridge and eat one ball a day.

Almond or cashew butter (unsweetened)
Honey
2 parts powdered ginkgo
1 part powdered ginseng
1 part powdered gotu kola
½ part powdered lycium berries
¼ part powdered rosemary
Chocolate chips (optional)
Coconut (optional)
Raisins (optional)
Slivered almonds (optional)
Carob powder

Train Your Brain

■ Help for attention deficit disorder (ADD) could be as close as your nearest martial arts studio. That's because martial arts, such as aikido, karate, and tai chi, demand a special kind of concentration that forces coordination of the attention centers in the brain. If you have ADD, your ability to coordinate these centers is naturally erratic. With training in these ancient practices, you can improve it.

EUREKA!

INTENSE AEROBIC EXERCISE—a brisk three-mile walk—as opposed to a two-block stroll—is one of the best ways to combat ADD because it stimulates the release of endorphins (brain chemicals that lift your mood and turn down the noisy static in your brain) and bumps up brain levels of calming serotonin. The key to success is to exercise hard enough to quicken your heart rate and breathing for 30 to 45 minutes at least five times a week.

Good-for-You Trail Mix

Snacking on junk food and empty calories can impede brainpower and hamper your nervous system. But healthy snacks don't have to be fancy or take a lot of time to prepare. Put together this tasty trail mix at the beginning of the week, and fill one ziplock plastic bag for each day. Then grab a bag in the morning and munch on the mix whenever you feel like your brain needs a boost.

Carob chips
Dried apricots
Dried cranberries
Pumpkin seeds
Raisins
Sunflower seeds
Walnuts

➤ Mix together your choice of ingredients, using organic versions whenever possible. Store the trail mix in an airtight container in a cool, dark place.

Fish for Focus

■ Cold-water fish, such as salmon and sardines, are the richest sources of docosahexaenoic acid (DHA), a type of omega-3 essential fatty acid that helps to improve focus, and possibly reverse memory loss. Not keen on fish? Then try this: As long as you're not taking blood-thinning medications, check your health-food store for fish-oil capsules that contain DHA, and take 1 to 3 grams (1,000 to 3,000 milligrams) daily. Be sure to buy fish oil that's certified free of heavy metals and pesticides.

Eat Italiano Style

■ A daily splash of olive oil will help keep your mind healthier and your memory sharper. A study found that cognitive impairment was less common among elderly people who ate a diet including lots of olive oil, a monounsaturated fat.

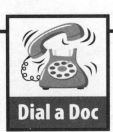

Dial a Doc

✚ If you have trouble performing the steps of a familiar task, such as serving a meal, are confused about time and place, or have forgotten the names of close friends or family members, or if your memory lapses are getting worse, ask your doctor for an evaluation.

Onion Poultice

Like garlic, onions contain the volatile oil allicin, which can help open your airways by relaxing your bronchi. But you don't have to eat the tangy bulbs to reap the benefits. In fact, this old-time fixer will do the trick even better.

Olive oil
Handful of chopped onions
1 tsp. of apple cider vinegar
Pinch of cornstarch

➥ Coat a cast-iron skillet with olive oil and add the chopped onions, apple cider vinegar, and cornstarch. Cook over low heat, stirring, to make a paste. Let the paste cool and place it on a cloth. Lay the cloth on your bare chest and cover it with plastic wrap. Add another cloth, and top everything with a heating pad set on low. The chemicals in the onion will be absorbed into your body—and you'll know it, because you'll have the onion breath to prove it! But you'll be breathing oh-so-much easier, too.

Skip the Sundae

■ It's fine to eat ice cream to soothe a simple tickle in your throat, but when you've been diagnosed with bronchitis, ice cream's a no-no. In this case, you want to avoid foods that produce phlegm, as well as those that cause inflammation. This means skipping not only dairy products but also wheat, soy, sugar, margarine, peanut butter, preserved meats, and processed foods. So what's left? Plenty. Namely fish, legumes, and green vegetables—all of which are rich in magnesium, which helps relax the muscles of your bronchial tubes so you can breathe easier. So just say no to dairy until your bronchitis has cleared up.

✚ **Call the doctor right away if you develop a low-grade fever that lasts more than three days; if you have a fever higher than 101°F; or if you cough up bloody, yellow, or green mucus. All of these are signs that your bronchitis may have turned into pneumonia. Discolored mucus could also indicate a bacterial infection, such as sinusitis, that needs medical attention.**

Dial a Doc

Triple-Threat Herbal Tea

When you have bronchitis, that bottom-of-the-well deep hacking or rasping cough that rattles your ribs feels like a tornado in your chest—and boy does it hurt! Make this soothing tea to clear out some of the junk in your lungs and take the edge off the cough.

2 tbsp. of dried
   marshmallow root
1 qt. of cold water
½ tsp. of dried licorice root
½ tsp. of dried thyme

➡ Soak the marshmallow root in the water overnight. Strain the mixture, and bring 1 cup of the tea to a boil. Add the licorice root and thyme, then cover the tea and let it steep for 15 minutes. Strain out the solids. Drink 3 to 4 cups per day. **Caution:** Licorice root should not be consumed by people with high blood pressure or kidney disease.

Eat Gobs of Garlic

■ One of garlic's key components—the volatile oil allicin—helps relax bronchi to allow more air to pass through them. Garlic also stimulates the immune system and reduces phlegm. So lace your chicken soup—a tried-and-true respiratory infection fighter—with lots of minced garlic.

Q: *I've noticed that my lungs just aren't working as well as they used to. Is there any way that I can get back some of my old wind power?*

A: As we age, our lung capacity decreases. When this happens, we become more vulnerable to respiratory ailments like bronchitis. Studies show that simply blowing up balloons 40 times a day for eight weeks can help decrease breathlessness. So volunteer for the next kiddie party, or sit around and blow up balloons on your own. What's a little dignity compared to the fun of breathing freely?

Take My Advice

Burn-Cooling Brew

If you're treating a burn with a topical remedy and want to boost the healing power, then this mixer's for you.

➡ To start your "inside job," combine equal parts of the herbs, then add 1 teaspoon of the mixture to the water. Steep for 15 to 20 minutes, strain, and sip. This tea will work wonders to help support your body as the burn heals. **Caution**: Don't take echinacea if you have an autoimmune disease, such as rheumatoid arthritis, lupus, or multiple sclerosis.

Dried calendula
Dried cleavers
Dried echinacea
Dried prickly ash
Dried red clover
1 cup of boiling water

Clean with Calendula

■ Calendula is an anti-inflammatory, astringent (cleanser), and antiseptic (germ killer) all rolled into one. Make a strong tea by adding 1 heaping tablespoon of calendula to 1 cup of boiling water. Cool and strain, then gently (and sparingly) apply the tonic to the burn several times a day to help heal and soothe tissues.

The Pizza Pizzazz

■ Oregano is not just for pizza—scorched skin loves it, too. Essential oil of oregano contains vitamins A and C and many minerals, including calcium, phosphorus, iron, and magnesium. Add 5 drops to 1 teaspoon of olive oil and apply to minor burns.

✚ **Contact your doctor immediately if you sustain any type of burn on your face, neck, genitals, the palms of your hands, or the soles of your feet, where nerves are close to the surface and may be severely injured; any blistering burn that's larger than a quarter; or any burn onto which your clothing has become stuck (don't attempt to remove it yourself). Likewise, head to the hospital for any type of electrical burn, a burn caused by caustic chemicals, or an inhalation burn from steam, vapors, or chemicals.**

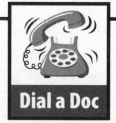

Dial a Doc

Cedar Soother

Try this burn-soothing salve made with dried white-cedar leaves. Its cooling properties are terrific, and white cedar is especially rich in minerals that calm skin irritations and burns.

➡ Chop the white-cedar leaves, and place them in the jar. Cover the pieces with the oil. Let the jar sit in a warm oven at 100°F for 12 hours. Then transfer the oil to a saucepan, and heat it on the stove over low heat. Stir in the grated beeswax, cocoa butter, and honey. Remove from the heat when the beeswax has melted, combine the ingredients thoroughly, and add the vitamin E oil before pouring the mixture back into the glass jar. Store the jar in the refrigerator, and use the salve in the days after getting a minor burn (but avoid putting oil of any kind on a fresh burn).

Handful of dried white-cedar leaves
1 pint of olive, almond, or sesame oil
2 oz. of beeswax (grated)
½ oz. of cocoa butter
1 tbsp. of raw honey
5 to 6 drops of vitamin E oil
Clean glass jar

Swab with Sweet Oil

■ Ever since French perfume chemist René-Maurice Gattefossé healed his burned hand by plunging it in a vat of lavender oil, this scented herb has been used to guard against infection and prevent scarring. Apply several drops of oil directly to the burned area throughout the day, but not if your skin is broken or blistered. For sensitive skin, dilute 5 drops of lavender essential oil with 1 teaspoon of olive oil.

EUREKA!

EVEN THOUGH YOU want to cool a burn as quickly as possible, leave the ice in the freezer because it'll probably just make things worse. It will make the area miserably cold and can even stick to the skin, which is mighty painful. Instead, just run some cool water (or milk, or a soft drink—whatever happens to be the closest thing that's cool but not frozen) over the area.

Saintly Salve

Whenever I get a little burn from working around the house, I reach for my jar of homemade St. John's wort salve in my kitchen so that I can treat it right on the spot! This elixir also works nicely on minor cuts and skin rashes.

Handful of calendula flowers
Handful of comfrey leaves
Handful of St. John's wort leaves and flowers
½ cup of vegetable oil
¼ cup of beeswax

➡ Place the fresh herbs and vegetable oil in a double boiler. Heat on low for about an hour, keeping an eye on the mixture to make sure that the oil doesn't boil. Lay a cheesecloth or muslin bag over a large stainless steel strainer set over a glass container. Carefully pour the herbal mix from the double boiler through the strainer into the container. Discard the solids. Now you're ready to make the salve: Add the beeswax to the herbal oil. Heat this mixture on the stove over low heat until the beeswax has completely melted. Remove the pan from the stove and pour the contents into tiny glass jars. Seal them with lids, and store away from direct sunlight and heat sources. The next time bacon grease splatters on your arm, quit your cussin' and reach for this soothing, healing salve.

Oil Well

■ St. John's wort oil can be applied to burns as long as the skin is not broken. You'll reap the double benefit of speedier healing and relief from the pain. Apply it two or three times daily.

What Would Grandma Do?

My Grandma Putt knew that aloe vera was especially made for burns. In fact, it's sometimes called the "burn plant" because it inhibits the action of a pain-producing peptide, and it helps healing and skin growth. Grandma Putt kept a big ol' aloe vera plant out on the porch. If we ever got burned in the kitchen, she'd just break off a leaf, split it open, and rub the soothing gel all over the burn.

Canker Sore Counterattack

In most cases, these irritating ulcers in your mouth lining clear up within a week or two, but stress or a weakened immune system may cause bothersome sores that just won't go away. If that's the case, try this herbal immune system soother.

1¼-inch slice of ginger
1 cinnamon stick
1 tsp. of echinacea
1 tsp. of goldenseal
1 tsp. of myrrh
2 garlic cloves, minced
4 cups of water
Honey and/or lemon

➡ Pour the water into a pan, and bring it to a boil. Add the herbs and simmer for 10 to 15 minutes. Remove the pan from the heat. Steep for 15 to 20 minutes. Strain out the solids and add honey and/or lemon to taste. Either drink the cool elixir or reheat it. Take up to 2 cups a day until your sores have vanished. **Caution**: Don't use echinacea if you have an autoimmune disease, such as rheumatoid arthritis, lupus, or multiple sclerosis.

Conquer Canker Sores with Cranberry Juice

■ Simply drinking cranberry juice between meals can help you relieve the pain of canker sores and heal them, too. Talk about a simple fix!

Relax, Already!

■ Just like other physical woes, canker sores can be caused by stress. So do yourself a favor and follow whatever stress-relief methods work best for you. Take up yoga. Spend more time walking and less time behind the wheel of a car. Put on a Mozart CD and curl up with a good book. Watch funny movies. Putter in your garden. You'll help your canker sores heal more quickly and help prevent new ones.

Nifty, Thrifty Tips

Get rid of a canker sore by coating it with a fixer you probably have in your medicine chest—milk of magnesia. Its alkalinity will counteract the acidic conditions in which the canker-producing bacteria thrive.

Flower-Power Rinse

Like most ailments, canker sores are easier to cure if you start treatment at the first sign of an eruption. Nip them in the bud with this fast fixer.

1 tsp. of calendula tincture
½ cup of water

➡ Mix the tincture and water together and store the liquid in a glass bottle with a tight cap. Rinse your mouth with it, then spit the liquid out. This elixir is a potent but harmless disinfectant, and you can use it as often as you like until your "owies" heal.

Try Tea

■ Every type of black tea imaginable, from a pricey imported Earl Grey to a store-brand orange pekoe, can help numb the pain of canker sores. Brew a cup of your favorite kind, let the tea bag cool, and squeeze it to reduce its size as much as possible. Then tuck it into your mouth to cover the distressed area.

Pick Some Plums

■ When painful canker sores break out in your mouth, they can make you feel like climbing the walls. But you can get relief fast with this classic remedy: Soak a piece of gauze pad in fresh plum juice, press it against the sore, and hold it in place for 10 minutes, or as long as you can. Repeat the procedure as needed until the nasty little bump is completely gone.

EUREKA!

ONE OF THE MOST EFFECTIVE fixers for canker sores is also one of the simplest: Eat yogurt twice a day. Stick with plain yogurt because sugar can worsen canker sores. And choose a brand that has live, active acidophilus cultures, because that's what kills the bacteria that often cause the sores.

Goldenseal Canker Sore Relief

There's nothing like a canker sore to remind you just how often your mouth moves. When one of these pesky sores erupts, the slightest movement—chewing, talking, yawning—can set off jolts of pain. To relieve the discomfort, use this antiseptic mouth rinse and you'll feel the pain fade away.

½ tsp. of goldenseal root powder
¼ tsp. of table salt
1 cup of warm water

➡ Completely dissolve the goldenseal powder and salt in the water. Take a swig of the rinse, swish it around, and spit it out. Do this four times a day, and you can kiss that bothersome canker sore good-bye in no time at all.

Swish with Soda

■ That same box of baking soda you use to cut odors in your fridge can also be used to reduce the acidity in your mouth. Just add 1 to 2 teaspoons of baking soda to a quart of warm water, swish it around in your mouth, and spit it out.

Turn to Myrrh

■ You may know myrrh as the herbal gift taken to biblical Bethlehem by one of the Magi, but herbalists view it as a highly effective treatment for mouth inflammations because of its astringent properties. Just mix a few drops of extract in a cup of warm water and rinse daily. Or open a myrrh capsule and dab the powder directly onto your canker sore. **Caution:** Do not use myrrh if you are pregnant or breastfeeding.

Nifty, Thrifty Tips

One of the best investments you can make for your own health is an aloe vera plant. For one thing, it can help heal canker sores. Just break off a couple of leaves, mash them up, and strain the juice into a glass. Then rinse your mouth with this juice three times a day to dull the pain and reduce bacteria. Just make sure you rinse with the juice, and not the gel.

Circulation-Boosting Solution

Unsightly, bulging varicose veins occur when veins weaken and cannot effectively move blood up the legs. The blood causes the veins to swell. Alternating hot and cold compresses soaked in this circulation-boosting mixer expands and then contracts the veins, providing a soothing pumping action.

Cypress oil
Geranium oil
Ginger oil
Juniper oil
Lavender oil
Rosemary oil

➡ Soak a cloth in a mixture of 10 drops of oil from each of these herbs and 1 quart of hot water. Press the cloth to your leg for 5 minutes. Then soak another cloth in a second batch of solution made with the same oils, but this time use cold water, and apply it for 15 minutes. Follow up by giving yourself a gentle massage (aided by a few of those aromatic, circulation-boosting oils), stroking your legs upward toward your heart.

Fire 'Em Up

■ Herbal formulas that include the classic vessel strengtheners like butcher's broom, horse chestnut, stone root, and yarrow may help tone veins and decrease inflammation inside them. The only catch is, you may need to stay on these formulas forever if you're prone to varicose veins in order to make sure the varicose veins don't return. **Caution:** Don't take horse chestnut if you're pregnant or breastfeeding.

What Would Grandma Do?

WHENEVER HER VARICOSE VEINS were going to pop out of her legs by the end of the day, Grandma Putt would turn to a common food found in her kitchen: onions. That's right—onion skin is one of the best sources of quercetin, a hardworking bioflavonoid that reduces capillary fragility. Grandma Putt would toss an onion—skin and all—into a soup or stew so the helpful bioflavonoids leached into the liquid. Then she would just discard the skin before letting anyone dig in.

Circulation Enhancer

Hawthorn, lime blossoms, and ginger are all recognized for their ability to reduce the stickiness of blood platelets and enhance circulation. As long as you're not taking any blood-thinning medications, it's your choice whether to use these herbs separately or in any combination.

Grated fresh ginger
Dried hawthorn berries
Fresh or dried lime blossoms
1 cup of hot water

➡ To use these herbs together, mix them in equal parts and add 1 heaping teaspoon of the blend to the water. Steep for 15 to 20 minutes and strain. You can drink up to 3 cups of this tea per day.

Berry, Berry Good

■ Colorful fruits and vegetables, especially dark berries, are a rich source of bioflavonoids, which strengthen your cardiovascular system. Eating 1 cup of blueberries a day will keep your circulation system running strong!

Grab Some Garlic

■ Raw garlic inhibits blood clots that can cause circulatory problems. It also lowers cholesterol, reduces blood pressure, and may even make your blood vessels more flexible. So toss some garlic into your food whenever you can.

Snappy Solutions

To help prevent atherosclerosis (hardening of the arteries), pick a pomegranate. If you live in a desert area with access to pomegranate trees, pick one, squeeze it, and sip the juice, or just eat the fruit as it is. Studies suggest that pomegranate juice prevents oxidation of the type of cholesterol that contributes to plaque formation— those artery-clogging deposits. These fruits appear seasonally in supermarkets, and you can find bottled pomegranate juice any time of year.

Herbal Leg Wraps

If you have poor circulation in your legs, every time you sit down you probably feel like you'll never get up again. To stimulate circulation in your legs, exercise your blood vessels with these chilling herbal wraps.

2 tbsp. of dried peppermint
2 tbsp. of dried yarrow
2 cups of hot water

➡ Make a strong infusion by steeping the herbs in the water, covered, for 15 minutes. Strain and chill. Meanwhile, prepare several lengths of gauze, muslin, or cheesecloth. When the infusion is thoroughly chilled, saturate the cloths, wring them out, and wrap them around your lower legs. Then relax with your legs elevated for 20 minutes. Do this daily for several weeks.

Garlic to the Rescue

■ Garlic is both a clot buster and cholesterol reducer. Its healing properties also make it a great circulatory tonic because it gets the blood moving to where it needs to be. Eat one raw clove per day to help alleviate leg cramps.

Take a Break

■ When you have intermittent claudication, it doesn't take a doctor to figure out that if you stop walking, you'll stop limping. And the pain in your lower leg that causes you to limp will subside after a period of rest. So when your legs begin to hurt, simply sit down for a little while and give them a break.

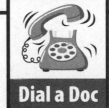

Dial a Doc

✚ How can you tell whether it's arthritis or intermittent claudication that's causing your leg pain? If you have arthritis, you limp when you begin to walk, and with continued walking—as your muscles and joints loosen up—your limp tends to go away. With intermittent claudication, you're fine when you start out, but the pain develops after you've walked for a while. If you still need help deciding which ailment is causing your pain, contact your doctor.

Meadow Mixer for Super Circulation

Keeping yourself healthy and your body's natural processes flowing freely can be as easy as going outside and picking ordinary plants you see every day. But since we're not all botanists, it's a whole lot easier to buy what you need at a health-food store. Either way, the end result is the same: Taking a mixer of these meadow herbs will keep your blood moving through your body.

Dried horsetail
Dried meadowsweet
Dried oat straw
Dried peppermint
Dried yarrow
1 cup of boiling water

➡ Combine equal parts of the herbs and add 1 heaping teaspoon to the water. Steep, covered, for 10 to 15 minutes, strain, and drink 1 cup twice daily. All of these herbs are rich in minerals that enhance circulation, and meadowsweet contains small amounts of salicylate for pain relief.

Get Going

◼ Exercise is good for your heart, and it's just as good for improving circulation in beleaguered leg muscles. So aim for at least 20 minutes of exercise every day. Swimming, cycling, and walking are all great choices no matter what your level of fitness is. The goal is to increase your heart rate and break a sweat.

Q: *Is there any type of vitamin or food that will help prevent blood clots and plaque from forming in my arteries?*

A: There sure is! You need adequate amounts of B vitamins, especially B_6, B_{12}, and folic acid, to clear excess homocysteine (an amino acid) from your system. If this amino acid builds up, it can encourage blood clots and plaque buildup. So take in plenty of Bs by eating beans, whole grains, orange juice, and leafy greens.

Take My Advice

A Royal Decongestant

There's nothing better for taking care of a stuffy nose than a little pennyroyal. When mixed in this fixer, it'll leave your nose running freely, and even take care of some of the stuff stuck in your chest.

1 cup of water
2 tsp. of dried eucalyptus leaves
2 tsp. of dried pennyroyal leaves and flower tops
2 tsp. of dried rosemary leaves

➡ Boil the water in a small saucepan, then add the herbs. Let the mixture simmer for 10 minutes and remove the pan from the heat. Place it on a heatproof surface, put a towel over your head to make a tent, and inhale the vapors to clear your congestion.

Swallow with Caution

■ When your throat is under siege from a cold, be wary of what you swallow. Avoid very spicy foods, hot soups and beverages, and any other edible irritant.

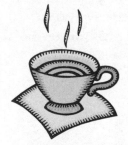

Gargle Galore

■ A red sage tea gargle can ease the mucous membranes of your throat and boost your immune system, allowing you to clear out the junk and fight the cold that ails you. To make the tea, pour 1 cup of warm water over 1 teaspoon of red sage, and let it steep for 10 minutes. Strain out the herb, then gargle until the tea is gone.

✚ Always pay close attention to how long your cold symptoms last. If there's no sign of improvement within a few days, or if your symptoms are worsening, call your doctor. If it's been one week or more and you still don't feel better, you could have a bacterial infection or more serious disorder that only your doctor will be able to diagnose and treat.

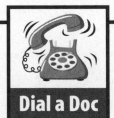

Dial a Doc

Cold (and Vampire!) Repellent

Garlic has long been used for its potent healing effects, and it doubles as a powerful cold preventive because it keeps people (and vampires) at a distance. Garlic tea is a great way to get garlic into your system quickly, and believe it or not, it's surprisingly tasty!

2 medium garlic cloves
1 cup of water
2 to 3 slices of fresh ginger
Honey (optional)
Lemon (optional)

➡ Chop the garlic cloves, and simmer them in the water for 10 to 15 minutes. Add the ginger to counteract the garlic's pungent flavor and increase the warming action. Add honey and lemon to taste. Drink 2 to 4 cups of this tea per day until your cold is gone. **Caution:** If you're taking blood-thinning medications, steer clear of large amounts of garlic unless your doctor gives you the green light.

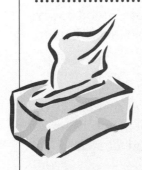

Turn Off the Drip

■ The pungent oval leaves of the sage plant aren't just for enhancing turkey stuffing—they can also nip a runny nose in the bud. At the first sign of a drip, steep 1 teaspoon of dried sage leaves in ½ cup of hot water for 10 minutes or so, then strain out the solids, and sip the tea slowly. **Caution:** Don't try this if you're pregnant or breastfeeding.

Nifty, Thrifty Tips

Instead of spending your hard-earned cash on various drug-related cold remedies, why not try a different approach entirely? It is now widely known among doctors that positive emotions can strengthen the immune system by increasing gamma interferon, an immune system hormone that activates other infection-fighting compounds. So the next time you have a cold, make your DVD rental a laugh-out-loud comedy, which will hopefully give your symptoms the cold shoulder.

Crooner's Delight

Believe it or not (as Ripley used to say), garlic is a terrific voice coach. If you're planning to sing or make a public speech, but you can feel your throat getting a bit ticklish, try this fixer to keep your vocal cords ready for the spotlight!

2 tbsp. of fresh lemon juice
1 tsp. of minced garlic
1 cup of boiling water
2 tsp. of honey

➡ Add the lemon juice and garlic to the water, then stir in the honey until it's dissolved. Do not strain out the garlic. Sip and relax as this terrific tea lubricates your larynx.

Elm Elixir

■ Slippery elm is used by professional singers and speakers to recover their voices and keep their laryngeal tissues in tip-top shape. Simply steep 1 heaping teaspoon of the dried herb in 1 cup of hot water for 15 minutes. Strain, add honey and lemon if desired, and drink 3 to 4 cups per day. If you can't find the herb itself, pick up a pack of slippery elm lozenges.

Thyme the Pot

■ An herbal steam facial can help soothe respiratory passages and alleviate laryngitis pain. Place 3 to 4 drops of essential oil of thyme in a pot of hot, steaming water. Bend over the pot—taking care not to get burned—and tent your head with a towel. Then breathe in the vapors deeply.

EUREKA!

A CARROT NECK WRAP may ease inflammation and help you recover from a cold more quickly. Start by grating a carrot onto a length of cheesecloth. Fold the cloth in half lengthwise, and moisten it with warm water. Wrap it around your neck, and then wrap a warm towel on top. Keep the wrap in place for 20 to 30 minutes. For extra heat, you can sprinkle a pinch of cayenne pepper on the grated carrot before wrapping it up.

Echinacea Tincture

When cold and flu season comes around, I like to head off problems before any symptoms appear. But why spend your hard-earned money at the drugstore, when you can make a preventive tonic yourself? I always like to keep some of this elixir on hand just in case I need it.

¾ cup of vodka or grain alcohol
1½ oz. of dried echinacea root

➡ Combine the ingredients in a jar. With the lid screwed on tight, give it a couple of good shakes. Then store it in a cool, dark place for two weeks. Remove the solid pieces of echinacea root by straining the liquid through a coffee filter. Add 60 drops of this tincture to a glass of water and sip three times a day. **Caution**: Don't take echinacea if you have an autoimmune disease, such as rheumatoid arthritis, lupus, or multiple sclerosis.

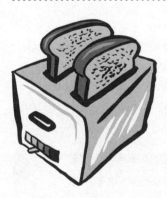

Garlic Toast

■ When you feel like you're coming down with a cold, you usually don't have much of an appetite, but take my advice: Pull out the toaster and whip up some pungent toast. Mash a raw garlic clove, spread it and some honey on a piece of warm toast, bagel, or English muffin, and munch away. If you do this two to three times a day, you'll be over your cold before you know it.

Snappy Solutions

Hardy cold viruses can live for hours on doorknobs, faucet handles, books, money—all the things we touch every day. But don't spend time and money on preventive medications; frequent hand washing is the single best way to avoid catching a cold or spreading your own. So wash your hands—often!

Essential Oil Solution

Congestion can be cleared up fairly quickly with a little steam power. You can either take a steam bath at the gym or turn on the shower and steam up your bathroom. But to unclog stuffy nasal passages even quicker, try this mixer.

2 drops of eucalyptus oil
2 drops of rosemary oil
2 drops of thyme oil
1 cup of Epsom salts

➡ When you're congested, climb into steamy bathwater that's been laced with these essential oils and Epsom salts. The steam will increase the flow of nasal mucus, and the molecules from the oils will dilate your small airways, helping to ease your breathing. The magnesium in the Epsom salts will be absorbed through your skin and help your bronchial passages relax. You'll be breathing freely again in no time at all!

Get Steamed

■ Steam will kill cold germs on contact if the water temperature is 110°F or more. Herbs, such as eucalyptus, add a penetrating scent and disinfecting properties. So put fresh leaves in a bowl, pour boiling water over them, and tent a towel over your head and the bowl. Lower your face over the bowl (carefully—you can scald yourself if the steam is too hot), and breathe the vapors in. For even more steamy strength, add a few drops of oregano oil to the water.

Nifty, Thrifty Tips

Before hundreds of cold medicines became available at the local drugstore, certain home remedies were probably a lot more fun to take. And if you sipped 'em enough, you certainly felt better because eventually you couldn't feel a thing! So try a hot toddy as a last-ditch effort to cure a cold; it's also a powerful way to ease the pain that cold remedies can inflict on your wallet. There are many variations on the hot toddy, but start with juice, honey, or tea, and add the liquor of your choice. Here's one simple recipe: Squeeze the juice from half a lemon into a mug of boiling water, pour in a shot of whiskey, and add honey to taste.

Ginger-Cinnamon Tea

There's something magical in the healing powers of this tea, and it's yummy, too! Plus, the warm, inviting smell as the aroma drifts through your house will make you feel much better instantly.

3 slices of fresh ginger
3 slices of fresh lemon
5 whole cloves
1 cinnamon stick
1 pint of water

➡ Combine the ingredients in a saucepan and simmer for 10 to 15 minutes. Strain out the solids and drink up to 4 cups a day at the first sign of the sniffles.

Menthol Steam

■ When you've got a nasty cold and your nasal passages are so blocked up that you can hardly breathe, reach for this guaranteed relief. Fill a bowl with steaming water, add 2 teaspoons of mentholated rub, and inhale the pungent vapors. Repeat every few hours, and before you know it, you'll be breathing freely again!

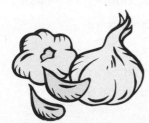

Garlic Cold Remedy

■ Keep this old-time remedy on hand during cold and flu season because it's a real lifesaver. Peel and mince six large garlic cloves, put them in a jar, cover them with olive oil, and put the lid on the jar. Let the mixture sit in the fridge for three days, but be sure to stir it every day. Strain it through cheesecloth into another clean jar. Then when you feel a cold coming on, rub a spoonful on your feet before climbing into bed.

EUREKA!

IF YOU'RE COMING DOWN with a cold, mix 10 to 20 drops of hot-pepper sauce or a big pinch of cayenne pepper in a glass of tomato juice, and drink to your good health. Bringing on the heat like this three to four times a day should kick the cold to the curb.

Herb Steamer

Old-time healers understood how herbs affect the body, and knew what to mix to make power-packed ailment fighters, including those for relieving nasal congestion. Here's a cold-stopping steamer made with common herbs that are often used in traditional folk medicine.

1 tbsp. of dried eucalyptus
1 tbsp. of dried rosemary
1 cup of boiling water

➡ Put the eucalyptus and rosemary into the water, place a towel over your head to make a tent, and inhale the aroma for five minutes or so. (Be careful not to scald your face—lower it very slowly over the steam.) Your congestion will soon be history.

Suppress the Cough

■ The more you cough, the more you irritate your sensitive larynx and the rest of your throat. When your cough is dry and unproductive, use a cough-suppressant medication to keep your larynx from further harm.

Tepid Is the Answer

■ Drink lots of water, but keep it tepid—not too hot or too cold, either of which might further inflame your vocal cords. Or enjoy a few cups of tepid tea with lemon and honey, which is very soothing for your throat.

Snappy Solutions

You can do your throat a lot of good when you have a cold simply by protecting it. Place a warm, wet cloth compress on your neck for two to three minutes. Then replace it with a cold one and wrap a wool scarf around your neck to keep it in place for 30 minutes. Your throat should soon feel better and loosen up enough to get you on the road to recovery.

Herbal-Oil Rub

Hacking, coughing, and stuffed-up congestion can ruin anyone's day, and difficult breathing makes you downright miserable. But there's hope! Get yourself to the health-food store for some essential oil of fennel. It's the key ingredient in this congestion-clearing chest rub.

10 drops of eucalyptus oil
10 drops of fennel oil
10 drops of thyme oil
4 oz. of sunflower oil

➡ Add the eucalyptus, fennel, and thyme oils to the sunflower oil. Using your fingers, massage the oil mixture gently onto your chest, using all of it. Cover the area with a flannel cloth and a hot-water bottle, and relax.

Rub On the Oil

■ Using poultices when you have a cold is a comforting way to get some rest. You can make a foot rub by adding 3 to 4 drops of an essential oil (try eucalyptus, lavender, or thyme) to 1 tablespoon of olive oil. Apply it liberally to your feet, put on a pair of clean cotton socks, and settle into a comfy chair with a good book.

Ginger Will Root It Out

■ The oil in ginger is similar to capsaicin in peppers—it is slightly irritating and thins out mucus. So you can clear your head with fresh ginger in several ways. First, cut the ginger into pieces, brew a tea, and then inhale the vapors as you sip. Or maybe you prefer to grate it up and toss it into a salad dressing. And you can even chop it and add it to a super sinus-clearing stir-fry.

What Would Grandma Do?

🦋 GRANDMA PUTT KNEW that the secret to stopping her eyes from watering while she was chopping onions was to hold the onion close to running water. But she also knew that the chemicals in onions could help her fight a cold. She would just peel an onion and hold it close to her face. The fumes would clear up her congestion in no time.

Hot-Mustard Plaster

A popular remedy for chest congestion that's been around for generations is a hot-mustard plaster, which helps break up stubborn mucus in the lungs by bringing heat to the area. Black mustard seed powder releases a potent oil when mixed with water that clears the gunk out of your chest and lungs.

**10 parts flour
1 part black
       mustard powder
Tepid water
Olive oil**

➡ Mix the flour and mustard powder with enough tepid water to make a paste. Spread a thin layer of the paste onto a cloth. Coat your skin with some olive oil and a layer of cloth *before* you place the plaster cloth on your chest—mustard side out. Leave it on for no more than 10 minutes, but remove it sooner if your skin begins to redden, or you may end up with blisters.

Add Some Spice to Your Life

■ Spicy foods like hot peppers and chili contain capsaicin, a substance that can help reduce nasal and sinus congestion. Try garlic, turmeric, horseradish, and other pungent spices for a similar effect. You can add these spices to chicken soup, but any hot soup or strong spice will get your eyes and nose running.

Snappy Solutions

Do you have a cold that you can't seem to get rid of, even though you're taking medicines that are supposed to clear up every possible symptom? Well, your continued suffering may be coming from something else you're putting into your system. When you've got a cold, you should stick to drinking diluted juices, water, and hot beverages. Avoid milk and milk products because they promote mucus formation. If you consume dairy products while you have a cold, not only will you get a milk mustache, but you'll also wind up even more congested, making your potential recovery time a whole lot longer.

Immune System Stimulant

Every day, your immune system takes hit after hit. If it's able to roll with the punches and recover, then you will ward off disease. But sometimes, it just can't quite recover from one punch before another hit comes along and a virus—like a cold—sets in. So give your body a boost to bounce back after a virus sets in. These immune-stimulating and astringent herbs pack their own punch that'll help clobber a cold quickly.

Dried eyebright
Grated fresh ginger
Dried lemon balm
Dried licorice root
Dried rose hips
Dried yarrow
1 cup of boiling water
¼-inch slice of fresh ginger

➡ Combine equal parts of these herbs in a jar. Stir 1 heaping teaspoon of the mixture into the water, then add the ginger. Steep for 20 minutes, strain out the solids, and enjoy. Drink 2 to 3 cups daily. **Caution:** Don't take licorice root if you have high blood pressure or kidney disease.

Slip In Some Elm

■ If you're coughing so much that your chest and back ache, try sipping some slippery elm tea. This time-honored expectorant will help break up sticky mucus. Look for it at health-food stores and follow the directions on the label.

Q: *Does vitamin C really cure colds the way they say it does on TV?*

A: I love to drink gallons of OJ when I have a cold. But while no one has yet proven that vitamin C can cure a cold, some say it acts like a body chemical that helps stop the growth of the virus. Vitamin C also has an antihistamine effect, so drinking citrus or taking a supplement may help reduce nasal symptoms.

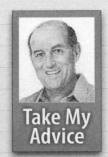

Take My Advice

Minty Tea

The best way to treat a cold? "With contempt," according to one of modern medicine's founding fathers. But if that's not your cup of tea, try this one to ease nasty cold symptoms.

1 to 2 tsp. of dried peppermint leaves
Honey
1 cup of boiling water

➤ Mix the ingredients well, strain out the solids, and sip to calm a cough, loosen congestion, or relieve a headache.

Stay Lubricated

■ Whenever you're in artificially controlled environments with really dry and constantly recirculated air, such as office buildings, airplanes, airports, and shopping malls, your nasal membranes dry out, and tiny cracks that invite viruses tend to form in your nasal passages. Your best defense? Avoid these places as much as you can! When avoidance is not an option, drink plenty of fluids and use saline nasal spray often to hydrate the tender membranes in your nose.

Mine Some Zinc

■ Some research indicates that zinc may cut the duration of colds by about two days. It can act as a physical barrier to prevent viruses from entering the cells that line the nose and throat. So take zinc lozenges within 24 hours of your first symptom. Look for zinc gluconate tablets or lozenges that are not flavored with citric acid, tartaric acid, or sorbitol. When these ingredients mix with saliva, they can prevent zinc from acting.

What Would Grandma Do?

As my Grandma Putt used to say, the graveyards are filled with people the world couldn't get along without. When a cold strikes, do yourself—and your coworkers—a favor: Stay home, get into your jammies, and use whatever remedies you choose to banish your germs before you plunge into the fray again.

Natural Nasal Balm

A good nasal balm can keep your airways clear and your breathing light. The only problem is that there can be loads of chemicals in store-bought varieties. So make your own that's all natural and ready for immediate use. Just follow this simple recipe.

¼ cup of petroleum jelly
10 drops of eucalyptus oil
10 drops of peppermint oil
10 drops of thyme oil

➡ Place the petroleum jelly in a small saucepan, and warm it until it melts. Remove it from the heat, and stir in the oils. When the balm has cooled to room temperature, pour it into a clean jar for storage. Apply a small amount to your nostrils one to three times daily. The balm works because the petroleum jelly prevents the other ingredients from being absorbed into the skin. That way, you can breathe in the volatile oils for a prolonged period and let them do their stuff.

Oh, Go Blow Your Nose!

■ During the first three days of a cold, the average adult blows his or her nose 45 times a day. And it's an important task—after all, sniffling the stuff back in can only prolong your discomfort. But pay attention to how you blow. An improper technique won't do you much good and will put extra pressure on your already achy ears and sinuses. Here's how to get the job done the right way: Press one nostril closed and gently blow through the open nostril into a paper tissue. Then switch to the opposite nostril and repeat the process.

EUREKA!

THIS ANCIENT FOLK REMEDY is hard to beat to fend off early cold symptoms. Boil a large whole apple in a quart of water until the apple falls apart. Strain out the solids, and add a shot of whiskey and about ½ teaspoon of lemon juice. Then hit the hay and drink ½ cup of the warm toddy. If you've acted in time, by morning, those germs will be history!

Old-Time Mustard Plaster

Before the days of antibiotics and other miracle drugs, folks treated chest colds, flu, bronchitis, and even pneumonia with this fixer. It still works like a charm—but use it along with, not instead of, your doctor's orders.

⅛ to ¼ cup of dry mustard
¼ cup of flour
3 tbsp. of molasses
Thick cream or softened lard
Piece of cotton flannel
Warm water
Thick cotton T-shirt

➤ Have the cold-sufferer put on the T-shirt and lie down. Then mix the mustard and flour together, and stir in the molasses. Add enough cream or lard to get an ointment consistency. Dip the cotton flannel in the water, wring it out, and lay it on the throat and upper chest, on top of the T-shirt. Apply the mustard mixture to the damp cloth, and leave it on for no longer than 15 minutes. Check the skin every five minutes, and if the skin has started to turn red, remove the cloth immediately. **Caution:** This stuff is hot, so wear rubber gloves as you work with it, and make sure it doesn't touch any bare skin.

Supercharged Chicken Soup

■ Chicken soup is a time-tested weapon in the fight against cold and flu germs. Here's how to add even more oomph to your favorite recipe: Heat some chicken soup or broth, and stir in 1 tablespoon of apple cider vinegar, 1 crushed garlic clove, and hot sauce to taste. Then sip yourself to better health.

What Would Grandma Do?

WHENEVER I CAME DOWN with a cold, the first thing Grandma Putt did was put a pot on the stove and simmer up a batch of chicken soup. Nobody knows exactly why it works, but chicken soup really does help relieve cold symptoms. Most doctors believe that the steam from the hot soup promotes drainage. There must be something to it because chicken soup's been used as a home remedy since the 12th century.

Stuffy Nose Spritzer

Every morning I wake up, take a big, deep breath, and welcome the new day. But when I wake up with a stuffy nose, it puts me in a bad mood before I even get out of bed. Instead of heading off to the doctor for a prescription, I head to my pantry to make this quick and easy nasal elixir.

¼ tsp. of baking soda
¼ tsp. of salt
1 cup of warm water

➡ Dissolve the baking soda and salt in the water. Use a medicine dropper to squeeze the liquid twice into one nostril while you gently pinch the other nostril shut. Inhale, then repeat the procedure in the other nostril. Since there are no drugs involved, you can use this mixture as often as you need.

Mix a Bloody Mary

■ To make a congestion-loosening drink, start with a glass of tomato juice, then add some lemon, a celery stalk, and horseradish, and drink it quickly. Tomato juice is full of vitamin C, but it's the horseradish that really does the trick. Its powerful fumes will clear out the crud.

Horseradish to the Rescue

■ Horseradish contains allyl isothiocyanate, which stimulates the nerve endings in your nose and makes it flow like a faucet. Plus, the herb has anti-viral properties. So when you've got a cold, take a teaspoon of grated horseradish up to three times a day to clear out your airways. Spread it on a cracker to help ease it down.

EUREKA!

APPALACHIAN HEALERS make the following cold remedy: Mix a dash of cayenne pepper and a pinch of salt into 1 ounce of apple cider vinegar, and drink it three or four times a day. Another remedy some folks rely on is mixing 1 tablespoon each of honey and lemon juice. Stir them into a cup of hot water and sip it three times a day.

Get-a-Move-On Mix

Having your bowels all stopped up can make you feel irritable, heavy, uncomfortable, and downright miserable. But why be unhappy when you can clean out your system overnight with this classic mixer?

½ cup of applesauce
4 to 6 prunes, chopped
1 tbsp. of bran

➤ Mix all of the ingredients together, and eat the concoction just before you go to bed. Drink a tall glass of water and by morning, things should be on the move again so you can get back to your happy, comfortable life!

Root for Regularity

■ Fresh dandelion roots (not leaves or stems) can have a mild laxative effect. Three times a day, either toss some rinsed roots into a salad or steep them in a cup of boiling water for 10 to 15 minutes, then strain out the solids and drink the hot liquid. Just be sure to use only dandelion plants that you know have not been treated with pesticides or other chemicals. **Caution:** If you're taking diuretics or potassium supplements, check with your doctor before taking dandelion.

Pop Some Prunes

■ Ounce for ounce, prunes are packed with more fiber than almost any other fruit or vegetable—including dried beans. Down a glass of prune juice before bed to encourage a morning movement, then nibble on dried prunes (or figs and raisins), and drink plenty of water during the day.

Snappy Solutions

Instead of wasting your time with expensive laxatives or prescription drugs, experts agree that the simplest way to wake up your colon is to drink water—lots and lots of it. Try to drink half your body weight in ounces within 24 hours (e.g., a 140-pound person would drink 70 ounces every day). Need to get things moving right away? Drink a large glass of water twice in one hour to encourage elimination.

Nutty Sipper

If you've got a bad case of constipation or hemorrhoids (which can be just as bad, if not worse), don't just sit there and take it. Go absolutely nuts with it instead. Not with the discomfort, but with nutmeg, a time-honored Ayurvedic remedy for curbing constipation and healing hemorrhoids.

¼ tsp. of ground nutmeg
¼ tsp. of lemon juice
1 cup of water

➡ Add the nutmeg to a glass of warm water that has the lemon juice already mixed in. Lemon water is an astringent that will help tone blood vessels. Drink it twice daily to help your lower half heal and flow more freely.

Strawberry Fields Forever
■ Here's an old Native American remedy for constipation that's a pleasure to try: Eat fresh strawberries. Fruit is a soluble fiber, which eases waste through the colon.

Rub It Out with Olive Oil
■ Treat a case of constipation by taking 1 to 3 tablespoons of olive oil. If this mild laxative doesn't do the trick in a few days, see your doctor. **Caution:** Avoid this remedy if you have gallbladder problems or liver disease.

Nifty, Thrifty Tips

Americans spend millions of dollars a year on laxatives, not realizing that some of them work by irritating the bowel. Over time, they cause your bowel to wait for artificial stimulation to do its business, rather than responding to body signals. Store-bought herbal remedies aren't much safer—they may contain senna, an irritant in many over-the-counter laxatives. Compounds containing mineral oils are a poor choice, too, as they interfere with the absorption of fat. Citrate magnesia and milk of magnesia both draw large volumes of fluid into the intestines in an attempt to get things movin'—this is too drastic for your body's sensitive system. So save your money and stick with homemade remedies.

Rhubarb Laxative

Go ahead, have another slice of pie. Just make sure it's rhubarb—one of the yummiest natural laxatives around. Rhubarb stimulates mucus production in the large intestine to ease elimination within 6 to 10 hours. Eat it stewed or whip up this lip-smacking smoothie.

3 cups of raw rhubarb stalks
1 cup of strawberries
¼ cup of honey
1 cup of water

➤ Juice the raw rhubarb stalks and the strawberries (fresh or frozen will do) in a blender. Add the honey and water, then sip and go! You'll be moving right along again in no time. **Caution:** Be sure to use only the rhubarb stalks, not the leaves, which are poisonous. Don't take rhubarb if you have arthritis or gout.

Praise the Plants

■ The best diet for beating constipation is the same one that doctors recommend for preventing heart disease, cancer, and dozens of other serious health problems: a lot of plant foods and very little, if any, junk food. It's easy—just eat as though processed food had never been invented. Instead, aim for a diet that's high in fiber and complex carbohydrates, like fruits and vegetables, whole grains, and legumes, as well as high-fiber cereals like oatmeal and oat bran.

Snappy Solutions

Sometimes it just takes too long for your body to move things along naturally, so you need to take matters into your own hands. A gentle belly massage will wake up your intestines and send them the message that it's time to get a move on! Using your favorite massage oil, start at your belly button, and begin to massage in little circles in a clockwise pattern. Gradually, let the circles get bigger, until you are massaging along the edges of your entire abdomen.

Root-It-Out Tea

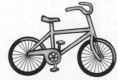

When constipation gums up the works on your body's "exit hatch," you may feel like the only way to get better is to run a plumber's snake through your entire system. But since that isn't the smartest or safest way to get things moving, make this anti-constipation elixir instead.

1 tsp. of dried burdock root
1 tsp. of dried dandelion root
2 cups of boiling water
1 tsp. of dried peppermint

➡ Simmer the burdock root and dandelion root in the water for 20 minutes. Remove it from the heat and add the peppermint. Cover and steep the tea for another 10 minutes. Strain out the solids and sip ½ cup of the brew first thing in the morning and before each meal. If your constipation is stress related, try adding 1 heaping teaspoon of catnip or lemon balm to the mixture. **Caution:** Dandelion is rich in potassium and should not be taken with potassium tablets. Check with your doctor.

Move Often

■ Any kind of physical activity—walking, lifting weights, riding a bicycle—helps the intestines work more efficiently. In fact, it's not uncommon for people who have been consti-pated for years to get completely regular once they start exercising for 20 to 30 minutes every day. It doesn't take much, folks—so get moving!

Dial a Doc

If feelings of discomfort or bloating linger after a bowel movement, or if constipation persists after you've tried to treat it, call your doctor. Persistent abdominal pain or fever, a change in the color or consistency of your stool, or blood in the stool could all be signs of an obstruction or disease. If constipation goes on too long, stools can become so hard and impacted that they won't budge without medical help.

Slippery Soother

While turning your large intestine into a slip-'n'-slide may not be the healthiest thing to do, getting a little slippery with your constipation can really lighten the load. Sip this concoction to soothe and ease inflamed intestinal tissues and soften stools.

Flaxseed
Dried marshmallow root
Dried slippery elm

➡ Grind equal parts of the flaxseed, marshmallow root, and slippery elm in a coffee grinder. Stir 1 rounded teaspoon of the mixture into an 8-ounce glass of water, and drink immediately. Repeat once or twice a day, following each dose with another full glass of plain water. For an added benefit, mix in unfiltered apple juice; its pectin content will soothe the bowels.

Hot, Cold, and Go!

■ Get things moving from the outside in by alternating hot and cold packs on your lower abdomen. First, heat a damp cloth in the microwave, remove it with tongs, and wrap it in a towel. Place the towel over your lower abdomen. Be careful not to burn yourself! After three minutes, replace it with an ice pack wrapped in a towel. Leave the cold pack on for 30 seconds, then repeat the sequence three times. Your blood vessels will expand and contract, initiating a natural pumping action that will spur elimination.

EUREKA!

IF YOU'RE RELUCTANT to use a public restroom even when you urgently need to, you're setting yourself up for uncomfortable trouble. Resisting the urge to have a bowel movement—whether you're in a restaurant or at home—can make it difficult to go later on. In fact, delaying bowel movements can make your large intestine lazy and it will start to ignore its natural urges. You'll be a lot more regular and save yourself a lot of pain if you go as soon as possible whenever you feel the need.

A Honey of a Cure

When you just can't stop coughing, don't worry if you don't have a bottle of cough syrup on hand. As long as you have a few healing staples in your cupboard, you can mix up a batch of this homemade soother right in your own kitchen!

1 cup of honey
1 tbsp. of apple cider vinegar
Juice of half a lemon

➡ Mix the honey, vinegar, and lemon juice. Use 1 to 2 teaspoons per dose, and refrigerate any leftovers. Use within a couple of days. **Caution:** Never give honey to a child under 1 year of age.

A Poultice That Pleases

■ Traditional healers swear by herbal oil poultices for easing coughs. To make one, add a few drops of thyme or eucalyptus essential oil to a teaspoon of olive oil. Rub the mixture on your chest and the outside of your throat, and cover the area with an old towel or a clean piece of flannel. Leave the poultice on for about 20 minutes to soothe your irritated airways and reduce the urge to cough.

Snappy Solutions

A lot of coughs are caused by obvious things, such as upper respiratory infections, air pollution, or secondhand smoke. But if you can't figure out what's making you cough, do some detective work. People can be sensitive to certain plants, perfumes, detergents, solvents in cleaning supplies, or any number of things. The only way to find out for sure why you're hacking is to make notes about what you're doing and where you are when coughing fits strike. Granted, this will take a little time on your part, but sooner or later you'll have a good idea of what's causing the trouble and you'll be able to take steps to avoid it. And that will save you a whole lot of downtime—and discomfort—over the long haul.

All-Purpose Cough Syrup

Coughs annoy the cougher—and everyone else who's within earshot. So try this old-time elixir to quiet any cough that comes your way.

2 large sweet onions
2 cups of dark honey
2 oz. of brandy (optional)

➡ Peel the onions, cut them into thin slices, and spread them out in a single layer in a shallow bowl. Pour the honey over them evenly, and cover the bowl with wax paper. Let the bowl sit for eight hours or so, strain off the syrup, and mix it with the brandy. Take 1 teaspoon every two to three hours, or as needed, to stop the coughing.

Warm Your Wine

■ A friend from Belgium told me that her mother's cough remedy was hot red wine with lemon, cinnamon, and sugar added. She said it puts you right to sleep, so you don't know if you're coughing (and probably don't care, either!). Alcohol is a component of many cough medicines, but use it cautiously—too much can weaken your immune response, which you need to fight infection.

Pass the Salt and Pepper, Please!

■ When you're coughing up a storm, you need relief—NOW! Here's a simple cure that you can whip together in a pinch. Just cut a fresh lemon into four wedges. Then sprinkle the cut side with salt and ground black pepper, and suck the juice out of the seasoned lemon. Your cough will calm down quickly.

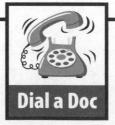
Dial a Doc

✚ If your cough really hurts, is accompanied by fever, is not improving, or gets worse after a week or so, see your doctor. Since we don't always know whether our coughs are just the first indication of a cold, or a symptom of something much worse, it's a good idea to get it checked out. You may have an infection like pneumonia that needs antibiotics. Coughing can even be a symptom of heart disease, so don't wait until it's too late.

Aniseed Syrup

Unlikely as it may seem, this simple fixer can solve two of life's more annoying problems: It can silence a hacking cough and (are you ready for this?) improve your memory. Just take some when you need it and you'll be in the pink of health in no time at all.

7 tsp. of aniseed
1 qt. of boiling water
4 tsp. of glycerin or
4 tsp. of honey

➤ Add the aniseed to the water. Reduce the heat to low, and simmer until the water is reduced to about 3 cups. Strain out the seeds, and while the brew is still warm, stir in the glycerin or honey. For cough relief, take 2 teaspoons of the syrup every few hours until your hacking stops. To give the old gray cells a boost, take 2 tablespoons three times a day as long as you feel the need. Glycerin can be found in most drugstores.

Forget the Fruit Juices

■ It's true that orange juice is loaded with vitamin C, so you'd think that drinking it when you have a cold or the flu would be a good thing. But drinking fruit juice when you have a cough may actually make it worse. Why? Because the acids in orange, pineapple, and grapefruit juices can irritate your throat and make a cough worse. So make veggie juice your drink of choice until you're well again.

Cleave to Cloves

■ To relieve a cough, pop a whole clove into your mouth, and suck on it. The clove oil helps to numb the tickle in your throat better than flavored cough drops or sweetened syrups.

What Would Grandma Do?

🦋 IF YOU EVER CAME DOWN with any type of cough around Grandma Putt, the first thing she'd have you do is put up your feet. After all, since most coughs are caused by upper respiratory infections, your first line of defense should be to help your body heal itself. And the best way to do that is to kick back and take it easy.

Healin' Honey

Honey mixed with onion juice was widely used as a healing tonic during the Great Depression, when few folks could afford drugstore remedies. Honey or sugar is used in this tonic to draw the juice from the onion, forming an effective cough syrup. The onion also stimulates saliva flow, which helps clear your throat and reduce inflammation. So give this mixer a whirl to get rid of a nasty cough.

1 medium onion
2 cups of honey
½ cup of sugar (optional)

➧ Slice the onion into rings, and place them in a deep bowl. Cover them with honey, and let the concoction stand for 10 to 12 hours. Then strain out the onion and take 1 tablespoon of the syrup four or five times a day. Or you can chop the onion finely, add about half as much honey, and mix with ½ cup of sugar. Let it stand overnight. Take 1 tablespoon of the resulting syrup every four to five hours. **Caution:** Never give honey to a child under 1 year of age.

Drink Your Veggies

■ Fresh vegetable juice is packed with nutrients that will feed your immune system. The advantage of drinking juices over eating solid foods when you're sick is that your body is able to absorb the nutrients quickly and easily. So unpack the juicer you got for your birthday five years ago, and crank it up. Green leafy vegetables are the best choices for juicing, and be sure to always use organic veggies so you don't ingest any pesticides.

Nifty, Thrifty Tips

Instead of spending your cold, hard cash on fancy cough syrups and lozenges, try keeping yourself hydrated. Any time, but especially when you've got a cough, is the right time to drink lots of fluids. So enjoy a cup of hot tea or a tall glass of lemonade with honey— they'll both soothe a cough, loosen up mucus, and taste delicious, too!

Horehound Candy

Horehound helps relax the smooth muscles in your lungs while clearing mucus out. Try this family recipe for horehound candy.

2 cups of fresh horehound leaves
4 cups of water
3 cups of brown sugar
3 cups of granulated sugar

➤ Put the horehound leaves in a pot with the water. Slowly bring the mixture to a boil, then let it simmer for 15 minutes. Remove the pot from the stove, and strain out the leaves. Add the sugars, stirring with a wooden spoon until they're completely dissolved. Put the pot back on the stove, bring the syrup to a boil, then pour the "batter" into a greased 9- by 13-inch baking pan and let it sit at room temperature. As soon as the candy hardens, break it into bite-size pieces, and wrap each one in waxed paper.

Reach for Radishes

■ To relieve a cough, make a batch of radish syrup. Just cut six or eight radishes into thin slices, spread them out on a plate, and cover them generously with sugar. Loosely place wax paper on top, and let them sit overnight at room temperature. In the morning, the slices will be swimming in rich syrup. Drain the syrup off into a glass bottle, and take a teaspoonful whenever you feel the need.

Q: *I've noticed that my cough is worse first thing in the morning after a full night's sleep. What can I do to improve this?*

A: When your chest is congested and you're coughing up a lot of mucus, pile on several pillows or sleep on a foam wedge. Sleeping with your head raised 6 to 8 inches off the mattress will prevent the mucus from pooling in your bronchial passages, thus easing your coughing and promoting more peaceful sleep.

Take My Advice

Hound Away Cough Syrup

If you're looking for a natural way to silence a nagging cough due to a cold, bronchitis, or even whooping cough, make this concoction part of your morning regimen. Since horehound is one of the main ingredients found in cough drops and syrups, it should work like a charm.

1 tsp. of dried coltsfoot leaves
1 tsp. of grated fresh ginger
1 tsp. of dried horehound leaves
1 cup of boiling water
Honey (optional)

➡ Blend all three herbs and scoop a teaspoon of the mixture into the water. Let it steep for about 10 minutes, then strain out the herbs. Add a teaspoon of honey, if you like, and sip your cough into silence!

Take a Bite Outta Your Bark!

■ How often do you use those little packets of hot mustard that accompany Chinese takeout? Well, don't throw the extras away—they can come in handy when you have a cough. Just work the super-hot mustard into a salad dressing or add it to chicken salad to loosen up mucus and stop your barking right quick.

Snappy Solutions

Whatever you do, don't try to hold back your cough while you wait for the medicine to kick in. Instead, allow yourself one long, strong hack. A strong cough is your body's equivalent of a bouncer: It tosses out all the potential troublemakers in the exclusive nightclub of your respiratory system. Coughing strongly will help drive out germs and eliminate irritating substances like smoke, pollen, and clouds of cologne. If possible, cough outside, away from people, so you don't have to cover your mouth. Covering up can be as harmful as it is helpful, since germs linger on your hand and get back into your system. If you must cough near others, cough into the crook of your elbow instead of your hand.

Old-Time Cough Stopper

Coughs can last for days at a time, showing no sign of leaving. Even when you have no other symptoms to indicate that you've got a cold or the flu, you end up feeling miserable all day long. So if you have a cough that just won't quit, try this elixir.

**1 cup of honey
Juice of 1 large lemon**

➡ Combine the ingredients in a saucepan. Heat the mixture for five minutes (don't boil it!), then stir it vigorously for two minutes. Pour the elixir into a bottle, and take 1 teaspoon every two hours. Before you know it, your cough will quit nagging you, and you'll be feeling much better.

Take Thyme Out

■ This familiar kitchen spice is great for fighting off a nagging cough because it inhibits bacteria and reduces cough-causing inflammation in your respiratory system. Thyme is also an effective expectorant: It makes mucus thinner, so you don't have to cough as hard to get rid of it. You can make thyme tea by steeping 1 teaspoon of the dried herb for 10 to 15 minutes in 1 cup of hot water. Or visit your local health-food store, pick up a bottle of thyme tincture, and take 10 to 20 drops in a cup of warm water up to four times daily. Add a teaspoon of honey or a squeeze of fresh lemon to your tea, if desired.

EUREKA!

EVEN THOUGH HOME REMEDIES are great for helping clear up the problems that ail us, sometimes they just aren't enough. Nature packs lots of vitamins and minerals into its healing herbs, but even if you get all of the essential nutrients in your diet, your body still needs extra vitamins and minerals when you're fighting an upper respiratory infection. Taking a daily multivitamin is an easy way to ensure that you get all the nutrients you need to help your body heal quickly.

Sweet 'n' Spicy Cough Syrup

If you're looking for a reliable cough medicine that won't make you drowsy, look no further. This fixer will even knock out dry, hacking coughs that seem to hang on long after your cold has flown the coop. But be forewarned: This stuff tastes awful. Truly awful, but boy, oh boy, does it do the job.

1 tbsp. of apple cider vinegar
1 tbsp. of honey
½ tsp. of ground ginger
¼ tsp. of cayenne pepper
2 tbsp. of water

➤ Mix the ingredients thoroughly in a plastic container with a lid. Take 1 teaspoon as needed. And don't say I didn't warn you about the taste!

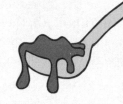

When to Encourage Coughs

■ The chest-racking cough that accompanies pneumonia can be agonizing, but you don't necessarily want to block it with a cough suppressant. Coughing is your body's way of expelling the gunk that's clogging your lungs. The more mucus you cough up, the better you'll feel, and the more quickly you'll recover.

Of course, there are times when a cough is so severe that it interferes with your sleep or causes intense pain. In fact, some folks have even broken ribs during coughing attacks! So if your cough is really bad—pneumonia or not—go ahead and use a cough suppressant, following the label directions.

What Would Grandma Do?

WHENEVER SHE'D GO SHOPPING, Grandma Putt would always bring home some catnip for the family cats. She would also get some extra for us because she knew that when it was brewed into a tasty tea, it helped get rid of nasty coughs. Make catnip tea by steeping 1 or 2 teaspoons of dried catnip leaves in 1 cup of boiling water for 10 to 15 minutes. Add honey to taste. You can drink up to 3 cups a day until the cough subsides.

Blues-Beating Tonic

Sometimes, in the ocean of life, the surf is calm and steady. Other times, it's so savage that it takes your breath away. For an herbal mood lifter, try this happy mixer.

Dried betony
Dried kava
Dried passionflower
Dried St. John's wort
Dried vervain
1 cup of hot water

➡ Combine equal parts of the five herbs, then steep 1 teaspoon of the mixture in the water for 15 minutes. Strain out the solids, and drink 2 cups daily. **Caution:** Kava has been linked to liver toxicity, so don't take this tea without consulting a qualified health practitioner first—especially if you're taking antidepressant or anti-anxiety medications. Also check with your doctor before taking St. John's wort if you are taking antidepressant or anti-anxiety medications.

Hold the Thistle

■ Blessed thistle is an old-time remedy for melancholy. To make an infusion, use 1 teaspoon of dried thistle per 1 cup of boiling water. Steep for 10 minutes, and drink 1 to 2 cups per day.

Seek Out St. John

■ Today, many people take St. John's wort for mild depression. Unlike some psychotropic drugs, it's not addictive, but you must take it regularly for three to six weeks to feel its full effect. Check with your doctor about whether this herb is safe for you—especially if you are already taking antidepressant medication.

EUREKA!

INSTEAD OF TEAS AND DRUGS to fight the doldrums, try faking yourself out and lifting your mood all by yourself. Put on your favorite music, dress in your best clothes, stand up straight, and go about your business as if it were the best day of your life. But if your depression is severe, be realistic. Putting a happy face on a serious problem is denial—and that's unhealthy.

Flower-Full Tea

Flowers do more than simply make our world a more beautiful place: Their fragrance, color, and chemical makeup can also lift our moods. To beat the blues, try making a tea with two or three of these beauties to give yourself the boost you need.

Fresh or dried borage
Fresh or dried lavender
Fresh or dried passionflower
Fresh or dried rosemary
Fresh or dried skullcap
Fresh or dried vervain
1 cup of boiling water

➡ These pretty purple and blue flowers can be just the thing for chasing the blues away. Combine equal parts of the herbs of your choice, and steep 1 teaspoon of the mixture in the water for 10 minutes. Strain and drink 2 to 3 cups per day, and watch your mood blossom into something lovely.

Discover Your Roots

■ Roots are what keep us grounded in reality and hold us to our center. To help give yourself some solid ground to stand on, be sure to include some roots in your diet, too. So if you're really feeling like you can't find your footing, make a tea of burdock and dandelion roots by simmering ½ heaping teaspoon of each of the dried roots in 1 cup of water for 20 minutes. Strain, and drink 1 to 2 cups daily. **Caution:** Dandelion is rich in potassium and shouldn't be taken if you're already taking potassium tablets.

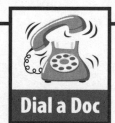

Dial a Doc

✚ It is important to distinguish between a passing feeling of sadness and the symptoms of a major or clinical depression. Untreated depression can lead to suicide, which is the third-leading cause of death for teenagers and the seventh-leading cause of death in adults aged 25 to 64. If you have any thoughts of suicide, are depressed for more than two weeks, can't concentrate, feel guilty, can't sleep or sleep too much, or have a noticeable change in weight, get professional help immediately.

Fragrant Bath Crystals

Even if you're not clinically depressed, a bad mood can ruin an entire day (or days), and sometimes it can seem like you'll never break out of it. So mix up a batch of this beautiful blend at the end of a bad day, and soak your troubles away for a fresh start tomorrow. While you're at it, prepare a few more batches of the crystals to give away as presents.

½ cup of Epsom salts
½ cup of sea salt
½ cup of fresh lavender, chamomile, or rosebuds
¼ cup of baking soda
15 drops of fragrance oil (any kind you like to match or complement the flowers' aroma)
Food coloring (optional)

➡ Blend the salts, flowers, and baking soda in an old blender or food processor. Let the mixture sit for 30 minutes to dry a bit, then add the oil and food coloring. Pour the mixture into small jars. Add 2 to 3 tablespoons to your bathwater, then sink in and melt your cares away.

Get Some Space

■ Although taking a vacation is not a cure-all for depression, a few days off and a change of scenery may help. Sometimes you can think things through more easily when you're away from your usual surroundings. You can take stock of the situation that has you down and plan more useful strategies. From a distance, you may even find that you see things more clearly.

Snappy Solutions

You could try some of the depression medications that are on the market and take them for weeks on end, or you could try exercising for 30 minutes. A Duke University study revealed that people with major depression who exercised aerobically for 30 minutes three times a week experienced the same relief from depression as people who took antidepressants. And the benefits of exercise won't stop at your depression—your entire body will thank you for the effort!

Happy Times Bubble Bath

Feeling down in the dumps? Try one of Grandma Putt's no-fail pick-me-uppers—a nice long soak in a good old-fashioned bubble bath. This was her favorite recipe, which makes enough for one very relaxing bath.

½ cup of Dr. Bronner's
   Peppermint Liquid Soap
1 tbsp. of sugar
1 egg white

➡ Mix all of the ingredients together, and pour the mixture under warm running water. Then ease into the tub, sit back, and say "Aaahhh." If you can't find Dr. Bronner's (or don't like peppermint), you can substitute ½ cup of liquid hand soap and a few drops of your favorite scented oil.

Feel Better with Fish

■ Cold-water fish, such as salmon and tuna, are packed with omega-3 essential fatty acids, which help the brain receive serotonin. Eicosapentaenoic acid (EPA) is a component of fish oil that has been shown to help reduce feelings of worthlessness. So go pick up some fish, or try taking fish oil to help get your mood back on track. Make sure the fish oil is certified free of heavy metals and pesticides like PCB.

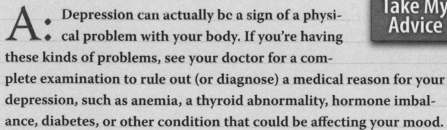

Q.: *My depression has been hanging over me for a while now, and the rest of my body is not exactly feeling great, either. What is causing my body and mind to go downhill like this?*

A.: Depression can actually be a sign of a physical problem with your body. If you're having these kinds of problems, see your doctor for a complete examination to rule out (or diagnose) a medical reason for your depression, such as anemia, a thyroid abnormality, hormone imbalance, diabetes, or other condition that could be affecting your mood.

Take My Advice

Herbal Cheer Tea

Old-time healers have always known exactly what herbs and other natural ingredients can be used to fix the things that ail the body. Here's a basic herbal cheer mixer that's perfect for beating back the blues.

Dried devil's club bark
Dried passionflower
Dried St. John's wort

➤ Combine equal amounts of each herb in a glass jar, mix well, seal, and keep it handy for whenever you're feeling low. To make the tea, put 1 teaspoon of the mixture in a mug, add boiling water, cover, let it steep for 10 minutes, and then strain out the solids. Relax as you drink 2 cups a day. **Caution:** If you are taking antidepressant medications, consult your doctor before using St. John's wort.

Talk About It

■ Depression is far more common in women than in men (or maybe, women just own up to it more readily). In our culture, women are encouraged to talk about their feelings. Thankfully, these days, more men are learning to do this, too. So don't deny your pain—that'll just keep you in an emotional prison. Seek advice from a trusted friend who can help you run a reality check on your complaints. Or see a counselor for a more objective view. What happens when you bottle it up? For men, unexpressed emotional problems are likely to manifest themselves as substance abuse or violence.

✚ Depression is a biological disease, not a sign of weakness—and you should never hesitate to get help. If you are clinically depressed, your doctor may prescribe an antidepressant and refer you to a professional for one of many "talk therapy" options, ranging from in-depth psychoanalysis to group therapy, behavioral therapy, and a variety of new technologies. But make sure that you use the antidepressant in combination with cognitive therapy or interpersonal therapy to maximize results.

Dial a Doc

Lifting Lemon Balm Sauce

When you're fighting a bout of depression, it's easy to slip into bad habits. A common side effect of depression is a nasty eating binge. If a gloomy mood has you headed down the grocery store's junk-food aisle, lemon balm and its mood-lifting properties could get you back on the right diet track.

2 cups of fresh lemon balm leaves
3 garlic cloves
½ cup of olive oil

➥ Chop up the lemon balm leaves, peel and crush the garlic cloves, and mix them together with the olive oil. What do you have? A great pesto sauce! Keep it handy to dribble over broiled or grilled seafood or poultry. It'll boost your mood and keep your eating habits headed in the right (healthy) direction.

Talk Turkey

■ Don't wait until the holidays to get your dose of tryptophan, an amino acid that's converted into serotonin in the body. In one study, when women ate turkey, fish, dairy products, nuts, and other foods high in tryptophan, their dark mood lifted. When you're eating a tryptophan-rich food, pair it with a lower-fat carbohydrate, such as whole-grain bread, brown rice, or mashed potatoes. Carbs trigger the release of insulin, which allows tryptophan to enter your brain so that your serotonin levels rise.

Nifty, Thrifty Tips

Before you turn to drugs and other expensive remedies to cure mild depression, think about this: Many people with depression have a vitamin B deficiency. The B vitamins help deliver oxygen to the brain, turn blood sugar into energy, and keep feel-good brain chemicals in circulation. So instead of emptying your wallet, check out the labels on your grocery store shelves for foods that give you a good dose of B vitamins, including fish, meat, poultry, eggs, milk, legumes, and whole grains.

Rekindle Your Fire Bath

Even mild forms of depression, such as temporary burnout, rob your body of essential electrolytes. So recharge those energizers—and soothe your spirit at the same time—with this tub-time mixer.

2 cups of Epsom salts
2 cups of kosher salt
2 tbsp. of potassium
1 tbsp. of vitamin C crystals

➥ Pour all of the ingredients into the tub while the water is running (at a temperature of your choice). Then ease yourself in and soak your troubles away for as long as you like.

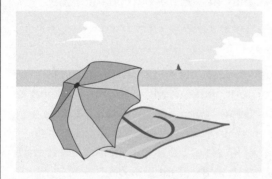

Change the Scenery

■ Sometimes all it takes to rev up your engine and renew your zest for life is to let your eyes feast on a new landscape for a little while. Are you surrounded by tall gray buildings or endless suburban sprawl? Head out into the country for a day or two, and gaze at fields of green. Likewise, if you're bored with a rural landscape, take yourself to a gritty, up-tempo city. And there's nothing like getting out on the water—lake, ocean, river, or stream—to give you a new perspective on the stresses in your life.

What Would Grandma Do?

🦋 *WHEN GRANDMA PUTT was feeling down in the dumps, she turned to one of the tried-and-true ingredients she used most in her kitchen: apple cider vinegar. This old-time treatment often relieves mild cases of depression. Just mix 1 teaspoon of apple cider vinegar with about ½ cup of water. Drink up once a day for a week or so, and your spirits should perk right up.*

Restore the Roar

Many herbs are used for their restorative actions, especially when it comes to lifting a bad mood. And when they're used together, the effects can be even greater. If you want to restore your mood to something happier, use a combination of two or more herbs.

Dried chamomile
Dried lemon balm
Dried lime blossom
Dried passionflower
Dried rosemary
Dried vervain
1 qt. of boiling water

➡ Steep 1 heaping tablespoon of your choice of herbs in the water for 15 minutes. Strain and let the mixture cool, then sip it throughout the day. Your mood will rise in no time at all, and you'll be back in action quick as a wink. **Caution:** People with ragweed allergies may be sensitive to chamomile.

Healing Rays

■ If you exercise outdoors, you may enhance the natural antidepressant effect of your workout without even realizing it. You see, exposure to sunlight—even on dim, overcast days—helps boost levels of vitamin D in your body, which in turn may help your body maintain higher levels of serotonin. In fact, even in a downpour, outside light is 30 times brighter than the light indoors.

EUREKA!

WHEN YOU CRAVE warm temperatures and sunny skies, the urge to huddle by the fireplace all winter long can be irresistible. But turning into a couch potato is the worst thing you can do to combat your cold-weather blues. If you're not up to joining winter-sports lovers on the slopes or frozen ponds, head for the warmth and light of your local gym, or maybe an indoor skating rink. Get 30 minutes of regular exercise a day to keep those endorphins circulating, and you'll more easily combat the depression of a long, cold, dark winter.

Smell the Roses Room Spray

Misting the air and inhaling aromatic herbs can provide a quick trip back to your center of calm. Try this essential oil combination to give every room in your house a refreshing smell, and lend your mood a refreshing lift.

➡ Fill a handheld sprayer bottle with the essential oils and salt. Fill the balance of the bottle with water, and allow the salt to dissolve. Spray some of the mixture into the air whenever you're feeling down, and you'll quickly get back to your center. All of these oils are made from calming and stimulating herbs and can be found at health-food stores.

5 drops of bergamot oil
5 drops of chamomile oil
5 drops of clary sage oil
5 drops of geranium oil
5 drops of lavender oil
5 drops of lemon balm oil
1 tsp. of salt
Water

Take a Deep Breath

■ Scent has a powerful effect on our mood because the olfactory nerve connects our nose to the limbic system—the part of the brain that rules our emotions. So find a scent that appeals to you, and experiment with ways to incorporate it into your life, via a body lotion, perfume, atomizer, candle, or bath oil.

Snappy Solutions

Instead of dosing yourself up with depression-fighting medication that can take too long to kick in and leave you waiting and waiting for its effects, try getting a massage. Preliminary studies indicate that massage may help reduce symptoms of depression, perhaps by combating a buildup of the stress hormone cortisol. To enhance the feel-good effect, use some mood-boosting herbal oils, such as bergamot, geranium, jasmine, neroli, or ylang-ylang, all of which are available at health-food stores.

Soothing Tea

There are plenty of teas on the market, and most simply offer a nice way to relax. But some are great for eliminating the problems that can plague your body and mind. Here's a recipe for a super-soothing elixir to sip when the blues start dragging you down.

1 part fresh or dried lavender blossom
1 part fresh or dried lemon balm leaf
2 parts fresh or dried green oat straw
2 parts fresh or dried dried St. John's wort blossom
1 qt. of boiling water

➡ Combine the first four ingredients, and steep 1 heaping teaspoon of the mixture in the water. Strain out the solids, then let the liquid cool. Sip the tea throughout the day. This blend will help your body cope with stress while easing your troubled mind.

Lighten Up

■ If seasonal affective disorder (SAD) is a problem for you, try what's called a dawn simulator—essentially a bedside lamp that gradually glows from dim to more intense light, mimicking a natural mid-May sunrise. Just program the fake dawn to start one to three hours before you awaken, and your body will detect the changing light through your closed eyelids. Look for 250-lux models on the Internet and in catalogs and stores that sell personal health-care products.

What Would Grandma Do?

🦋 WHEN GRANDMA PUTT *was feeling a little blue, she knew the best, and fastest, way to drag herself out of it was to spend some time with her friends or neighbors. And, once again, she was right. Studies indicate that when a woman spends time with another woman, her body releases a brain chemical called oxytocin that counters the kind of stress that can contribute to depression. So get together with a buddy, and hopefully, you'll feel better just like that.*

Take a Whiff Air Freshener

Since fragrance has a mighty powerful effect on mood, it makes perfect "scents" to find one you love and incorporate it into your daily routine. Here's an uplifting air freshener made with essential oils that are bound to make everything smell better.

➥ Combine all of the ingredients in a clean, 4-ounce handheld sprayer bottle that's got a fine-mist setting. (Do not use a bottle that previously held cleaning products or products like hair spray.) Spray, sniff, and smile!

1½ oz. of distilled water
1½ oz. of high-proof alcohol (vodka is suitable; rubbing alcohol is not) or 3 oz. of distilled water
20 drops of lime essential oil
14 drops of bergamot oil
4 drops of ylang-ylang oil
2 drops of rose oil

Flax to the Max

■ People who are depressed often have low levels of essential fatty acids. Taking 1 tablespoon of flaxseed oil once or twice daily can often help beat the blues. This simple fixer can be especially effective for folks who suffer from seasonal affective disorder (SAD). So spoon it up, and clear out the dark clouds.

EUREKA!

BURNOUT IS YOUR SOUL'S WAY of telling you that it's hungry. So feed it in whatever way you know will satisfy its appetite. Take some time away from the daily grind and visit an art gallery or museum—or several. And while you're at it, buy a painting to add to your collection (as long as the expense won't worsen your woes). Stroll through a botanical garden—being sure to stop and smell the roses. Or rent a place at the beach for a few days and watch the waves crash on the shore. In other words, take time to enjoy yourself, even if you only have an hour or two to spare.

Bilberry Brew

Ask anyone with diabetes, and chances are they'll tell you the biggest hassle of having the disease is being more disciplined about their diets—all the time—than most celery-stick-thin supermodels. The biggest problem that people with diabetes face is the challenge of keeping the condition under control. Well, here's a terrific tea that can be used to treat diabetes.

Dried bilberry
Dried devil's club
Dried fenugreek
Dried goat's rue
1 cup of boiling water

➡ Combine equal parts of the herbs, then steep 1 heaping teaspoon of the mixture in the water for 15 minutes or so and strain. Drink the tea as desired between meals. **Caution:** When using any therapies that may alter blood sugar, you must monitor your blood sugar levels more frequently than normal. Before you try this tea, check with your doctor if you are taking any blood-sugar-altering medications.

Get More Shut-Eye

■ Getting a good night's sleep will enhance your beauty and help keep your blood sugar levels in line. In fact, studies show that if you're shortchanging yourself by as little as two and a half hours of sleep a night, you may be 40 percent less sensitive to insulin than you would be if you got a full eight hours of rest.

Berry Good Tincture

■ Bearberry has been traditionally combined with bilberry in a tea to treat diabetes. Just add 2 parts of bilberry tincture to 1 part of bearberry tincture. Stir 10 to 20 drops of the mixture into a glass of water, and sip it between meals. Be sure to monitor your blood sugar levels carefully.

✚ **If your blood sugar levels soar too high or dip too low, it can be an emergency. So if you feel sluggish or begin to feel like you've been drugged, get emergency medical help immediately.**

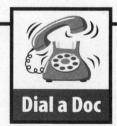

Dial a Doc

Cinnamon Tea

Studies suggest that cinnamon can help lower blood glucose levels in people with type 2 diabetes. Sprinkle the delicious spice on toast or stir it into your morning oatmeal. Or try this warming elixir to get your day off to a healthy start.

1 cinnamon stick
1 green tea bag
    (either regular or decaf)
1 cup of boiling water
Artificial sweetener (optional)

➡ Put the cinnamon stick and the tea bag in a cup, add the water, and let it steep for three minutes. Add artificial sweetener to taste, if desired. Then drink up!

Dunk Your Spuds—in Vinegar

■ Gram for gram, potatoes are converted to sugar faster than any other food—including sugar sprinkled on cereal. If you're a spud lover, opt for potato salad made with unpeeled potatoes and vinaigrette dressing. The acid in the dressing will reduce the effect on your blood sugar. And if it's French fries you crave, simply eat them the British way—doused with malt vinegar.

Bump Up Your Fiber

■ Getting 50 grams of fiber daily—double the amount normally recommended—may lower insulin resistance, studies show. Those fiber-rich psyllium powders sold in drugstores and grocery stores can help you meet that quota, but be sure to select brands without sugar or laxatives, follow the package directions, and consult your doctor before using them.

Nifty, Thrifty Tips

A high intake of high-fructose corn syrup—now the leading sweetener in packaged foods—may put you on the high road to insulin resistance. Stay away from foods that have ingredients ending in "-ose" at or near the top of the list. Besides being bad for you, those processed foods usually cost more than naturally sweet treats like fresh fruits.

Dilly of a Diarrhea Remedy

As unpleasant as it is, diarrhea is your body's way of getting rid of some things that shouldn't be there—you know: bacteria, parasites, and spoiled food, to name a few. But all of those trips to the bathroom can leave you feeling dehydrated and weak, and this is one herbal fixer that can make you better, just like that.

1 tsp. of slippery elm powder
1 tsp. of ground ginger
1 cup of warm water

➤ Mix the slippery elm powder and ginger into the water. Sip up to 4 cups per day to help relieve the symptoms. Before you know it, the only slippery thing will be the elm in your drink.

Pick the Right Liquids

■ When you have diarrhea, your intestines are temporarily impaired in their ability to digest milk and other dairy products. So you'll need to give up milk and other dairy products until you're feeling better. Likewise, avoid citrus, acidic vegetable juices, alcohol, and caffeine, which also tend to make things worse.

Be a BRAT

■ This acronym helps you remember a diet of bland and binding foods—bananas, rice, applesauce, and toast—that are widely recommended to eat while you recover from diarrhea. It's also a good idea to eat chicken-and-rice soup to replenish the sodium and potassium you've lost.

Snappy Solutions

*G*ot a bad case of diarrhea that bland foods and lots of water just can't stop? You've spent all that time trying different remedies when the problem could just be your choice of chewing gum. Many brands of sugar-free gum are made with the artificial sweetener sorbitol, which can cause diarrhea. If you want to chew gum, read the labels first to find a sorbitol-free brand.

Hydration Formula

Even a brief bout of vomiting or diarrhea will whisk crucial fluids and electrolytes right out of your body quick as a wink. But this simple elixir will put them back where they belong and have you feeling better in no time.

4 tsp. of sugar
1 tsp. of sea salt
1 qt. of water

➡ Mix the ingredients together in a pitcher until the sugar and salt have completely dissolved. Then drink 2 cups of the mixture every hour until you're in tip-top shape again. Both the salt and sugar will replace the right nutrients that the diarrhea made off with.

Tame Your Sweet Tooth

■ For some people, sugar in any form—whether it's the fructose in fruit or the lactose in milk—is simply not well digested and can cause intestinal distress. So cutting back on your sugar intake might just curb your diarrhea.

Barley Can't Be Beat

■ Bland though it may be, this grain can slow intestinal motion and put a stop to diarrhea. To give it some flavor, prepare pearl barley according to the package directions and add it to 1 cup of beef broth. The mixture will replace lost fluids and electrolytes, in addition to taming your tummy's turmoil.

EUREKA!

YOU CAN DO A LOT to prevent diarrhea from ever becoming an issue if you're just a little cautious about what you eat. For example, watch out for seafood. Fish sold in markets and restaurants is not necessarily safe to eat. Regulations differ from one part of the world—or the country—to another. Very often, fish, especially shellfish, is contaminated by pollution in the lake, bay, or ocean in which it was caught. So educate yourself, and always ask where the fish came from before you indulge.

Remedy for the Runs

Ugghhh. An attack of the runs. It's no fun now, and it was no fun in Grandma Putt's day. Fortunately, she had a great-tasting fruity fixer that was as close as one of her backyard apple trees.

1 apple, peeled and cored
1 tsp. of honey
1 tsp. of lime juice
Pinch of cinnamon

➡ Puree all of the ingredients in a blender or food processor, pour the mixture into a bowl, and dig in. **Just a few words of caution:** Never give this concoction—or anything containing honey—to a baby under 1 year of age. Babies with diarrhea should be seen by a doctor. And if your diarrhea lasts more than a day or two, call your doctor.

Take Away the Burn

■ If you have burning diarrhea, marshmallow tea can minimize the irritation by soothing your intestinal walls. Look for marshmallow tea or powder at a health-food store. Make the tea according to package directions, and drink a cup several times a day. To use the powder, add a teaspoon to a flavored gelatin product and snack on it throughout the day.

Pamper with Peppermint

■ Try a cup of calming peppermint tea to relax the muscles of your digestive tract and relieve the spasms that trigger diarrhea. Just stir 1 teaspoon of leaves (fresh or dried) into 1 cup of boiling water and let it simmer for 10 minutes or so. Strain out the leaves and drink as many as 3 cups a day after meals until your symptoms clear up.

✚ Diarrhea usually takes care of itself, but sometimes it signals serious problems, such as food poisoning, a digestive disorder, or even thyroid disease. Call your doctor if your bout lasts more than 48 hours—or immediately if you have bloody diarrhea, pain, or a fever.

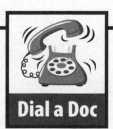

Dial a Doc

Run Relief

Try this fruity-flavored tea the next time diarrhea has you on the run. It's a good-tasting mixer that will replenish lost fluids and prevent you from becoming dehydrated.

1 tsp. of dried marshmallow leaves
1 tsp. of dried meadowsweet leaves
1 tsp. of dried strawberry leaves
1 cup of boiling water

➥ Blend the herbs together and scoop a teaspoon of the mixture into the water. Let it steep for 15 minutes, then strain out the herbs before sipping. You can drink up to 3 cups a day.

Rice-Is-Nice Water

■ The next time you've got tummy turmoil, prepare a batch of rice and add an extra 1½ cups of water to the pot. When the rice is cooked to the texture you want, drain off the extra water, chill it if you like, and drink it as a hydrating, binding tonic. You can add a small amount of sugar or honey for even sweeter relief.

Q: *I've heard that garlic is a good way to fight an infection that can cause diarrhea. But the extra garlic in my food doesn't seem to be doing the trick. Why is that?*

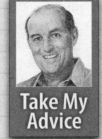

Take My Advice

A: Garlic is definitely one of the best ways to fight infection internally. So if your diarrhea is caused by bacteria or the flu, adding garlic to your meal is a good choice. But don't add the garlic until the food's already off the stove because its immune-boosting powers are most potent when garlic is raw. If eating raw garlic doesn't appeal to you, pick up some garlic capsules at a local health-food store and take them three times a day until your diarrhea subsides.

Diverticulitis Diverter

A diet made up of highly processed, low-fiber foods can finally catch up with you and cause a painful condition called diverticulitis. Constipation can cause irritated pouches in the colon, which in turn lead to pain and swelling. One of the best fixers I've found is this wild yam tea.

2 tbsp. of dried wild yam
1 qt. of boiling water
½ tsp. of dried black haw
½ tsp. of dried peppermint
½ tsp. of dried valerian

➡ Put the wild yam into the water. Reduce the heat and let it simmer for 20 minutes. Enhance the brew's medicinal might by adding the black haw, peppermint, and valerian. Strain out the solids, then drink up to 3 cups daily.

Eat More Fiber

■ Soluble fiber, found in apples and other fresh fruit, keeps your stool soft for an easier passage through your colon. Insoluble fiber, found in whole grains and vegetables, adds bulk, which decreases the pressure on your colon walls. So bulk up your diet with these good-for-you foods.

Fill Up on Fluids

■ A high-fiber diet requires lots of liquids to wash it all down and out. Fiber, you see, acts as a sponge in your large intestine. If you don't drink enough liquids, you could become constipated. So aim to drink at least eight glasses of water every day to keep things moving along.

Nifty, Thrifty Tips

Before you buy a lot of fiber supplements and foods that supposedly are high in fiber, try finding a secret fiber source. Actually, it shouldn't be such a secret. But unless you read nutrition labels in the cereal aisle, it's a big one. Although most cereals—including whole-grain varieties—have only a few grams of fiber per serving, there are a few out there that have 13 or 14 grams per serving. Which ones? You'll have to read the labels to find out!

Get Going—Gingerly

The pain of diverticulitis can be downright debilitating. But don't let it get you down. Ease your woes—or better yet, head off trouble—with this gentle elixir.

2 gal. of water
4½ tbsp. of grated fresh ginger
Cheesecloth bag

➡ Add the water to a pot, and bring it to a boil. Put the grated ginger into the cheesecloth bag, dunk it in the water, and remove the pot from the heat. Let the pouch steep until the water cools to a comfortable (but still warm) temperature. Then dip a clean towel into the brew, and lay it over your abdomen until the compress cools. Repeat the process four more times, reheating the water and applying a fresh compress each time. You'll find that things will soon be on the move again.

Easy Does It

■ When you add fiber to your diet, do it gradually to avoid uncomfortable bloating and gas. A high-fiber diet helps form bulkier stool, which requires less contraction and pressure to move through your bowels. It's much the same as a tube of toothpaste. When the tube is full, you don't have to squeeze as hard to get the stuff out as you do when it's nearly empty.

✚ A diverticulitis attack can develop without warning. Call your doctor immediately if severe abdominal pain strikes suddenly, along with tenderness in the left side of the lower abdomen. Fever, nausea, chills, and other symptoms may also occur. Unless the infection is treated with antibiotics, an abscess may form and lead to further complications, including peritonitis and emergency surgery.

Dial a Doc

Inside-Out Tea

A dry vagina often is the result of diminishing levels of estrogen at menopause. It doesn't mean that your love juice is gone forever—just that you need to help it along. These herbs have been used to reduce most perimenopausal symptoms, so try this mixer to put some moisture back where you want it.

Dried black cohosh
Dried chastetree berry
Dried partridgeberry
Dried red clover
1 cup of boiling water

➡ Combine equal parts of the herbs, then place 1 heaping teaspoon of the mixture in the water. Cover the mixture and let it steep for 15 minutes, then strain out the solids. Drink 2 cups daily. This is a toning tea, so for best results, it should be taken for several months.

Vaginal Dryness Remedy

■ As its name implies, when tissue-soothing slippery elm is moistened, it becomes slick. Simply mix 2 tablespoons of slippery elm powder (available at health-food stores) with enough water to make a paste and add a dab of pure aloe gel (you can either purchase it at your local health-food store or scoop it straight out of a leaf). Use clean hands to spread the slick stuff over your vulva and inside your vagina.

Sweeten Up!

■ Good, old-fashioned honey can be used to gently moisturize vaginal tissues. While you may need to use it daily at first, over time, you should be able to decrease the frequency of use. For ease of application and extra benefit, add several drops of vitamin E oil to it.

EUREKA!

IF YOU NEED a lubricant now and can't dash off to the pharmacy, help is in the fridge. Yogurt is a vaginal lubricant that's nonallergenic for most people. Use only in a pinch when you have no lubricant on hand.

The Flower Factor

Calendula flowers have a gentle healing effect on the skin and mucous membranes. Soaking in this soothing elixir could be all it takes to put your sex life back on the high road to happiness.

1 cup of fresh
 calendula flowers
1 qt. of water

➡ Bring the water to a boil, reduce the heat to simmer, and add the flowers. Steep for 15 minutes, strain, and pour the brew into a warm sitz bath. Immerse yourself up to your belly button. After soaking for 5 to 10 minutes, get out of the tub and apply a cold, wet towel like a diaper. Leave the towel on for 3 to 5 minutes. This may be repeated two to three times a session. The greater the contrast between the hot and cold, the greater the toning effects.

Use It or Lose It

■ Try to stay sexually active as you age. It helps keep your vagina more elastic, flexible, and lubricated. According to those famous sexologists Masters and Johnson, intercourse at least once or twice a week over a period of years will keep a woman of any age wonderfully slick. The stimulation encourages the production of mucus secretions, helps maintain muscle tone, and preserves the shape and size of the vagina. (Even if you've been celibate for a while, your vagina will quickly adjust to renewed sexual activity, so "lose it" isn't as dire as it sounds.)

Snappy Solutions

When you don't have the time or patience to whip up homemade concoctions or experiment with commercial lubricants, try this ultra-simple trick: Use vitamin E capsules as vaginal suppositories. You don't even have to break open the capsule—the outer coating will dissolve naturally. For quicker results, use a pin to poke a hole in the capsule before insertion. Insert one capsule daily for a week, then once or twice a week to keep things moist.

Ginkgo Tea

Ginkgo is used to increase circulation and may be helpful in some cases of erectile dysfunction. Combine it with two other male-helping herbs for a tea that can get you rarin' to go, and turn you back into the man your wife always knew you were.

Dried false unicorn root
Dried ginkgo
Dried saw palmetto
1 cup of boiling water

➥ Combine equal parts of the herbs and add 1 heaping teaspoon of the mixture to the water. Steep for 10 minutes and strain out the solids. Drink 1 to 2 cups daily. Tonic herbs are slow acting, so you may need to drink the tea for several weeks. **Caution:** If you are on blood-thinning medications, do not take ginkgo without checking with your doctor first.

The Ginseng Option

■ Ginseng has had a reputation of being an aphrodisiac, so why not try it as a tonic? Drink 1 cup of ginseng tea daily, using 1 heaping teaspoon of the dried herb per 1 cup of hot water and steeping it for 15 to 20 minutes. Before using ginseng, check with your doctor, especially if you have high blood pressure.

Q: *I've noticed that my erectile problems have been getting worse over the last few years. My lifestyle hasn't changed much; I've just gotten more comfortable around the house. What's my deal?*

Take My Advice

A: Maybe your comfort has come with a price. If you've gained a fair amount of weight, or your diet has changed, then you've found your culprit. Just as high-fat foods clog the arteries to your heart, they also clog the arteries to your penis. Because the latter are a lot smaller, they tend to clog up quicker. Good health and good sex go together hand in hand, so cut out the fats to keep your blood circulating to all the right places.

The Carrot-Combo Cure

As wacky as it may seem, the combination of carrots, eggs, and honey has been widely used to treat impotence. What's more, this quick fixer makes a tasty snack.

1 hard-boiled egg
¼ cup of honey
¼ cup of finely
    shredded carrot

➡ Dip the egg in the honey, then into the carrot, and eat up. Enjoy this treat once a day for a month or two, and you may see your performance improve considerably.

No More Blazing Saddles

■ In the 19th century, horseback riding was nailed as a prime ED culprit. Today, riding a bike (both moving and stationary) claims that dubious distinction. That's because bicycle seats, like saddles, can compress the arteries and nerves that feed the penis. If you've noticed numbness, stop biking for six weeks and purchase a wider, padded seat or a style that has a hole in the middle of it. When you return to the saddle, point the seat downward, and hop off every 10 minutes or so to encourage blood flow.

Order Pizza to Go

■ Italian men are reputed to be great lovers well into their 70s and 80s. It turns out they owe their sexual prowess largely to the fact that they eat plenty of foods with lycopene-rich tomato sauce. Studies show that increased lycopene levels help maintain prostate health, which, in turn, promotes performance. So to soup up your sex drive, eat five servings of cooked tomato products a week.

What Would Grandma Do?

🦋 IN GRANDMA PUTT'S DAY, *Grandpa Putt and his cronies swore by oysters as the ultimate aphrodisiac. Well, it turns out they were right—in part. Oysters are rich in zinc, which the prostate needs to manufacture seminal fluid. You can also load up on this helpful mineral by eating other shellfish, poultry, wheat germ, vegetables, grains, and yogurt.*

Antioxidant-Activity Enhancer

You know the old joke: How many folks does it take to change a lightbulb? If you increase the microcirculation to your eyes and enhance antioxidant activities, you may help prevent the onset and slow the progression of macular degeneration. That way, the answer to the lightbulb-changing question will always be: just one.

Dried bilberry
Dried ginkgo
1 cup of hot water

➥ Make an elixir of bilberry and ginkgo by steeping 1 heaping teaspoon of each herb for 15 minutes in the hot water, then strain the tea. Drink 2 to 3 cups daily. **Caution**: If you are on blood-thinning medications, do not take ginkgo without checking with your doctor first.

Try Nature's Sunglasses

■ Your macula contains pigment that's made up, in part, of lutein. This pigment helps filter out the light that's implicated in macular degeneration and also fights oxidation. So to get more lutein in your system, eat plenty of leafy green vegetables like kale, spinach, and chard.

Learn to Love Orange Food

■ You've always known that carrots are good for your eyes. But so are other orange and yellow fruits and vegetables. They are all rich sources of beta-carotene, the plant-based building block for vitamin A. So add plenty of carrots, squash, pumpkin, and cantaloupe to your menu, along with lots of greens.

EUREKA!

SMOKING CIGARETTES INCREASES YOUR RISK of developing macular degeneration by a factor of two to six times. This ugly addiction deprives the retina of oxygen and constricts blood vessels, making it more difficult for nutrients to be carried through those vessels to your eyes. So kick the habit now, and don't be afraid to ask for help if you need it.

Instant Eye Relief

Aside from its other debilitating effects, macular degeneration can cause extreme eyestrain. Try a warm compress to relieve the discomfort quickly.

1 cup of water
1 tsp. of dried chamomile
Gauze pads

➥ Heat the water until it's almost boiling, add the chamomile, and let it steep for 10 to 15 minutes. Strain and let it cool, then saturate the pads with the solution. Lie down, put the pads over your eyes, and rest for 20 minutes or so. **Caution:** Avoid chamomile if you have ragweed allergies.

Through Glasses Darkly

■ When you're shopping for sunglasses, make sure the ones you choose provide 100 percent protection from ultraviolet light. And to provide even more protection from the sun's rays, buy the darkest-possible lens color. Brown and tan offer the best balance of comfort and protection, with gray and green second best.

Get Milk

■ Sore, swollen eyelids may not rank as a major health problem, but they sure are uncomfortable! Fortunately, relief is as close as your refrigerator. Just soak a couple of cotton pads in ice-cold whole milk, lie down, put one pad over each eye, and rest for 5 to 10 minutes.

What Would Grandma Do?

🦋 To treat a stye or cyst on the eye, doctors often prescribe a hot compress, applied three or four times a day. As usual, Grandma Putt had her own clever take on that approach. She simply hard-boiled an egg, wrapped it (still in its shell) in a washcloth, and held it against the sore eye for 10 minutes. Then, when it was time for the next treatment, she'd put that same piece of "hen fruit" back in a pot of water and reheat it.

Blah-Bustin' Bubble Bath

When fatigue's got you down, there's one surefire way to make yourself feel better on the inside and out—just climb into a nice hot bubble bath. And you couldn't find a smoother or simpler mixer than this one to put your troubles to rest.

2 cups of vegetable oil
3 tbsp. of mild shampoo
¼ tsp. of perfume or scented oil

➥ Pour all of the ingredients into an old blender, mix them at high speed, and store the mixture in a capped bottle at room temperature. Come bath time, pour about ¼ cup of the mixture under running water. Watch the bubbles start to build, then climb in and soak your cares away.

Bet on Bran

■ All of the B vitamins can help improve energy levels, but vitamin B_1 is needed to break down and release energy from carbohydrates. To make sure you get enough B_1, stir some wheat germ into your yogurt. And eat a bowl of rice bran cereal for breakfast to jump-start your day. But one word of warning: Too much B_1 can cause nerve damage, so don't take any high-dose supplements of it.

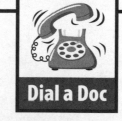

Dial a Doc

✚ If you've been feeling tired for quite a while, and no amount of rest or remedy seems to be making any sort of impact, it may be time to see your doctor to rule out thyroid or adrenal diseases, lingering infections, mononucleosis, arthritis, lupus, cancer, and depression as possible causes. Once your doctor gets to the bottom of your problem, he or she can determine the best course of treatment to help you beat the fatigue and get back to your normal self.

Chilling Spray

On those scorching, humid summer afternoons, anyone who spends time outdoors runs the risk of overheating. If you ignore the symptoms, you can develop a much more dangerous condition—heatstroke. So before you suffer from the first hot blasts of summer, make like a Boy or Girl Scout and BE PREPARED. Whip up this cooling medicinal fixer, and keep it handy, just in case.

2 tsp. of witch hazel tincture
12 drops of lavender oil
10 drops of peppermint oil
Distilled water

➡ Fill an 8-ounce handheld sprayer bottle almost to the top with distilled water and add the ingredients. Then give the bottle a couple of good shakes. When the weather heats up, keep yourself and others cool, calm, and fatigue-free by occasionally misting your faces, arms, necks, and legs.

Shop Till You Drop
◼ When you're feeling fatigued, go shopping for something that will make you feel special, unless, of course, it will add to your worries by causing you financial stress. If a tight budget is a barrier, keep the treat inexpensive, but meaningful to you.

Get a Date
◼ Fatigue won't get you down if you make a date with dates. Simply soak seven dates overnight in 1 cup of water, then crush the dates in the water the next morning (removing the pits), and drink to good health. Follow this routine at least twice a week until you're feeling better.

Nifty, Thrifty Tips

Fatigue can be your body's way of telling you that it's short on electrolytes. If you feel like you're running on empty, grab an electrolyte sports drink that's loaded with sodium and potassium, or try soaking in a soothing bath that's got salts and potassium added to it. Your body will bounce back once it's balanced out.

Easy Energizing Bath

There certainly is a lot of outdoor fun to be had during the warm summer months (or all year round, depending on where you live). But as much fun as it is to be outside, the sunshine can really drain you of energy. So when hot, muggy weather lays you flat (or anytime you need a quick pick-me-up), pour this mixer into your bathtub.

½ cup of baking soda*
½ cup of lemon juice
½ cup of lime juice
5 to 6 drops of lemon extract

➡ Mix all of the ingredients in a bowl, pour the solution into tepid bathwater, and ease into the tub. When you get out, you'll be revitalized and ready to take on whatever comes your way. **Caution:** Don't use this bath mix if you have any open wounds or skin abrasions.

* Add the baking soda only if you have hard water.

Sleep Well

■ Most people feel they can't afford to indulge in a good night's sleep because they have too much to do during the day. But sleep is the most efficient way for the body to restore itself to working order, and allows your brain time to recharge itself. This is why you feel brighter and smarter in the morning—even without that first jolt of java. So make sure you establish a sleep routine, and get seven to nine hours of z's every night.

Nifty, Thrifty Tips

When you're feeling burned out from a variety of tiring circumstances, a little exercise might be just what you need. Sometimes that tired feeling is just that, a feeling. Your body may be telling you it's tired, but it actually has plenty in the tank. It may simply be mental fatigue from everyday life. So take 30 minutes to go for a nice walk or bike ride. The exercise is good for you, it'll take your mind off your troubles, and best of all—it's free!

Electrolyte Recharger

Grandma Putt knew the secret to bringing a dead-tired body back to proper working order as quickly as possible. So whenever she was feeling exhausted, she soaked in this fixer that perked her up and quickly helped her bounce back to life.

**2 cups of Epsom salts
2 cups of kosher salt
2 tbsp. of potassium
    chloride**

➡ Mix the ingredients together in a bowl, and pour the mixture under the warm running water of your bathtub's tap. Once the solids start to dissolve, climb in. The sodium in the salts and potassium will recharge the minerals that your body has lost throughout the day. Plus, you'll feel more relaxed and energized than you ever thought possible!

Control the Phone

■ Nothing can be more tiring than picking up the phone, expecting a pleasant conversation with a friend, only to hear another sales pitch or crank call. So screen your calls with caller ID or an answering machine, and respond only when you feel up to it. Constant interruptions add stress and make you feel defeated. If you establish a routine of returning phone calls when you're not busy or exhausted, you'll eliminate lots of unnecessary stress.

Snappy Solutions

Instead of spending weeks, months, or even years trying to figure out what's causing your fatigue, and trying every conceivable cure on the market, see if simplifying your life doesn't do the trick. This may be the time to delegate housekeeping or line up more babysitters. If you have a spouse and children, work out a plan to share the chores. If you can afford to hire some help, spend some money on that, and cut back on things that matter less. Your body will thank you for the reprieve.

Energizing Elixir

Long before flashy sports drinks came on the market, folks took a break from hard work or play by sitting under a shady tree and drinking this restorative beverage. It gave their bodies exactly what they needed to keep going strong, and it can do the same thing for you.

2½ cups of sugar
1 cup of dark molasses
½ cup of apple cider vinegar
1 gal. of water

➡ Combine all of the ingredients in a big jug, and drop in a couple handfuls of ice cubes to cool the mixture down. Then get your team out of the sun, and pour everyone a nice tall, refreshing glass. They'll be ready to get back to action in no time!

Lavender Oil

■ Lavender is lovely, and it's a wonderful restorative for the soul. Aromatherapists say it relaxes and calms, banishing your blues and putting the blahs on the back burner. Try using it in an at-home spa. Just fill the tub with warm water, then add several drops of lavender essential oil—enough so that you can smell its clean, fresh floral fragrance. Light a candle or two, turn off the bathroom light, and slip into the soothing water.

What Would Grandma Do?

🦋 WHEN GRANDMA PUTT'S TIRED SPELLS went on for days at a time, she would turn to her trusted healthy helper—apple cider vinegar—for a little pick 'er up. We now know that constant fatigue may be caused by a lactic acid buildup in your system. So do what Grandma did and drink 3 teaspoons of apple cider vinegar mixed with ⅛ cup of honey each night before bed to rebalance the acid level. Continue this nightly routine until your energy has completely returned to normal.

Fatigue Fighter

When you're feeling tired and downright drained, the power of herbs can be exactly what you need to get your engine firing on all cylinders again. Combining restorative, relaxant, and tonic herbs may just help ease your fatigue and improve your immune system over time.

Dried lavender
Dried lemon balm
Dried licorice root
Dried skullcap
Dried vervain
Dried wood betony
1 cup of hot water

➥ Combine equal parts of all these herbs to create a perfect restorative tea. Steep 1 heaping teaspoon of the mixture in the water for 20 minutes. Strain and drink 2 cups a day to get yourself back into tip-top shape. **Caution:** Licorice root shouldn't be taken by people with high blood pressure or kidney disease.

An Apple a Day

■ To prevent fatigue from making your metabolism drag, load up on apples. This fantastic fruit provides malic acid, which helps energize your cells and gets your body rarin' to go. And one a day keeps the doctor away!

Fighting Avocado

■ If you've been feeling tired and achy lately, whip up a salad that includes plenty of avocado in it. Avocado is a great source of magnesium, which is the mineral used by your body to stave off fatigue and ease muscle pain. Plus, it tastes great, too!

EUREKA!

THE BEST WAY to keep your energy level high is by loading up on carbohydrates. And there's no better source than beans, which release carbs into your bloodstream slowly. If you want to fight fatigue, beans will sustain you longer than foods like potatoes, which quickly release carbohydrates into your bloodstream. Potatoes will give you a sudden burst of energy, but it won't last. So stick with beans to keep you humming along at peak capacity.

Get Up 'n' Go Tonic

My Grandma Putt taught me the value of taking homemade fixers for a general head-to-toe feeling of goodness. Here's one of my favorites she passed down for getting your body up and running even when it's been dragging you down.

➡ Mix all of the ingredients together in a container, seal it with a lid, and let it stand for about two weeks. Strain out the solids and pour some of the liquid into a small glass. Drink ¼ cup a day, and you'll soon feel A-okay!

2 pints of red wine
1 oz. of ground
    ginseng root
8 almonds
5 dried apricots

Don't Cut the Carbs

■ Sometimes it's hard to relax, especially after a long, hard, tension-filled day. So chill out by eating plenty of carbs at dinner. Foods that are high in carbohydrates, like pasta, crackers, and bread, stimulate the release of chemicals that promote relaxation. If you eat a hearty meal, then you'll be able to release the day's stress and enjoy an energy-restoring night of sleep.

Q: *My tiredness seems to carry over from one day to the next because I can't stop worrying about my problems. What can I do to get it to go away, even for just a little while?*

Take My Advice

A: Try taking a break and feeding your soul. Do something that you love to do, and spend a whole day doing it, whether it's riding a bike, reading a good book, or vegging out with a movie marathon. I have a friend who spends the afternoon at art galleries and museums whenever he's feeling overwhelmed. Find something that shifts your focus and helps you get away from it all—you'll feel much, much better.

Gin-Zing Tea

Need to get your motor running, but you're tired of the same old cup o' joe? Here's an energizing elixir that'll really add some pep to your step!

1 tsp. of ground ginseng root
5 cups of water
1 tsp. of dried borage leaves
1 tsp. of dried mint leaves
10 to 20 drops of ginkgo biloba tincture

➡ Let the ginseng simmer in a pot of the water for 30 minutes or so, keeping a lid on it at all times. Then add the borage and mint and let the blend steep for another 15 to 20 minutes. Finally, add the ginkgo biloba. Strain out the dried herbs, and sip up to 3 cups a day. The tea has a parsley-like flavor, so you can add honey to sweeten it to taste. **Caution:** If you take blood-thinning medications, check with your doctor before taking ginkgo.

Create a Sanctuary

■ We're so busy balancing our work, home lives, and other interests that we rarely have time for ourselves. If this sounds like your life, here's some friendly advice on how to carve out some space. One way to recover is to create a restful place in your home as a private retreat. Even a quiet corner with a simple screen and comfortable armchair will do. Whatever area you choose, make it a welcoming place to rest and relax after a long, hard day.

Snappy Solutions

Fatigue is one of the most common complaints people have nowadays. Our lives are so busy and filled with activity that there never is any time to calm down and get back on track. So if your life is a little hectic, eat more cauliflower. It provides a bunch of pantothenic acid, which is critical for keeping your adrenal glands in good working order whenever stress puts a strain on them.

Luxurious Bath Oil

After a long, hard day in the yard (or even a short, easy one), nothing feels better than sinking into a tub full of hot water and this terrific toddy for the body.

2 cups of milk
1 cup of honey
1 cup of salt
¼ cup of baking soda
½ cup of baby oil

➡ Combine the milk, honey, salt, and baking soda in a large bowl. Fill the tub with water, pour in the mixture, and then add the baby oil (and, if you'd like, a few drops of your favorite fragrance). Ease into the tub, and you'll soon feel your fatigue float away.

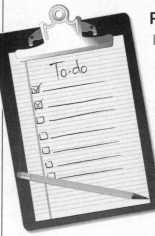

Plug Away at What You've Put Off

◼ Most of us start many projects that we never seem to get around to finishing, like sorting jumbled photos, researching the family genealogy, redecorating the bedroom, or planning a trip to someplace special. The pressure of to-do lists left undone can add to feelings of fatigue at the end of an already long day. To solve this problem, chip away at your list one task at a time—and be sure to do things you enjoy as well as what you consider to be chores. Being involved in something you like will recharge your batteries.

Snappy Solutions

You can save yourself a lot of time, frustration, and fatigue if you're smart about nutrition. Eating healthy food may be the single most important strategy for whipping fatigue. When you're fatigued, your immune system is functioning at less than an optimum level, so it makes good sense to focus on "nutrient-dense" or unprocessed foods—typically roots, tubers, grains, beans, fish, and poultry.

Sports Rehydrator

While they may just seem like overpromoted and overpriced flavored water, sports drinks have a science behind their creation. But don't spend your money on these high-priced beverages when you can make this rehydrating herbal mixer at home.

Fresh dandelion leaves
Grated fresh ginger
Fresh nettle
Fresh oat straw stems
Fresh peppermint leaves
1 tbsp. of lemon juice
1 tbsp. of pure maple syrup
1 cup of hot water

➡ Mix equal parts of the first five ingredients together, and steep 1 heaping teaspoon of the mixture in the hot water for 15 minutes. Strain out the solids, and pour the tea into a 1-liter jug along with the lemon juice and maple syrup, then fill the jug to the top with water. **Caution:** Use only dandelion plants that you know have not been treated with pesticides or other chemicals. If you take diuretics or potassium supplements, talk to your doctor before taking dandelion leaf, and remember to wear gloves when handling fresh nettle to avoid its stinging hairs.

Feel Your Oats

■ Oats, specifically the oat "straw," are rich in minerals that can help restore a tired nervous system. When you're feeling low, make a cold oat infusion by soaking 2 tablespoons of oat straw in 1 quart of cold water overnight. Strain and drink the soothing sipper throughout the day.

EUREKA!

MANY TIMES, IT'S THE LITTLE THINGS that really tire us out (even if they shouldn't). So why not spend some time finding a way to make the little things easier? For example, invest in a wheeled suitcase or duffel bag, and buy a lightweight folding cart you can toss in the backseat and use for groceries or even as a briefcase. And have your groceries and other supplies delivered whenever possible, so you can conserve your strength.

Super Spring Tonic

Spring always marks new beginnings and the blooming of new life. Heck, it almost seems like it would be more appropriate for the year to begin in March rather than in January. This applies not only to nature, but also to your own body. So celebrate the onset of spring each year with this cleansing fixer to get your year off to a great start.

1 tsp. of dried alfalfa leaves
1 tsp. of ground
    dandelion root
1 tsp. of fennel seeds,
    crushed or mashed
1 cup of boiling water

➡ Combine the three herbs in a small bowl. Scoop a teaspoon from the mixture and add it to the water. Let the tonic steep for 10 minutes, then strain out the herbs and sip. It's a terrific kick in the pants that'll get you going! **Caution:** If you take diuretics or potassium supplements, talk to your doctor before using dandelion.

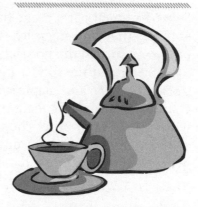

Soothing Sips

■ Ginseng is a whole-system tonic that helps increase endurance and improve mental performance. For a quick pick-me-up, make a revitalizing tea by steeping 1 teaspoon of the herb in 1 cup of hot water for 15 minutes, then strain. Drink 1 or 2 cups daily. Use with caution if you have high blood pressure.

Snappy Solutions

Feeling tired and out of sorts these days? Welcome to the club—millions of Americans go through life feeling a little fatigued, as though their zest for life simply left. To refresh your body and restore your vitality, try a peppermint oil foot rub. Add 3 or 4 drops of peppermint oil to 1 tablespoon of olive oil, then rub it into your clean feet.

Bee Balm Tea

Bee balm leaves contain a compound called thymol, which helps ease nausea, vomiting, and even embarrassing flatulence. So if you've got a bad case of gas, try mixing up some of this bee balm tea to get that end of your digestion on a better—and less embarrassing—track.

1 tsp. of dried
    bee balm leaves
1 tsp. of dried black
    or green tea leaves
1 tsp. of honey
1 cup of boiling water

➡ Combine the bee balm leaves with the black or green tea leaves. Put 1 teaspoon of the mixture into the water and steep it for 5 to 10 minutes, then strain out the solids. Sweeten the tea with the honey, and sip it until your gas is gone.

Fight the Fumes

■ Flatulence is a natural—albeit odoriferous and sometimes embarrassing—fact of life. You can't eliminate it entirely, but you can reduce gas levels by eating plenty of artichokes. They contain fructo-oligosaccharides (FOS), which are indigestible dietary sugars that feed the naturally present "friendly" bacteria that facilitate digestion.

Gas Reliever

■ If beans and other starchy foods tend to make you gassy, simply top your favorite dish with a sprinkling of basil. It's a carminative herb, which is a fancy way of saying that it helps reduce gassiness.

Nifty, Thrifty Tips

Everyone gets gassy from time to time. But there's no need to eliminate starchy food from your diet—simply sprinkle it with tasty carminative (gas-reducing) seeds, such as dill, fennel, or caraway. For more oomph, stir in some rosemary, oregano, or sage, all of which are also carminative. You can buy over-the-counter products that reduce gas, but the herbal approach may work just as well—and cost a whole lot less!

HERE'S TO GOOD HEALTH! **119**

Cent-Sible Stomach Settler

Do you have a problem with gas? Your family and friends will thank you if you try this terrific flatulence-taming tea. When teamed up with catnip and ginger, pennyroyal makes a potent elixir that'll get rid of excess gas—fast!

1 tsp. of dried catnip leaves
1 tsp. of ground ginger
1 tsp. of dried pennyroyal leaves
1 cup of boiling water

➧ Mix the herbs together, then infuse them in the water. Let the tea steep for 10 minutes, and strain out the herbs before drinking. This is a good tea to sip after a hearty meal, before you head off to sleep. **Caution:** Do not take pennyroyal if you are pregnant or breastfeeding.

Cast Off the Pain

■ When gas pains persist, help ease the discomfort with a good old-fashioned castor oil pack. To make the pack, saturate a clean cloth with castor oil, and place it against your skin, taking care to cover your abdomen completely. Cover the cloth with plastic wrap (castor oil stains clothing!), and then place a hot-water bottle on top—wrapped in cloth so it won't burn you. Leave it in place for one hour, or until the pains go away, then wash off the oil.

What Would Grandma Do?

WHENEVER I HAD DINNER at Grandma Putt's, she would pile the veggies on my plate. Like any normal youngster, I found myself opposed to eating veggies—especially because I thought they gave me bad gas. But she made me eat every last bite (which I didn't appreciate at the time, but now I do!). While cabbage, broccoli, and Brussels sprouts may seem to cause more than their fair share of flatulence, they actually don't. And you need them—their healthful nutrients prevent lots of serious diseases. So add more to your diet gradually, and with time, your body will thank you for the added benefits.

Fumigation Tonic

Sometimes the best way to get rid of bad gas is to simply let it all come out the way it's supposed to. Try this elixir, and it'll help the entire uncomfortable ball of gas escape from your body.

½ tsp. of black pepper
½ tsp. of honey
¼ cup of fresh onion juice

➡ Mix the black pepper and honey with the onion juice (an analgesic), then toss it back to ease stomach pain, as well as any flatulence or bloating. It may not produce the sweetest smell in the world, but it'll clear you out— and make you a lot more comfortable—in no time at all!

Take an After-Dinner Stroll

■ Regular exercise promotes good bowel function and helps ease the digestion of food. So put on a pair of walking shoes and take a nice long stroll after eating.

Don't Suck Up Bubbles

■ Always refresh yourself with a bubble-free beverage because carbonated drinks are full of extra air, which means extra gas. And when your beverage arrives with a straw, open one end of the wrapper, crumple it short, place it over one end of the straw, and blow it at your dinner companion. Then set the straw aside. Drinking through a straw pulls unnecessary air into your digestive system.

EUREKA!

BELIEVE IT OR NOT, most people release about 2 pints of gas a day, and half of that comes from swallowed air. There would be a lot less swallowed air—and expelled gas—if everyone would simply eat the way their mothers always told them: Take small bites, don't talk while you're eating, and eat slowly. Why? Because hurried eating increases the amount of air you swallow. So save your body the energy (and embarrassment) of expelling all that gas by slowing down and enjoying your meals.

Gas-Away Tea

A bad case of gas after a meal can put a damper on the rest of your day. You're worried about going out in public and feel like you have to stay isolated until it passes. When you need to relieve the bloated, gassy feeling you sometimes get after eating certain foods, try this surefire fixer.

1 tsp. of dill seeds
1 tsp. of dried
    peppermint leaves
1 cup of boiling water

➡ Mash the dill seeds by putting them in a plastic bag and hitting them with a rolling pin or wooden mallet. Then put the dill and peppermint in a big mug and pour in the water. Cover, and let it steep about 15 minutes. Strain out the herbs and then sip slowly. You'll be feeling better in no time at all!

Snack On After-Dinner Seeds

■ Native American healers advise that chewing ½ teaspoon of fennel seeds at the end of a meal will make you feel less gassy. They also recommend chewing aniseeds or dill, caraway, or coriander seeds to ease digestion. For a refreshing after-dinner (and anti-gas) drink, steep 1 teaspoon of aniseeds in 1 cup of hot water for 10 minutes or so, and enjoy.

De-Gas Strong Foods

■ Whenever you're cooking "gassy" vegetables such as Brussels sprouts, broccoli, and cabbage, add some anise, fennel, or ginger to the food. Along with enhancing the veggies' flavor, these herbs offset their gas-producing properties so that you can enjoy them without any aftereffects.

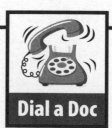

Dial a Doc

✚ If you have persistent flatulence accompanied by abdominal pain that lasts for more than three days, it could be a more serious problem, like appendicitis, gallstones, an ulcer, or a malabsorption problem. So call your doctor immediately if either condition persists.

Gas Turn-Off Tea

For centuries, people of many cultures have used natural gas-fighting, or carminative, herbs to tame the effects of poor digestion. You can take advantage of these natural gas busters by whipping up this after-dinner tummy-taming mixer.

Aniseed
Caraway seed
Fennel seed
1 cup of boiling water

➡ Combine equal amounts of the three seeds, then crush 1 teaspoon of the mixture and add it to the water. Steep for about 20 minutes, strain out the seeds, and sip. Your gas leak will be history!

Visit the Tropics

■ Relief from gas problems may be as close as the nearest pineapple. Along with papaya, pineapple contains natural enzymes that improve digestion and help reduce excess gas. As little as one or two rings a day can help clear the air.

Avoid the Big Offenders

■ Deep-fried foods and other fatty dishes are difficult to digest and thus, cause gas. So choose a healthy, low-fat diet of fruits, vegetables, and whole grains, along with fish and lean meat. Also avoid sorbitol, a common sugar substitute.

Q: *I need a quick remedy for my gas that doesn't require a whole lot of prep time or effort on my part. Got any ideas?*

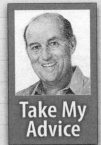

Take My Advice

A: Lemon water jump-starts your stomach into action and helps your digestive system work more efficiently. When you're having trouble with gas caused by poor digestion, squeeze the juice from a slice of lemon into a glass of water and drink it before and after meals. It'll take you a minute to prepare, but the benefits will last for hours.

Good-Bye, Gas Massage Oil

Sometimes all the teas and little eating tricks to prevent gas are just a hassle to pull together before every meal—especially when you're going out with friends or having a snack at the office. But there's a way to help yourself from the outside, too. Just try this abdominal massage to get things moving and clear out the gas.

4 to 6 drops of catnip tincture
4 to 6 drops of lobelia tincture
2 tbsp. of olive oil

➡ Add the catnip and lobelia tinctures to the olive oil. Then gently massage the mixture into your abdomen in a clockwise pattern. The lobelia and catnip are anti-spasmodic herbs that will help relax the muscles of the digestive tract and allow gas to pass through much more comfortably.

Sweeten with Cinnamon

■ To make a sweetly spiced, gas-busting after-dinner drink, steep a stick of cinnamon in a cup of boiling water for about 10 minutes, then let the tea cool slightly. Discard the cinnamon and sip the tea.

Be Bitter

■ Bitter herbs have been used for thousands of years to improve the digestive process, but you don't have to eat pounds of arugula or dandelion to get the benefits. Instead, add a splash of Angostura® bitters to a glass of water. This aromatic flavoring, which is used in food and beverages, is available in most supermarkets and works wonders at keeping things moving along.

Nifty, Thrifty Tips

The best way to get your digestion on the right track is with a little culture. Live cultures, that is. Yogurt with live cultures breaks down milk sugars and keeps a balance of healthy bacteria in your digestive channels. But don't just buy any old yogurt; check the label first to make sure it contains live cultures. At only about 60 cents per serving, this is one healthy remedy that won't break the bank!

Flee, Flu Formula

It's always been my philosophy that you should be prepared for absolutely anything. That's why I like to head off something nasty, like the flu, before it even has a chance to settle in. So before cold and flu season starts, arm yourself with this fixer and you'll be able to fend off nasty diseases all winter long.

> ¾ cup of vodka
> 2½ tbsp. of dried
> echinacea root
> ¾ cup of distilled water

➡ Mix the vodka and echinacea root in a glass jar that's got a tight lid. Store the jar in a cool, dark place for two weeks, then strain out the root, add the water, and pour the mixture into a glass bottle. At the first sign of cold or flu, mix 20 to 30 drops in a glass of water, and drink up! **Caution**: Don't take echinacea if you have an autoimmune disease, such as rheumatoid arthritis, lupus, or multiple sclerosis.

Suck Down the Fluids
■ Lots of liquids are in order when you're battling the flu. When you're not adequately hydrated, your symptoms feel worse, and your immune system won't function as well as it should. So try to drink at least eight glasses a day.

Super Surface Cleaner
■ To prevent passing the flu bug by hand-to-hand contact, clean frequently touched household surfaces like doorknobs, phones, countertops, and toilet handles often. You can disinfect them with a few drops of eucalyptus oil mixed with water in a handheld sprayer bottle.

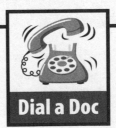

Dial a Doc

✚ Anyone with advanced heart disease, immune system problems, lung disease, or other serious health conditions should call a doctor at the first sign of flu symptoms. Even if you're in great shape, talk to your doctor if you don't start feeling better within a week.

Heirloom Flu Stopper

When Grandma Putt was growing up, antibiotics were few and far between—and vaccines lay decades ahead. So getting the flu was serious business. That's why, when anyone in the family showed signs of coming down with the Big F, Grandma pulled out the big guns in the form of this powerful fixer.

1 large tart, juicy apple
1 pint of water
1 shot of whiskey
½ tsp. of lemon juice
Honey (optional)

➡ Boil the apple in the water until the apple falls apart. Strain out the solids, and add the whiskey and lemon juice to the remaining liquid. Sweeten to taste with honey, if you like. Then get in bed and drink the toddy. If you've acted in time, by morning, those germs will be history!

Cool and Soothe

■ It won't affect your fever, but applying a cold compress to your skin will make you feel a lot more comfortable. Soak a washcloth in cool water, wring it out, and put it on your forehead or neck. When the cloth warms up, repeat the process.

Welcome a Fever

■ Nobody enjoys having a fever, but that high temperature is actually doing you a favor. An increase in temperature is one of the most potent defenses your body has against infections. In other words, lowering a fever with aspirin or other drugs may actually prolong your illness. So unless you're just too uncomfortable or the fever's very high (above 102°F), it's best to just leave it alone.

Nifty, Thrifty Tips

If you're very young or very old, have contact with the chronically ill, or just plain don't want the flu, then you need to get a flu shot. It's best to get it in the fall to give the vaccine time to take effect. And it probably won't cost you a thing. Many pharmacies at local supermarkets have free flu shots available to those who need them most. So keep an eye out for the signs when you're out and about in late fall.

Spicy Flu Fighter

The flu can leave you feeling down and out for days on end. The next time you come down with a cold or flu, show those nasty germs the door with this powerful and potent elixir. Before you know it, you'll be back in full swing!

1 cinnamon stick
3 to 4 whole cloves
2 cups of water
1½ tbsp. of blackstrap molasses
1 shot of whiskey
2 tsp. of lemon juice

➡ Put the cinnamon, cloves, and water in a pan, and bring the mixture to a boil over medium heat. Let it boil for three minutes or so. Remove the pan from the stove, and mix in the molasses, whiskey, and lemon juice. Cover the pan, and let it sit for about 20 minutes. Drink no more than ½ cup of the toddy every three to four hours, heating it up again before drinking it.

Get Well with Garlic

■ Garlic has immune-stimulating and antiviral properties. So if you don't mind the odor, you may want to try a garlic foot rub. Start by coating the soles of your feet with olive oil. (Better yet, have someone else do this for you, and enjoy a soothing foot massage!) Slice a clove of garlic in half, and rub the cut end on your well-oiled feet. Put on a pair of clean socks, and go to bed. **Caution:** The oils in garlic can cause burns, so it is imperative that you oil your feet well before applying the garlic to them.

EUREKA!

EATING BIG, HEAVY MEALS isn't a good idea when you're sick because your body will put more energy into digestion than into stomping out the virus. Nor do you want to go hungry, because your body needs nutrients in order to recover. A good compromise is to plan your menu around soups (homemade chicken with rice is my favorite), vegetable juices, and other easy-to-digest foods.

Appetite-Control Formula

Herbs that tune up and tone your digestive system can help normalize your eating patterns. If you find yourself reaching for unhealthy foods all too often, try this bitter elixir warmed up before meals.

Dried centaury
Dried chamomile
Dried dandelion root
Fennel
1 cup of hot water

➡ Mix equal parts of these herbs together, steep 2 teaspoons of the mixture in the water for 20 minutes, then strain. Drink ¼ to ⅓ cup before each meal, and your system (and your diet) will be rolling along. **Caution:** If you take diuretics or potassium supplements, talk to your doctor before taking dandelion. If you have ragweed allergies, steer clear of chamomile.

Give In

■ Whether a food craving is caused by repressing your feelings or a nutrient deficiency, denying the craving will only make you want it more. So go ahead, have a piece of candy or a small scoop of ice cream every now and then.

Chow Down on Chocolate

■ When you're stressed, your body uses more magnesium than it does under normal circumstances, leaving you feeling low. So have a little chocolate—it may regulate your mood and bring your magnesium level up to par. Don't eat it at night, though. The caffeine content may keep you up or disturb your sleep.

Snappy Solutions

Food cravings are often a reaction to stress. When you feel yourself tensing up, you can temper your taste buds and relax your mind with aromatherapy. Just rub a drop or two of a calming essential oil (like peppermint, chamomile, or lavender) into your temples. Because essential oils can irritate sensitive skin, you may want to apply a thin layer of vegetable oil to the area before massaging in the oil.

Red-Hot Fat Burner

This savory sauce makes an excellent fat-burning meal topper. You can grow your own tabasco peppers in your garden or in a container, or substitute dried ones that have been rehydrated. Other small, hot, fresh red chili peppers can also be substituted for the tabascos.

1 lb. of fresh red
   tabasco peppers,
   chopped
2 cups of distilled
   white vinegar
2 tsp. of salt

➡ Combine the peppers and vinegar in a saucepan and heat them up. Stir in the salt, and simmer for five minutes. Remove from the heat, cool, and place the mixture in a blender. Puree it until smooth, transfer to a glass jar, and let the sauce steep for two weeks in your refrigerator. Remove it, strain out the solids, and adjust the consistency by adding more vinegar, if necessary. Then try the hot sauce on meat, fish, poultry, and vegetables that need a tangy topping.

Pass the Pickles

■ The joke about pregnant women craving pickles or pizza in the middle of the night is not as far-fetched as it sounds. When women are pregnant, their digestion slows, which might create a craving for vinegar or spicy foods. So if you're pregnant and dying for a pickle or another very sour food, crunch away.

Detour Around Cravings

■ Try to anticipate your craving ahead of time, and you may be able to get around it. For example, if you know there is a certain time of day when you will crave chocolate, have a piece of fruit a few hours before then. Fruit can raise your blood sugar levels, so you won't crave the empty calories of sweets so intensely.

✚ Extremely bizarre cravings for nonfood objects, like laundry starch or paint chips, may indicate that you have a disease called pica. So if your cravings seem odd, check with your doctor immediately.

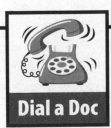

Dial a Doc

Ache-No-More Foot Formula

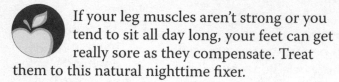 If your leg muscles aren't strong or you tend to sit all day long, your feet can get really sore as they compensate. Treat them to this natural nighttime fixer.

➡️ Combine all of the ingredients, and massage the mixture into your skin. Pull on a pair of clean cotton socks, and leave them on overnight. In the morning, remove the socks and rinse your tootsies with cool water. Your feet will be refreshed and ready to take on a new day.

¼ cup of coarsely
　　ground almonds
¼ cup of dry oatmeal
3 tbsp. of cocoa butter
2 tbsp. of honey

The Great Cucumber Cure

■ When your feet feel so tired and achy that you don't think you can stand up for another minute, reach for three or four cucumbers. Chop them up, toss the pieces into your blender or food processor, and whirl them into a thick pulp. Put an equal amount into each of two pans that are big enough to hold your feet. Then sit back in your easy chair, put a foot into each pan, and think lovely thoughts while the mix does its work. The next thing you know, you'll be ready to dance the night away—or at least take Rover for a walk around the block.

Splinter Savvy

■ Got a splinter in your foot that just won't budge? Well, don't dig into your skin with a needle. Instead, cover the sliver with a piece of adhesive tape, wait an hour, and pull it off. If the sliver stays behind, apply a fresh piece of tape, and keep it on overnight. When you remove the tape, the splinter should slide right out.

EUREKA!

WE'VE ALL BEEN THERE: You're on your feet all day, and there's a long evening ahead, with no time to sit down and rest your tired dogs— much less to soak them in a soothing elixir. Well, don't just grin and bear it. Instead, get instant relief by massaging lime juice into the skin on your legs.

A Treat for Sweaty Feet

Are you prone to sweaty feet—and the aroma that often comes with them? If your answer is "yes," then you know how self-conscious you are in any situation where your feet might come out. But if you're looking for a quick and easy way to get rid of the smell, then this heirloom remedy's right for you.

1¼ cups of rubbing alcohol
1 tsp. of alum
1 cup of water

➡ Mix the rubbing alcohol and alum (available at drugstores and health-food stores) in the water. Pour the mixture into a handheld sprayer bottle, and spritz those wet dogs as needed. You'll be amazed how quickly they dry out and how fast the smell disappears.

Pickle Your Toes

■ Good old-fashioned vinegar is an effective anti-fungal foot remedy. For best results, use distilled white vinegar. If your skin is broken or sensitive from irritation, begin with a diluted preparation of 1 tablespoon of vinegar per ¼ cup of water, washing the affected areas twice daily.

Take a Powder

■ While ointments that squish between your toes may be helpful at night, for daytime walking they're kind of icky. So use herbal powders instead of ointments. Powdered marigold and oregano can be combined in equal parts and sprinkled between your toes for soothing relief.

Nifty, Thrifty Tips

Tea tree oil is a cheap, safe, and effective alternative to expensive over-the-counter anti-fungal agents from pharmacies. Apply a light coating of tea tree oil to affected areas on your feet three or four times a day. Just keep in mind that it's important to continue these applications for two weeks after the infection disappears to make sure the fungus has hit the road for good.

Dry, Cracked Feet Fixer

Being on your feet all day long can lead to a lot of problems. Your feet can dry out and become cracked, which is not only unsightly, but can be painful as well. But there is help—treat your feet to Grandma Putt's favorite moisturizing mixer.

1 ripe, smashed banana
2 tbsp. of honey
2 tbsp. of margarine
1 tbsp. of lemon juice

➥ Put all of the ingredients in a bowl. Stir them together until the mixture is nice and creamy, then massage it onto your clean, dry feet. Pull on a pair of cotton socks, and head to bed for the night. In the morning, your feet should look and—more importantly—feel much better.

Sock It to Me

■ A pair of thick cotton socks can be the best pals your feet ever had—that is, if those dogs are prone to getting either dry and cracked, or tired and achy. Keep a couple of pairs close at hand, so when the nights get cold or the days get hot, your feet will be protected and stay in great shape.

Say Good-Bye to Rough Skin

■ You can use plain old banana peels, minus the fruit, to soften the skin on your heels. Just sprinkle the inside of a peel with a few drops of lemon juice, and rub it across the rough body part. It'll feel a little strange at first, but your dry feet will love it—guaranteed!

What Would Grandma Do?

🦋 WHEN GRANDMA'S FEET got a little too tough for her liking, she would sit in the bath and give them a good, hard rubdown. She didn't have a pumice stone, so she used her own DIY recipe. Grandma would moisten a handful of Epsom salts with a small amount of almond or olive oil, and then scrub her feet until the salts dissolved and the oil softened her skin. The next time you're in the bath, treat your feet to the same moisturizing salt rub.

Foot and Leg Refresher

When you do more walking or standing than you're used to, or you spent last night "cutting a rug," your legs need energizing relief—NOW! So give it to 'em with this refreshing gel.

½ cup of aloe vera gel
1 tbsp. of witch hazel
1½ tsp. of cornstarch
3 to 4 drops of peppermint extract

➡ Mix the aloe vera, witch hazel, and cornstarch in a microwave-safe container. Nuke it on high for one to two minutes, stirring every 30 seconds, until the mixture is about the consistency of honey. Let it cool, stir in the peppermint extract, and store the gel in an airtight container. Smooth it on your tired, aching feet and legs, wait 10 to 15 minutes, and rinse it off with warm water. Afterward, you'll feel like running a marathon! (Well, almost.)

Step Out of Your Rut

■ Have you been wearing the same type, or even the same brand, of shoes for years? It may be high time to switch to a style that's got more padding. As we age, the natural cushioning in our bodies wears out. So if you're wearing a shoe that has next to no padding in the heel, try getting a shoe with cork or gel padding and/or consider adding a gel insole for even more support.

Q: *I work all day, and then come home and have very little time before I have to get started on my evening chores. What can I do during my little break to help take the pain out of my feet?*

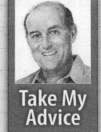

Take My Advice

A: Just sit back, relax, and prop up your feet. Raising your tired old dogs gives them a chance to rest, and allows gravity to drain away some of the swelling that's contributing to your discomfort. For it to be really effective, though, you must raise your feet higher than your head.

Foot Soother and Smoother

If your feet are rough and cracked, you know how unsightly they are and how painful it can be. You try to hide your feet whenever possible, but why hide them when you can fix them for good? Say good-bye to rough, dry, cracked skin on your feet with this soothing solution.

1 tbsp. of almond oil
1 tbsp. of olive oil
1 tsp. of wheat germ

➡ Combine all of the ingredients, and store the mixture in a bottle that's got a tight cap. Shake well before using, then generously rub the mixture into your feet and heels, especially the dry parts. Your tootsies will love you for it!

Keep It Clean

■ When the skin on your feet is chafed, it's more vulnerable to infection, so it's essential to keep the area clean. Wash with soap and warm water a few times a day, and be gentle because you don't want to rub off more skin. Then dry the area, and cover it with a bandage. Continue this routine until the skin is healed.

Wash and Wear

■ Chafing on your feet is usually caused by the friction of hard things rubbing against them, although sometimes the problem is more subtle. Accumulations of dirt, sweat, or chemicals in your clothes can aggravate your skin as much as simple friction. So take the time to wash your socks thoroughly after every use.

Snappy Solutions

Two great (and quick) soothing moves for tired feet are "ankle wobbles" and "toe boogies." To wobble your ankle, put your palms on each side of your foot, covering your ankle. Shake your palms while keeping them pressed against your ankle. To do a toe boogie, put one finger on either side of a toe, right where it's connected to your foot. Vigorously vibrate your finger back and forth for a few seconds, then repeat the movement for the rest of your toes.

Fruity Foot Reviver

Did you spend all day on your feet? Then the best way to get them back into proper working order is to give them a sweet treat, just like you'd do for your tummy as a midday pick-me-up. So try reviving your tired tootsies with this fruity fixer.

8 strawberries, mashed
2 tbsp. of olive oil
1 tsp. of sea salt or
   kosher salt

➤ Mix the ingredients together to form a paste. Massage the entire amount into your feet at the end of the day. Rinse it off, and dry your feet with a soft towel. By morning, your feet should feel better than ever and you'll be ready to take on a new day.

Toe the Line

■ If you tend to get cramps or aches in your toes or the balls of your feet, you need to exercise them. The best way is to lay a small towel on the floor, grip it with your toes, and pull it toward you. Or you can use your toes to pick up marbles—trust me, it's not as easy as it sounds!

Roll with It

■ To stretch your foot and leg muscles and get a foot massage at the same time, take off your shoes and roll a golf ball along the floor with the sole of your foot. If you want to get a slightly different stretch, alternate with a tennis ball for a good full-foot workout.

EUREKA!

INSTEAD OF GOING to lots of different shoe stores to find shoes that'll meet an individual activity's pain needs, try buying all your shoes at a store where the clerk actually measures both of your feet. Shoe sizes vary by brand, so always try the shoes on, even if you already know your size. You might also want to try shopping toward the end of the day, when your feet are naturally a little bit larger.

Herbal Foot Massage

Have you ever been out walking for a long time and realized at the end of your walk that you've got an ingrown toenail? Or maybe you're just naturally prone to those little buggers. This herbal foot massage can soothe that pain and protect the area from a potentially serious infection.

1 oz. of calendula oil
10 drops of lavender oil
10 drops of oregano oil
10 drops of thyme oil

➡ Combine the oils and apply the mixer all over your foot. The hands-on attention will make the area feel a lot better, and the oils will help reduce swelling and pressure around the sore nail. Soon enough, the nail will start to rise back to the surface, where you can properly clip it or do whatever you feel is best to solve the problem.

Soak It in Salt

■ An Epsom salts bath will help draw out the pain and infection of an ingrown toenail. To treat it, fill a basin with warm water, add a cup of Epsom salts to it, and soak your foot for 20 to 30 minutes. Not only will it help relieve the pain, but it will also soften the skin around your toe so you can draw the nail back to the surface and keep it growing out, instead of in.

What Would Grandma Do?

🦋 WHENEVER I WOULD GET an ingrown toenail, Grandma Putt wouldn't waste her time with different remedies. She would just pull out her secret weapon—cotton—to make that nail start growing out again. You can train ingrown nails to head in the right direction before they cause real trouble by taking a small piece of cotton and rolling it into a tight cylinder. Slip the cylinder under the nail right where it's touching the skin. The cotton will relieve the pressure and help the nail to grow out rather than in.

Sock It to Germs

A lot of different germs can accumulate on your feet, and since the bottoms of your feet are very sensitive, it's an easy place for germs to infiltrate your body. To reduce the risk of infection, change your socks two or three times a day. For additional protection, try this fast fixer to make your socks bacteria-proof.

**Lavender oil
Oregano oil
Thyme oil**

➡ Add a few drops of these three essential oils to a basin of water, and soak your socks in the solution overnight. Then let the socks air-dry. The germ-killing action of the oils will help ensure that your socks won't allow infection-causing bacteria to thrive.

Dry Each Digit

■ If you're prone to sweaty, stinky feet, make sure you dry each toe separately, then run a paper towel between them to absorb every last drop of moisture. Or use the blow-dryer on a low setting—it'll dry 'em fast and feel good, too!

Q: *I've heard that chlorine bleach can cure athlete's foot, so I'd like to give it a try. But is it really an effective treatment?*

Take My Advice

A: Footbaths of chlorine bleach used to be a remedy for athlete's foot. In fact, the recipe was printed right on the Clorox® bottle in the 1950s. Doctors say there is no basis for this treatment, but some people still claim it works. To try it, soak your feet in a mixture of ½ cup of bleach and 1 gallon of water twice a day. Using white vinegar instead of bleach is a better—and more environmentally friendly—remedy. (Reduce the water to 1 quart.) Caution: Folks with diabetes or peripheral vascular disease should not soak their feet without their doctor's OK. Do not use bleach if your skin is broken.

Tea for Toes

Oftentimes, the best way to get your feet back to 100 percent and allow your whole body to perk up is to just soak those toes. A foot soak can make your tired feet feel totally refreshed in a matter of minutes. So here's a tea treatment that's taken by foot, not by mouth.

1 cup of dried calendula flowers
½ cup of dried lavender flowers
1 tbsp. of dried thyme
1 qt. of water

➥ Put the water in a saucepan, then add the calendula, lavender, and thyme (all available at health-food stores). Simmer the mixture for five minutes, then let it cool to room temperature. Put it in a basin and soak your feet for about five minutes. This tea is guaranteed to reduce infection and painful swelling and make your feet feel a whole lot better.

Beach Sore Feet

■ If you live on or near a seacoast, take a barefoot walk along the edge of the water and let the surf wash over your feet when they're sore or have a rash. The highly saline environment has a cleansing effect and can speed up healing.

Rub It Out with Arnica

■ Native American healing traditions say you should rub your feet every morning and evening to ease the burdens they carry. How? By using 4 or 5 drops of arnica oil for your foot massage. Simply shake the oil into the palm of your hand and rub it in gently for a few minutes, moving from your toes up to your ankle and back down to your soles. **Caution:** Do not use arnica on broken skin.

EUREKA!

DON'T FORGET THE MENTHOL when your feet are sore or swollen. Any foot cream that has menthol in it will stimulate the flow of blood to your feet and wash away any inflammation that's causing soreness. It'll easily get your feet back into proper working order.

Tired Tootsie Soother

A warm footbath erases your cares and pampers your soul. It can also turn your tired feet into lean, mean, moving machines. Here are the right ingredients to get you back on your feet again.

½ cup of Epsom salts
1 tsp. of lavender oil
1 tsp. of dried lemon balm

➡ Add the ingredients to a basin of warm water, dip your feet in, and sit back. The Epsom salts will relax you, and the lavender and lemon balm will refresh your mind and calm your spirit. **Caution:** If you have diabetes, check with your doctor before soaking your feet in anything.

Chamomile Foot Soak

■ Another great way to relax your tired tootsies at the end of a long day is to soak them in water that's been spiked with Epsom salts and a few drops of chamomile oil. The oil reduces inflammation as well as muscle spasms.

Ease Away Foot Pain

■ Creams that include the herbs arnica, comfrey, or St. John's wort work well to increase circulation and reduce the inflammation that may be making your feet hurt. You can buy a ready-made cream or make your own by adding 6 to 12 drops of one of these herbal oils to an ounce of grapeseed, olive, or almond oil. **Caution:** Do not use arnica on broken skin.

What Would Grandma Do?

🦋 GRANDMA PUTT OFTEN SPENT *so much time on her feet that by the end of the day, her toes would be tender and sore. And it wasn't always just fatigue talking—sometimes the pain would be from a nasty ingrown toenail. So she would make an herbal foot massage to soothe the pain and protect against infection. She'd combine 1 ounce of calendula oil with 10 drops each of thyme, oregano, and lavender oils and rub the mixture all over her feet until they felt better.*

Dissolve and Conquer

There are plenty of herbs available that can help keep your gallbladder in proper working order. Herbalists have long recommended these herbs to people who are prone to developing gall-stones. **Caution:** If you have active gallbladder disease, consult your doctor before taking one of these remedies.

1 tbsp. of dried gravel root (a.k.a. Joe Pye weed)
1 tbsp. of dried pellitory-of-the-wall
1 tbsp. of dried stone root
1 qt. of hot water

➡ Make a tea by adding the herbs to the water. Steep for 20 minutes, strain, and let it cool. Drink it throughout the day. **Note:** If you plan to use the herbs for more than a few days, consult a naturopathic doctor, who can advise you about their benefits and risks.

Dandelion Salad

■ Old-timers used to pick young dandelion leaves in early spring to cure what ailed 'em. The powerful compounds in the leaves act like a mild laxative and digestion stimulator. And it's a long-held belief that these same compounds can bust up those painful little stones. So if you're prone to stones, it probably wouldn't hurt to toss a bunch of dandelion leaves with some salad oil once in a while and serve 'em up at dinner. **Caution:** Use only dandelion plants that you know have not been treated with pesticides or other chemicals. Also, if you take diuretics or potassium supplements, talk to your doctor before taking dandelion.

A gallbladder attack can often be mistaken for a heart attack. Gallstone pain begins in the lower right abdomen and shoots upward to the shoulder and around the back to the right shoulder blade. If you have any unusual abdominal pain that won't go away, fever, sweating, chills, yellowish skin, yellowing of the whites of your eyes, or clay-colored stool, then you need to see your doctor immediately.

Dial a Doc

So Long, Spasms

Many herbs have long been known for their ability to tone, relieve inflammation, and release spasms in the liver and biliary tract. But don't take my word for it. Try an elixir made from any of the herbs listed below, and see if you don't feel better fast.

Dried artichoke
Dried butterbur or
  dried peppermint
Dried dandelion root
Dried milk thistle
1 cup of hot water

➡ Put 1 teaspoon of any one of these herbs into the water. Steep for 15 minutes, strain, and drink the warm beverage between meals. **Caution:** If you take diuretics or potassium supplements, talk to your doctor before taking dandelion.

Get Going, Girls!

■ Overweight, middle-aged females are more prone to gallstones than any other demographic group. In fact, women have twice the risk of developing gallstones than men do. But studies show that women who increase their exercise routine to two to three hours a week are much less susceptible to the problem than their sedentary sisters. Need more motivation? Then think about 20-20 (not the TV show!). Walk briskly for 20 minutes a day, five to seven days a week, and you'll reduce your chances of developing gallstones by 20 percent.

Diet Smart

■ Even though shedding excess weight will help reduce your chances of developing gallstones, rapid weight loss actually increases your risk. So instead of embarking on a crash diet, aim for a gradual, long-term weight goal.

Snappy Solutions

A traditional way to help the gallbladder work more efficiently is to drink vegetable-juice cocktails that include celery, parsley, beets, carrots, radishes, and lemon. (Grandma Putt would mix and match ingredients to suit her taste.) Drink two 8-ounce glasses a day.

A Sage Solution

This excellent elixir couldn't be easier. And you can't find a better way to tone gum tissues and protect them against infection. It'll make your breath clean and fresh, too!

Calendula tincture
Myrrh tincture
Sage tincture
Warm water

➡ Two or three times a day, add 5 drops of each tincture to a small amount of warm water, swish the liquid around in your mouth for several minutes, then spit it out.

Something to Chew On

◾ Double your pleasure, double your fun—while reducing inflammation and helping slash gum bleeding by half. How? Simply by chewing gum that contains French pine bark extract, or Pycnogenol®, after each meal. You can find this gum-protecting gum at health-food stores.

Splurge on a Sonic

◾ Available at most drugstores, sonic toothbrushes are three times faster than ordinary electric toothbrushes and have been shown to reverse gingivitis and help shrink gum pockets. They can be pricey—often costing anywhere from $75 to $100—but if you have the beginnings of gum disease, or come from a family that's prone to the condition, a sonic brush will be well worth the investment. **Note:** You may be able to buy a sonic toothbrush from your dentist for much less than you'd pay for the same brand at a retail store.

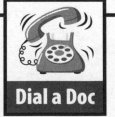

Dial a Doc

✚ If you have chronic bad breath, tooth sensitivity to hot or cold, and red, shiny gums, you may have gingivitis. Left untreated, this condition progresses to chronic infection and bone degeneration. Watch for loose, shifting teeth, receding gums that leave the root exposed, gum pain, and inflammation and pockets of pus between teeth and gums. If you spot any of these conditions, get to your dentist ASAP.

Goldenseal Gargle

Goldenseal should be in everyone's medicine cabinet because it not only reduces inflammation and fights bacteria, but it also contains a host of minerals, including calcium, phosphorus, potassium, and vitamins that keep gums healthy. A goldenseal gargle can be just what the dentist ordered to keep your gums healthy.

¼ tsp. of goldenseal root powder
½ tsp. of baking soda
¼ cup of warm water

➡ Combine the goldenseal powder and baking soda, then add the mixture to the water. Take a swig, swish it around, and spit it out. In no time, your sore gums will thank you. Also, look for toothpastes that already have goldenseal in them to give your mouth a little extra help.

Make a Paste

■ If you want to clear up a persistent case of gingivitis, try this inexpensive, yet very effective, gum paste. Shake about 1 teaspoon of baking soda into a small dish, and drizzle in just enough hydrogen peroxide to make a paste. Then work it gently under the gum line with your toothbrush. Leave the paste on for a few minutes, then rinse well.

Be an Apple Polisher

■ Apples contain compounds that inhibit the gum-destroying enzymes secreted by oral bacteria. So crunching an apple a day will help keep the dentist away. If you don't like apples, look for apple extract, which, believe it or not, provides the same protective action.

Nifty, Thrifty Tips

Sometimes preventing a nasty case of gingivitis is as economical and easy as taking a trip to the sink. Water stimulates the production of saliva that you need to fight excess mouth bacteria. If you drink 8 to 10 glasses a day, your chances of coming down with any sort of mouth condition will be drastically reduced.

Tooth-Repair Paste

Gum disease can put your entire mouth in serious danger. If it's not taken care of quickly, the problem can spread to your teeth. And if you've never lost a tooth as an adult, why not keep it that way? If you've got a tooth that's suffering from gum disease, try to save it by packing it with this mixer, then see your dentist soon.

Goldenseal powder
Powdered myrrh
Hydrogen peroxide

➡ Mix equal parts of goldenseal and myrrh together, adding enough hydrogen peroxide to the powders to make a paste. Apply the mixture around the tooth one to three times daily. When pain is an issue, add a pinch of ground cloves—and call for a dental appointment today!

Paint with Goldenseal

■ Goldenseal helps protect against infection, while strengthening the gum and mouth tissues. So if you're having problems, get a cotton swab, and use it to paint your gums with a tincture of goldenseal once or twice daily. Goldenseal can irritate inflamed gums, so test it first by dabbing a spot on your gums.

Swish with Salt

■ Plain salt is a wonderful all-purpose gum healer. Dissolve ¼ teaspoon of salt in ¼ cup of warm water. Use it as a mouthwash two or three times daily.

EUREKA!

BRUSHING YOUR TEETH is the best way to keep your mouth happy. But it's important to pay attention to how long you brush them. Generally, brushing for at least two minutes is optimum. Some electric toothbrushes have a built-in mechanism that reminds you to work on all four areas of your mouth for 30 seconds each. If you don't use this style of toothbrush, set a timer or sing a two-minute-long song in your head. My choice? "Fun, Fun, Fun," by the Beach Boys.

Anti-Migraine Tea

Migraines can be devastating. I know, because my grown-up children still suffer from them occasionally. But they fight off the throbbing pain and other debilitating migraine symptoms with this tasty, easy-to-make fixer.

Dried feverfew leaves and flowers
Dried lemon balm flowers
1 cup of boiling water

➡ Combine the herbs and scoop 1 heaping teaspoon of the mixture into the water. Let it steep 5 to 10 minutes. Strain out the herbs, and sip away until your headache is gone. Keep drinking the tea if one cup isn't enough to get rid of the pain completely. **Caution:** Feverfew is a uterine stimulant, so if you are pregnant or nursing, don't take it. Feverfew may cause mouth irritation in sensitive people.

Cushion Tension Headaches

■ Did you know that the lack of good head and neck support while you sleep may bring on tension headaches? Some pillows do an excellent job of supporting your head and neck, while others are so soft that you might as well be sleeping on air. Firm pillows are usually best for preventing tension headaches, but you'll have to experiment to find the type that works best for you.

Snappy Solutions

Studies show that if you rub peppermint oil—a proven anesthetic—on your forehead, you may be able to relieve the pain and reduce the sensitivity associated with tension headaches. What's more, if you use the oil daily, you may even be able to sidestep future headaches. Simply mix peppermint oil with an equal amount of rubbing alcohol and apply no more than a couple of drops to your forehead and temples once a day.

Exotic Herbal Elixir

A headache can show up in the middle of an otherwise perfect day and stay for hours, or even days. For tension headaches, combine these gentle pain- and stress-relieving herbs for fast relief.

Ginger tincture
Jamaican dogwood tincture
Kava tincture
Wood betony tincture

➤ Combine equal parts of all four herb tinctures, and take 15 to 20 drops of the mixture every 30 minutes for relief of acute pain, up to four times in 24 hours. **Caution:** Kava has been linked to liver damage, so check with your doctor before taking it.

Willow Works

■ Willow bark contains salicin, which metabolizes in the body like aspirin, its synthetic sister. So the next time your head hurts, chew some fresh willow twigs to ease the pain. If there's no willow tree nearby, try the more powerful willow bark tea or tincture (available at health-food stores) per the package directions.

A Little Night Oil

■ The night-blooming herb evening primrose contains phenylalanine, which is one of the best natural sources of pain relief. The powerful medicine in this herb is found in the seeds' oil. Because the seeds are tiny and the oil is almost impossible to extract, you'll save yourself another headache by simply purchasing oil capsules at a local health-food store. Be sure to follow the directions on the label.

Nifty, Thrifty Tips

Do you find that most of your migraines come immediately after a stressful situation has passed? Don't buy a bunch of different medicines to counter the pain. Instead, take up regular aerobic exercise for 15 to 20 minutes a day. It'll help you reduce stress, and once you do, you'll reduce your headaches. But stay consistent: Any change in routine will likely trigger another round of migraines.

Gillyflower Syrup

As early as Mr. Shakespeare's time, the sweet-smelling blooms that we call pinks, carnations, and sweet William were all known as "gillyflowers," or sometimes "gilloflowers." And, like most other plants back then, they earned their keep. For instance, they formed the prime ingredient in this headache mixer from my Grandma Putt's youth.

¼ lb. of fresh
    gillyflower blossoms
    (any variety will do)
2½ cups of distilled water
2½ cups of sugar

➡ Put the flowers in a heat-proof container. Bring the water to a boil, pour it over the blooms, and let sit for 12 hours. Strain the liquid into a pan, and heat it on low, mixing in the sugar until it's thoroughly dissolved. Store the syrup in a tight-lidded container in the refrigerator, and take a teaspoon or two at the first sign of a headache. The syrup will keep for up to two weeks in the refrigerator.

Quit Smoking

■ If you're hooked on nicotine, then the next time you're flattened by a migraine or cluster headache, say these words to yourself: "Smoking triggers my headaches and makes them harder to treat." Repeat this mantra until you feel well enough to get to your doctor's office—where you're going to ask for help in quitting this nasty habit.

✚ Sometimes a headache can be caused by some underlying disease, such as a brain tumor or meningitis. Sudden, intense, or chronic and worsening head pain should always send you running to the nearest emergency room.

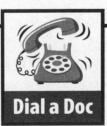

Dial a Doc

Headache Tea

Some headaches seem to gather in certain areas of your head and leave you with an intense pain that's localized in one spot. If you have episodes of this type of excruciating head pain, known as ice pick headaches, you can make this analgesic elixir to take the edge off.

1 tsp. of dried feverfew
1 tsp. of ground ginger
1 tsp. of dried lemon balm
1 cup of hot water

➡ Combine the herbs and add 1 teaspoon of the mixture to the water. Steep for 10 minutes, strain out the herbs, and sip. Your ice pick headache should disappear fairly quickly. **Caution:** Feverfew is a uterine stimulant, so if you are pregnant or nursing, don't take it. Feverfew may cause mouth irritation in sensitive people.

Try the Caffeine-Aspirin Fix

■ The combination of two cups of coffee and two aspirins relieves a headache 40 percent better than the pain reliever alone does. In addition to starting your motor in the mornings, caffeine helps your body absorb medications. The full effects are felt in approximately 30 minutes and can last for three to five hours.

Q: *I always seem to get a headache right after dinner a couple days a week, and my menu on those days is pretty consistent from week to week. Is my meal causing me more pain than pleasure?*

Take My Advice

A: Many people do in fact find their migraine attacks connected to what they eat. Watch your menu to see if it contains things like alcohol, aged cheese, smoked fish, sour cream, yogurt, or chocolate. These are all trigger foods, and if your menu remains fairly constant, it should be easy to tell if your diet is causing your pain.

Give Heartburn the Slip

Tame the burning sensation quickly with slippery elm lozenges. You can buy them in health-food stores, or make your own.

¼ cup of slippery
   elm powder
3 tbsp. of honey
4 drops of vanilla
   extract
Flour

➡ In a small bowl, mix the slippery elm powder and the honey together and form it into a nonsticky dough. Then mix in the vanilla. On a cutting board dusted with flour, roll the dough into a long, thin shape. Cut the roll into bite-size pieces and put them on a baking sheet. Bake for an hour at 250°F. Cool, then place the lozenges in an airtight container. The next time you feel the burn, just pop one in your mouth.

Mellow Meadowsweet

■ Meadowsweet is a digestive herb that protects and soothes the stomach lining while reducing excess acidity. So if you suffer from heartburn, sip a cup of meadowsweet tea between meals. To prepare the tea, steep 1 heaping teaspoon of the dried herb in 1 cup of hot water for 15 minutes, strain, and sip.

Don't Eat Before Bedtime

■ Whatever you do, don't eat a big meal and then head off to bed. Always wait two to three hours after eating to go to sleep. This delay gives your food a chance to digest, so it won't cause you discomfort when you lie down.

What Would Grandma Do?

🦋 I USED TO LOVE racing through my dinner to get back to playing as fast as I could. But Grandma Putt would always tell me to slow down and chew my food, instead of just inhaling it. Once again, Grandma was right. You should always sit down and relax, then chew your food thoroughly. This routine increases your saliva production and improves the entire digestive process, preventing the acid production that causes heartburn. So don't eat and run or gulp your food.

Heartburn-Relief Remedy

When you get that nasty chest pain that's associated with heartburn, you feel like your chest is on fire. So when the fire starts burning, try this marvelous mixer to douse the heat and give you a dose of nutritious garden veggies at the same time!

2 to 3 sprigs of parsley
2 garlic cloves, peeled
1 angelica stalk
1 medium carrot
1 celery stalk
Water

➡ Put all of the solid ingredients in a blender or food processor, and liquefy them. Add enough water to get the consistency you prefer. Pour the potion into a glass, and sip it slowly. Note that for some people, garlic makes heartburn worse. Feel free to leave it out.

Root Out the Heat

■ Licorice root soothes stomach fires and increases circulation for healing at the same time. Place 1 teaspoon of the herb in 1 cup of hot water. Let it steep for 15 minutes, then strain out the root and enjoy. **Caution:** If you have high blood pressure, talk to your doctor before you take anything that contains licorice root.

Don't Lie Down on Dinner

■ Try to restrain yourself from flopping down on the couch after you've just indulged in a too-big, too-heavy meal. Bending over after overeating can also result in heartburn. So the moral is: Stay upright and walk off the calories—and the heartburn—with some much-needed exercise.

✚ The pain you believe is heartburn could be something more serious, like gallbladder inflammation or even a heart attack. Amateurs can't tell the difference. So if you have chest pain, particularly if it radiates into either arm or your jaw and is accompanied by nausea, fever, or chills, call an ambulance—and let the paramedics figure out what's going on.

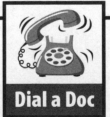

Dial a Doc

Soothing Papaya Potion

Heartburn occurs when the acid content in your stomach backs up into your food pipe (a.k.a. your gullet or esophagus). Eliminating acidic foods like tomatoes and citrus fruits from your diet will help stave off trouble, but if you don't want to give 'em up, reach for this effective elixir instead.

1 cup of papaya juice
1 tsp. of organic sugar (available at health-food stores and some supermarkets)
2 pinches of cardamom

➡ Mix the ingredients in a glass and drink up as soon as you feel the onset of that all-too-familiar burning sensation, or anytime you're in the mood for a cool, tasty beverage.

Pepperoni Pizza Protocol

■ Fiery-food fans, take heart. Studies show that a post-meal session of progressive muscle relaxation (alternately tensing and releasing one group of muscles at a time, starting with your feet) and deep belly breathing may help you dig into hot delights like pepperoni pizza without feeling the burn afterward. Plus, you'll have fewer reflux episodes in the future. You can learn these techniques from videotapes, or ask your doctor for a referral to a stress-management center.

Snappy Solutions

If your on-the-go schedule leaves little time for brewing tea or whipping up other potions to ease your heartburn, head to your local health-food store and buy some 380-milligram tablets of deglycyrrhizinated (DGL) licorice. Chew two tablets 20 minutes before each meal to calm the indigestion that triggers acid backup. More good news: For those of you with high blood pressure, DGL is a safe form of licorice, so you can take it without worry.

Garlic-and-Brandy Blood Pressure Tamer

For generations, health-conscious folks have used this elixir to lower their blood pressure and keep their hearts ticking merrily along. My Grandma and Grandpa Putt both swore by it, and I do, too!

1 lb. of garlic cloves
1 qt. of brandy

➡ Peel the garlic cloves, and soak them in the brandy for two weeks, shaking the mixture a few times a day. Then strain it, pour the liquid into bottles with tight stoppers, and take up to 20 drops a day.

Yes, Please Have a Banana

■ Have a banana today. As a matter of fact, have a banana every day. The potassium in the mellow yellow fruit helps prevent thickening of the artery walls and works in conjunction with sodium, an electrolyte, to regulate your body's fluids—keeping your heart healthier in the process. Other good potassium sources to include in your diet are apples, string beans, peas, beans, and skim milk.

EUREKA!

SOMETIMES IT TAKES only a few simple changes to whip your body into better shape than it was just 24 hours ago. In terms of heart health, chronic stress increases the levels of cortisol, a hormone secreted by the adrenal glands. Along with depression and anxiety, extra cortisol can have a harmful effect on your heart. Stress hormones may spike your cholesterol level, raise blood pressure, and promote heart disease. So fight stress with a heart-healthy diet, regular exercise, deep breathing when something upsets you, and relaxation techniques.

Let's Hear It for Hawthorn

For centuries, hawthorn berries have been widely used to help lower blood pressure. Combining them with other herbs and relaxants can increase their effect. If your blood pressure is higher than it should be—or you simply want to head off trouble—treat yourself to this first-class fantastic fixer.

Hawthorn berries
Dried motherwort
Dried passionflower
Dried skullcap
1 cup of hot water

➡ Combine equal parts of the herbs, steep 1 heaping teaspoon of the mixture in the water for 15 minutes, and strain. Drink 2 or 3 cups daily.

Mind Your Mood

■ If you think the state of your heart has nothing to do with the state of your mind, think again: Researchers at Johns Hopkins University found that depressed people were four times more likely to have heart attacks than those who said they were not depressed. What's more, a study of middle-aged women found that those who had depressive symptoms (sleeping problems, lack of energy, frequent boredom, and crying) and who felt unsupported by their families had low levels of high-density lipoprotein (HDL)—the "good" cholesterol that helps prevent heart disease. The moral of the story: If you have even an inkling that you may be suffering from clinical depression, get professional help—*today*.

✚ If you wear dentures, the last thing you would expect is to have a "toothache" in your lower jaw. Don't ignore it—you could be having a heart attack. If you have what seems to be tooth pain in your lower jaw, call 911 immediately.

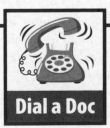

Dial a Doc

Terrific Ticker Tonic

Let's face it: Your heart is the single most important organ in your entire body. If it stops working properly, so do you—permanently. So why not do every little bit that you can to help your ticker last as long as possible? These herbs are rich in compounds called bioflavonoids, which help boost the strength of your heart.

Dried ginkgo
Dried hawthorn
Dried lime blossom
1 cup of hot water

➡ Combine equal parts of the herbs and add 1 heaping teaspoon of the mixture to the water. Steep for 10 minutes and strain. Drink 2 cups a day for your continued good health. **Caution:** If you are on any blood-thinning medications, do not take ginkgo without checking with your doctor first.

Remember the Reds

■ Lycopene is a compound known to protect the heart, and the richest sources of it are red fruits: tomatoes, guavas, and red and pink grapefruits. Even watermelon contains some of this substance. Lycopene is a carotenoid that's believed to have powerful antioxidant properties. A red that isn't so good for you? Red meat—which is high in saturated fats and thus a risk to your arteries. So go easy on the beef and round out your menu with fish or lean poultry instead.

Nifty, Thrifty Tips

One of the easiest things you can do to save money on your grocery bill is also one of the best things you can do to protect the health of your heart—and the hearts of those you cook for. That is to read all food labels carefully and avoid anything that contains the words *hydrogenated* or *partially hydrogenated*. Either term indicates that the product contains artery-clogging trans fats. These potential killers are found in many fast foods and packaged snack foods—just about all of which are a whole lot more expensive than fresh fruits or anything you could make at home from fresh, natural ingredients.

Hemorrhoid-Healing Tonic

If nasty little pains in the rear, also known as hemorrhoids, are making your life uncomfortable, try this tea. The herbs are all tonics for your venous system. And taken over time, they can help strengthen your blood vessels and may relieve hemorrhoids.

Dried butcher's broom
Dried horse chestnut
Dried rose hips
Dried yarrow
1 cup of hot water

➡ Combine equal parts of each herb, then add 1 heaping teaspoon of the mixture to the water. Let it steep for 10 minutes and then strain. Drink 2 to 3 cups per day. Soon those pains in the you-know-what will be out of your life for good.

Put a Potato Poultice Where?

■ To reduce the pain and swelling from hemorrhoids, place a potato poultice where "the sun don't shine" and leave it on overnight. To make the poultice, grate 2 tablespoons of raw potato, wrap it in cheesecloth, chill for an hour, and apply.

Horseradish Poultice

■ Whoa, Dobbin! When it's time to mount an attack on those itchy, burning hemorrhoids, use a homemade horseradish poultice, which can speed up the healing process by drawing blood to the area. Apply a thin layer of grated fresh horseradish to a wet cloth, and place the cloth on the hemorrhoids for 5 to 10 minutes. You can protect the surrounding skin from any burning effects by applying olive oil to the sensitive area first.

EUREKA!

WITCH HAZEL IS WELL KNOWN for its drawing action, which reduces swelling and helps ease the discomfort of itching. To make your own witch hazel infusion, put 1 heaping teaspoon of the fresh or dried leaves in 1 cup of hot water, and steep for 15 minutes. Soak a clean cloth in the solution, and apply it three to four times a day until your 'rhoids disappear.

Hemorrhoid Helper

Most hemorrhoids are caused by nothing more than constipation. So if you make an anti-constipation/anti-hemorrhoid decoction, you can get rid of both problems in one fell swoop. Use this recipe to clean out your insides, and help your outside heal up quickly, too!

1 tsp. of dried burdock root
1 tsp. of dried dandelion root
1 tsp. of dried peppermint
2 cups of boiling water

➡ Simmer the burdock and dandelion in the water for 20 minutes. Remove from the heat and add the peppermint, then cover and steep for another 10 minutes. Strain and sip ½ cup of the tea first thing in the morning and before each meal. This will loosen up your stool, get things moving, and clear up both of your annoying problems. **Caution:** If you take diuretics or potassium supplements, talk to your doctor before taking dandelion.

Baby Your Hemorrhoids

■ Ease the pain and itch by using baby wipes instead of toilet paper. (Just remember to toss them in the trash afterward—they're not flushable!)

Q: *I spend a lot of time sitting at my desk, and by the end of the day, my hemorrhoids are killing me. Got any discreet solutions?*

A: I sure do! Thanks to a nifty invention called a doughnut cushion, you can treat your hemorrhoids while you're sitting at your desk or in your favorite easy chair, or even while driving your car. The pillow's strategically cut-out design prevents pressure from being put on the affected area. The doughnut shape not only relieves pain but also helps the hemorrhoids heal. Look in your local pharmacy or in a health-products catalog for these handy helpers.

Take My Advice

The Cranberry Cure

Believe it or not, there is a tasty and nutritious drink that can actually help stop the bleeding that often accompanies hemorrhoids. If you're suffering from these major pains in the neck, er, lower parts, give this fabulous fixer a try.

1 part cranberry juice
1 part pomegranate juice

➡ Mix the juices together, and drink a glass between meals. Both fruits are hemostatic, which in layman's terms means that they help stanch bleeding. **Caution:** If you take warfarin (Coumadin®), check with your doctor before drinking cranberry juice.

Stop Straining

■ Sitting on the toilet for long periods of time puts pressure on hemorrhoids and only compounds the problem. So let your bowels move in their own sweet time, without trying to rush things along. You can also make things move more easily by drinking at least eight glasses of water a day and by adding fiber to your diet.

Root 'Em Out

■ Check your local health-food store for powdered elderberry root, which contains vessel-strengthening bioflavonoids. Mix it with warm water to make a paste, smear it on a piece of gauze, and hold it against your hemorrhoids for 10 minutes once or twice daily.

Nifty, Thrifty Tips

Don't worry about buying creams, astringents, and other pricey products to heal your hemorrhoids. Instead, just go to the freezer and find a bag of ice to sit on. A large plastic bag filled with crushed ice and covered with a towel may not be suitable as a long-term seat, but it can numb the pain and swelling for a while and help you feel more comfortable. You can do this two to three times a day, but limit your time on the ice to no more than 10 to 20 minutes.

Poppy Seed Paste

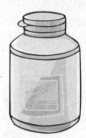 As anyone who's broken out in hives knows all too well, those annoying—and unsightly—red welts are a lot more troublesome than a simple skin itch. Whether the culprit is an allergy, contact with a toxic plant, or stress (the most common causes of hives), this seedy mixer will help cool the burn, ditch the itch, and reduce the swelling.

3 tbsp. of poppy seeds
1 tbsp. of lime juice
1 tbsp. of water

➡ Grind the poppy seeds in a food processor or coffee grinder. Pour the powder into a small bowl, and mix in the lime juice and water. Apply the paste to the affected areas. **Caution:** Do not apply this paste to broken or irritated skin.

Find Out Who Dunnit

■ When hives first hit, try to remember everything you've recently eaten and any new medications you've just started taking. If you can identify the trigger early, especially if you suspect a medication, you can avoid a more serious recurrence. Drawing a blank? Keep a daily food diary until you're sure whether or not something in your diet might be triggering the hives.

Axe the Aspirin

■ You might be surprised to learn that this common analgesic is a frequent cause of hives. If you're allergic to aspirin, you should also try eliminating foods that contain its active ingredient, salicylate. These include apricots, berries, grapes, raisins and other dried fruit, and tea.

Snappy Solutions

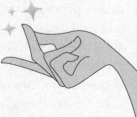 Foods that are processed with vinegar, such as pickles, cause hives in some people. So give up the sour stuff for a while, and see if it helps clear things up.

Ayurvedic Elixir

A bad case of indigestion can ruin your whole day. Your stomach feels like it's being eaten from the inside out (reminiscent of that scene from *Alien*), and you can't concentrate on anything other than trying to get rid of the pain. For acute indigestion, try this old-time elixir from Ayurveda, the traditional medicine of India.

¼ of a lime
1 cup of warm water
½ tsp. of baking soda

➡ Squeeze the juice from the lime into the water, and just before drinking it, add the baking soda. Then down the mixture quickly to avoid any of the sour taste from the lime. You'll soon be bidding that nasty feeling in your stomach a not-so-fond farewell.

Skip the Starbucks®

■ Coffee promotes stomach acid production, and so do tea and cola drinks. The amount and acidity of the stomach acid you produce varies, but in most cases, cutting back on coffee, tea, and colas can help prevent indigestion—and it won't hurt your smile, either (all three drinks can stain your teeth).

Heavenly Angelica Tea

■ Say a quick prayer of thanks for the lovely herb angelica and its power to ease indigestion. This herb, which tastes a bit like celery, can be made into a tea by putting 1 teaspoon of the dried herb (or 3 teaspoons of crushed fresh leaves) in 1 cup of boiling water. Steep for about 10 minutes, strain out the herb, and enjoy a cup after every meal.

Nifty, Thrifty Tips

If you're suffering from a bad case of indigestion, then good ol' water is one of the quickest, cheapest, and best remedies because it dilutes the burning acid and flushes it back into the stomach. So as soon as the indigestion starts up, slowly drink a couple of large glasses of water to ease the pain.

Berry Nice Tea

It's not just food that can bring on a bad case of indigestion. Sometimes, having a cold or the flu can mess up your stomach just as much as those jalapeño poppers. So if your indigestion is being caused by other health issues, tackle them one at a time. In the meantime, try this fixer to relieve indigestion and put a stop to the sniffles.

1 tsp. of dried alfalfa leaves
1 tsp. of dried blackberry leaves
1 tsp. of dried hibiscus leaves
1 tsp. of dried rose hips
1 cup of water

➡ Crumble all of the herbs together in a bowl. In a small saucepan, bring the water to a boil, then add 1 teaspoon of the herb mixture. Reduce the heat and let it simmer for about 15 minutes. Strain out the herbs and pour the tea into a cup. After a few sips, your tummy should start to feel better—and if it's a cold you have, you'll feel like less of a drip!

Stand Up to the Pain

■ You can't fight the law of gravity—whatever goes up must come down. It was true for Isaac Newton's apple, and it's equally true for stomach acid that inadvertently splashes upstream. To help gravity do its job, stand up at the first pangs of indigestion. You'll feel better as soon as the acid drains back down into your stomach and settles where it's supposed to be.

Snappy Solutions

Believe it or not, indigestion can be made worse by tight clothing, which can press on your stomach and push the acid uphill. So when the gnawing begins, make sure you're comfortable. Loosen your belt a few notches, untuck your shirt, or undo a few buttons. Less pressure means less indigestion. But whatever you do, don't get so comfortable that you head right over to the sofa and lie down after eating. Stay upright after a meal to give your stomach time to settle.

Ginger to the Rescue

 Here's an old-time elixir that grandmas everywhere swore by. It is safe and effective and stops indigestion in its tracks.

Fresh ginger
Boiling water
1 teaspoon of honey

➡ Take a piece of the ginger and steep it in the water for five minutes. Add the honey and relax while sipping the brew slowly. It'll tame a restless tummy in no time.

Aid from Aniseed

■ It's near the start of the alphabetic lineup on the spice aisle, and it should be near the head of the line in your anti-indigestion kit, too. To put this powerful fixer to work, just place about 7 teaspoons of aniseed in a pan with 1 quart of boiling water, and bring it to a boil. Reduce the heat to low, simmer until the water has reduced to about 3 cups, and strain out the seeds. Then drink 2 cups of the potion once or twice a day, sweetened to taste with honey if you like. You'll be feeling better in no time at all.

Q: *I get terrible stomachaches. I've taken antacids and tried walking them off, but nothing seems to work. What's causing this discomfort, and how can I deal with it?*

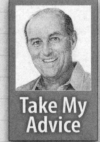

Take My Advice

A: If the usual fixes haven't done the job, you may simply have some trapped gas. So burp it up! Mind you, there's a good reason mothers "burp" their babies; it happens to be one of the best ways to relieve a stomachache that's caused by trapped gas. To burp properly, stand up straight and swallow a little air slowly so the valve between your esophagus and stomach relaxes and opens. This allows the gas to come up and escape instead of going down and becoming painfully trapped.

Terrific Tummy Tamer

What can I say? Sometimes a meal just tastes so good that I'm guilty of putting away much more than my fair share. Of course, I always pay for it later. So when my three-alarm chili and turkey club sandwich start to turn on me, I treat my troubled tummy to this tasty tea.

1 tsp. of dried catnip
1 tsp. of dried lemon balm
1 tsp. of dried peppermint
   (or spearmint) leaves
1 tsp. of dried sweet marjoram
1 cup of boiling water

➡ Combine all of the herbs thoroughly in a bowl. Then scoop out 2 teaspoons of the mixture and add it to the water. Let it steep for 15 minutes. Strain out the herbs and sip the tea slowly. Keep the rest of the herbs in an airtight glass container for the next time your tummy has a tantrum. **Caution:** If you have acid reflux disease, you should avoid mint.

Get Ginger

■ This pungent root is the jack-of-all-trades for stomach ailments, but it's especially good for relieving pain, since the gingerol it contains helps stop intestinal contractions. Best of all, you can take ginger in capsule form, drink it as a tea, or gnaw on a fresh slice, so there's no excuse not to try it. Check your supermarket or health-food store for ginger in all its forms and follow the label directions when given.

What Would Grandma Do?

🦋 WHEN GRANDMA PUTT had a bout of indigestion, she eased the discomfort in a flash by eating a few sprigs of fresh parsley. When there's no fresh parsley on hand, scoop ¼ teaspoon of the dried version out of the jar, mix it into a glass of warm water, and drink up. Your tummy will feel better in a hurry.

Tummy-Care Tea

Does your stomach do somersaults every time you eat stuffed peppers or other spicy food? Sometimes it's hard to say no. So when you get to the point where you never want to eat anything again—*ever*—tame your tummy with this herbal tea blend. And remember that flip-flop feeling the next time you think about indulging.

1 tsp. of dried bay leaves
1 tsp. of ground ginger
1 tsp. of dried mint leaves
Honey
1 cup of boiling water

➡ Combine the herbs and scoop 1 heaping teaspoon of the mixture into the water. Let it steep for 5 to 10 minutes. Strain out the herbs, and add honey to taste. Drink this tea anytime your stomach starts acting up, to quell the pain. **Caution:** If you have acid reflux disease, you should avoid mint.

Ease the Ache with Lemon Balm

■ This sweet-smelling herb, also known as Melissa, can help relax muscles and calm a roiling digestive tract. Add 20 to 30 drops of lemon balm tincture (available at health-food stores) to a glass of water, and drink it three times a day.

Stick with Marshmallow

■ That's marshmallow root, not the gooey roasted treat. Marshmallow is an herb that helps coat and soothe the mucous membranes in your stomach. Try drinking at least a cup (preferably more) of marshmallow root tea a day. You'll find the tea at most health-food stores.

Nifty, Thrifty Tips

An easy way to relieve stomach pain at home without having to dip into your wallet is to rub it away. To relax tense, constricted muscles, push gently into the lower left side of your belly, or rub the area in circles for 30 seconds or more. You may even consider adding a few drops of fennel or peppermint oil to vegetable oil to enhance the effects of the massage.

Yummy Tummy Soup

If tea isn't your thing, but stomach pain has you on the ropes, try making this stomach-calming soup instead. It has the same power as any tea, but it adds a little more flavor and gives you another remedy for pain with ingredients you may already have sitting around your kitchen.

2 12-oz. cans of vegetable broth or bouillon
2 garlic cloves, minced
2 quarter-sized pieces of fresh ginger
¼ tsp. of soy or tamari sauce (optional)

➡ Mix all of these ingredients together in a big pot. Bring the mixture to a boil, then turn down the heat. Let the soup simmer for 30 minutes. Then pour yourself a bowl, and sip it slowly by the spoonful. Quicker than you can say "Bob's your uncle," your stomach pain will be gone.

Get Your Jaw Moving

■ It may not be polite at formal gatherings, but chewing on a stick of gum is a great way to stop indigestion and the pain that comes along with it. Chewing increases the flow of saliva, which acts as a natural acid neutralizer in your stomach, and eases your gastric distress.

Trim the Squares

■ Eating gargantuan meals all but guarantees a bout of indigestion because all that food in your stomach requires enormous amounts of digestive acids. One simple way to prevent this is to eat five or six small meals a day instead of gorging yourself on two or three large ones.

EUREKA!

A LOT OF PEOPLE GET INDIGESTION after going to bed because lying down puts their stomach at the same level as their vulnerable esophagus. An easy solution is to raise the head of your bed a few inches by putting boards or sturdy blocks under the legs of the headboard.

Bug-Bite Liniment

You couldn't ask for a more effective treatment for insect bites than this old-time herbal elixir. But that's not the extent of its virtues. It's also just the ticket for cleansing cuts and scrapes and reducing muscle inflammation.

1 oz. of echinacea powder
1 oz. of powdered myrrh
1 oz. of powdered Oregon grape root
¼ oz. of ground cayenne pepper
Rubbing alcohol

➡ Put the powders and pepper in a glass jar, and pour in the alcohol until it reaches 2 to 3 inches above the top of the herb layer. Cover the jar with a tight-fitting lid, set it in a warm location, and let it sit for four weeks, shaking the jar every now and then to keep the herbs from packing down on the bottom. Strain out the solids, and pour the liquid into a clean, fresh bottle. Clearly label the bottle "FOR EXTERNAL USE ONLY," and store it out of the reach of children. To use the potion, dab it onto the bitten area. (Or pour it onto a cotton pad to clean and disinfect wounds, or rub it into your aching muscles.)

Dress for Success

■ Many insects are drawn to bright colors as much as they are to sweet aromas. So do your body a favor—in addition to nixing the perfume or fragrant body lotion, wear dark or neutral-colored clothing when you venture into buggy territory. And avoid brightly colored jewelry, which also attracts biters and stingers.

Snappy Solutions

The most powerful bug repellent of all is knowledge. Learn as much as you can about the potentially harmful insects—and snakes—that inhabit your part of the world so that you can protect yourself (and your nearest and dearest, both two- and four-legged) and treat a bite or sting properly. When you're prepared, your close encounters of the buggy or slithery kind won't live up to their painful potential.

Sassafras Squish

Sassafras has long been known for its insecticidal properties. This potent bug repellent is a modern interpretation of an old Native American mixer.

Fresh sassafras leaves
1 charcoal tablet (available in health-food stores) or a small piece of charred wood*
Vegetable oil

➡ Crush the leaves and the charcoal tablet or wood chunk, then mix in just enough vegetable oil to make a paste. Before you venture out, dab the paste onto your forehead and nose and around your mouth and ears, then rub it in gently. Reapply frequently.

* Do not use a charcoal briquette from the barbecue!

After You've Scratched

■ When mosquito bites have you itching like crazy, reach for a bottle of antiseptic mouthwash. Moisten a tissue with it, hold it on the bite for about 15 seconds, and kiss that irritating itch good-bye.

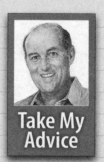

Take My Advice

Q: *We've just put in a new swimming pool, and we're starting to plan the landscaping around it. My husband insists that we stick to an all-green scheme to avoid trouble from bees. But I'd love to include some flowering plants. Is there anything we can plant that won't attract bees?*

A: There sure is! Bees won't go anywhere near feverfew, and you couldn't ask for a prettier plant. It grows about 2 feet tall, with lacy, light green leaves and delicate, daisy-like flowers that bloom from early summer all the way through to early fall, and it's hardy in Zones 5 to 9.

Soothing Sage Mash

No matter what kind of bug has sunk its business end into your body, this easy herbal fixer will make you feel better fast.

1 handful of freshly picked sage leaves
Apple cider vinegar

➡ Run a rolling pin over the sage leaves to bruise them. Put the leaves in a pan, cover them with the vinegar, and simmer on low until they soften. Remove the leaves and allow them to cool. Then carefully wrap them in a washcloth, and apply it to the afflicted site.

Remove the Weapon—Carefully

■ Unlike ticks and mosquitoes, stinging insects, such as hornets, bees, wasps, and yellow jackets, don't transmit disease, but they do inject venom, which the stinger continues to release even after the attacker has gone. So don't squeeze your flesh to get the stinger out; that will only force the venom farther in. Instead, keep your skin flat as you scrape the stinger out with your fingernail or the edge of a credit card, or pull it out with tweezers held flat against your skin.

Tenderize the Bite

■ Meat tenderizer is a classic fixer for treating insect bites and stings. Just mix it with a few drops of water and spread it on the stricken site. The tenderizer will break down the protein in the poison, thereby nixing its pain-producing properties. Meat tenderizer takes the pain right out of a jellyfish sting, so take along a shaker of the stuff whenever you head to the beach.

✚ In most cases, an insect sting is simply a minor nuisance in the overall scheme of life, but in some folks it can trigger a severe and life-threatening allergic reaction. If you have trouble breathing after being stung, you've received multiple stings, or (I hope this goes without saying!) you know you're allergic to insect venom, dial 911 immediately.

Dial a Doc

Chickweed Salve

Whether it's from a mosquito bite, a scrape, poison ivy, or some other skin irritant, an itch can drive you crazy. Chickweed salve is a reliable itch reliever.

1 cup of fresh chickweed leaves
Olive oil
1 vitamin E capsule

➡ Clean and chop the chickweed leaves and allow them to dry thoroughly, until they become slightly wilted. Place them in a glass jar, and add enough olive oil to cover the leaves completely. Break open the vitamin E capsule, and add the liquid to the jar. Cap the jar, and let it sit in a sunny window for one week, turning the jar end to end several times each day. Strain the mixture and pour the oil into a clean bottle. For best results, store it in your refrigerator, and apply to itchy areas as needed.

Take a Dip in the Ocean

■ Seawater can kill fungi, dry up poison ivy blisters, and relieve almost any skin condition known to man. And it's readily available—even to landlubbers! Just convert your tub into your very own ocean by adding salt to your bathwater. Use sea salt if you think it will feel more authentic, although it's a bit pricey.

Get the Starch Out

■ Cornstarch is another reliable itch reliever. Dust this satiny powder right onto your body, or add it to your bathwater for soothing relief. You'll be amazed at how fast you'll ditch the itch. **Caution:** Don't use cornstarch when the itch comes from a fungal infection.

EUREKA!

YOU MAY HAVE a bad winter itch, and nothing seems to be causing it. Before you waste a lot of time trying to figure it out, it may be that your indoor heat is sucking all the moisture from your skin. To fix the problem, buy a humidifier and set it up in the rooms where you spend most of your time.

Extinguish That Itch!

Even though warm water generally irritates skin and can make itching worse, when the right ingredients are added, it can be one of the best ways to stop the scratching. This mixer will relieve itching and restore the proper pH to your skin.

1 cup of apple cider vinegar
1 cup of barley flour
1 tubful of warm water

➤ Add the apple cider vinegar and barley flour to the tubful of water. Sink in and let the vinegar and barley flour get that itch right out of your skin. And don't worry—the vinegar smell will dissipate quickly.

Chill Out

■ Taking a cold shower when the itch gets the best of you is one of the simplest ways to calm it down. Cold water and ice reduce blood circulation, which in turn reduces swelling and inflammation. If you can't take that much cold all at once, put some ice packs on the itchy areas (for up to 20 minutes) until they chill out.

Soak It Out

■ Nothing ditches an itch like the quick relief of an oatmeal bath. You can buy colloidal oatmeal at a health-food store or drugstore and add it to a warm bath. Or fill an old sock with about a cup of plain, dry oatmeal, attach the open end of the sock to your bathtub faucet with a rubber band, and run warm water through it until the tub is filled. Then settle in for a nice long, soothing soak. **Note:** Whatever you do, don't simply toss regular oatmeal into the tub, or you'll wind up with a clogged drain!

Snappy Solutions

If your wintertime itch is due to the dryness of the weather and heated indoor air, help protect your skin by eating foods that are rich in omega-3 fatty acids, such as cold-water fish, nuts, and seeds. You should be getting at least one serving a day.

Rapid Relief

That nasty itch can be more annoying than it is painful. And stopping to scratch (especially if the itch isn't in the most flattering of places) isn't always an option. So zap your urge to scratch with a strong infusion of this itch-soothing fixer.

Dried balm of Gilead
Dried chickweed
Dried peppermint
¼ cup of witch hazel
1 cup of boiling water

➡ Combine equal parts of the dried herbs, and scoop 1 heaping teaspoon of the mixture into the water. Steep, covered, for 15 minutes. Add the witch hazel and chill. Then pour the concoction into a handheld sprayer bottle. Mist it onto your skin whenever you need relief.

Say "Nuts" to Itchy Skin

■ If your skin gets itchy in water, you probably need more fatty acids in your diet. Walnuts are loaded with these valuable fats, so dig the nutcracker out of the drawer and enjoy a few of these nuts each day. Your skin will probably feel better within a few weeks.

Baking Soda Soother

■ Baking soda has a major reputation as a powerful itch fighter. If your skin is especially irritated, try shaking some baking soda into your hand and rubbing it right onto your damp skin when you get out of the shower. The light, pasty film that forms will soothe your skin for hours.

Nifty, Thrifty Tips

If you want to save a little money on creams and ointments that are "guaranteed" to make itching disappear, then simply help your skin repair itself. How? By getting plenty of vitamins C and E, two nutrients that are critical for skin health. Pick up some juice that is naturally high in vitamin C and has some vitamin E added to it. Soon enough, your skin will be back to normal.

Lovely Lung Rub

There's almost nothing more miserable than the flu or a chest cold that keeps you tossing and turning all night long. When you've been laid low by nasty germs, reach for this old-time fixer.

**1 tsp. of olive oil
3 or 4 drops of
thyme oil**

➡ Combine the oils in a small bowl and rub your chest with the mixture. The warming vapors will keep your respiratory passages open and moist as they fight infection with their antiseptic action. Plus, they make it easier to get to sleep at night by helping mucus drain so you can breathe better.

Fight the Big C with Beta-Carotene

■ Researchers have long known that people who eat the most beta-carotene-rich fruits and vegetables have the lowest risk of lung cancer. One study of nonsmokers found that people who ate the most vegetables could lower their lung cancer risk by 25 percent. Sweet potatoes, carrots, kale, spinach, and winter squash (including pumpkin) all pack big doses of beta-carotene. So fill your plate with these and other colorful veggies, and eat to your good health!

Horse Around with Horseradish

■ The pungent root is packed with isothiocyanates, chemical compounds that seem to deactivate other chemicals before they can trigger cancer. Scientists think isothiocyanates may be especially helpful in staving off lung cancer.

✚ Most respiratory infections don't require an immediate trip to the doctor. However, that's not true for children, people over the age of 55, and anyone who has (or has a history of) lung disease. If you fall into one of these categories, get to the doc or emergency room—pronto. Even if you think you're in great shape, talk to your doctor if you don't start feeling better within about a week, or are getting worse at any time.

Dial a Doc

Thyme Out Tonic

Weak lungs can lead to a lot of breathing problems that could otherwise be avoided. And if you already have a breathing problem, like allergies or asthma, then weak lungs are especially troublesome as well as dangerous. Here's an elixir that'll tone up your lungs with restorative herbs, anti-inflammatory ginger, and vitamin C–rich rose hips.

Aniseed
Ground ginger
Dried ginkgo
Dried rose hips
Dried thyme
1 cup of boiling water

➡ Combine equal parts of the first five ingredients. Add 1 heaping teaspoon of the mixture to the water and steep, covered, for 15 minutes, then strain out the solids. Drink 2 to 3 cups per day. Before long, your lungs will be full of life and life-giving air, and you'll be less susceptible to breathing problems. **Caution:** Do not take ginkgo if you are on blood thinners.

Breathe More Slowly

■ If you're a wheezer, experts say that you're also an overbreather. That is, you breathe heavily or rapidly or inhale through your mouth—any one of which can promote irritation and inflammation of the airways and weaken your lungs. To slow your breathing, use your heart rate as a guide. For every seven heartbeats, breathe in once through your nose. For the next nine beats, breathe out through your mouth with your lips pursed until your air is gone. It may take a bit of practice, but you'll get the hang of it in no time.

Nifty, Thrifty Tips

If you suffer from asthma, allergies, or other respiratory woes, relief is as close as your bathroom—and it won't cost you a cent. Just turn on the shower and crank up the water temperature as high as it will go. Let the room get good and steamy, then sit back and relax for 10 to 15 minutes. The steam will thin the sticky mucus that's clogging up your breathing passages.

Hot Flash Tonic

If you're a woman over 50, then you've probably already had the talk with your doctor about menopause and the effect it will have on your body. The least comfortable side effects of this time in a lady's life are usually the hot flashes. These traditional herbs with hormone-balancing properties may help reduce the frequency and severity of hot flashes and help you keep your cool.

Dried black cohosh
Dried chasteberry
Dried dong quai
Dried motherwort
1 cup of hot water

➥ Combine equal parts of the herbs, and steep 1 heaping teaspoon of the mixture in the water for 15 minutes. Strain out the solids. Drink 2 cups of cooled tea daily for two months or longer to help ease menopause symptoms.

Edamame Poppers

■ Eating soy can provide blessed relief from hot flashes. And the soy fixers don't come much easier—or tastier—than this soybean-in-the-pod snack. Just add 2 cups of frozen edamame and ½ teaspoon of salt (if desired) to 2 quarts of boiling water. Reduce the heat and simmer for five minutes. Pour off the boiling water, then rinse the pods with cold water. One by one, gently squeeze the cooled pods and slurp the soybeans right into your mouth.

Cool Down with Alfalfa

■ Alfalfa contains plant sterols, which make it an ideal choice for treating hot flashes. Steep 1 teaspoon of alfalfa in 1 cup of hot water. Strain, and drink 1 cup of the cooled tea daily.

What Would Grandma Do?

🦋 WHEN GRANDMA PUTT'S *hot flashes were causing her a lot of discomfort, she knew how to keep herself cool. Her secret: Dress in layers of clothing. She'd just peel off a layer or two when she felt hot, and put them back on when she was cold. Also, wear silk or cotton underwear; the fabrics breathe and won't trap the heat as much as synthetics do.*

Menopause-Relief Capsules

Once menopause begins, the ovaries make fewer and fewer hormones, while the adrenal glands continue producing small amounts of estrogen until about age 70. But in many cases, a woman's adrenals have become prematurely worn out through stress and poor eating habits. The resulting symptoms, such as fatigue, mood swings, depression, and irritability, can make hot flashes seem like a stroll in the park. The herbal powders in these easy-to-make capsules will strengthen your adrenal glands and help get them back on the job.

2 parts kelp powder
2 parts licorice powder
1 part black cohosh powder
1 part ground ginger
1 part ginseng powder
½ part dong quai powder
Size 00 capsules

➡ Mix the first six ingredients together thoroughly, and put the powder into the capsules (available at health-food stores and drugstores). Take two or three capsules daily, as needed. **Caution:** If you have hypertension, avoid licorice and ginseng. If you have a history of breast cancer, take black cohosh only under a doctor's supervision.

Get With the Program

■ Some of the classic woes of menopause can be attributed to dramatic hormonal changes. But many of these signs of "ungraceful aging" are a direct result of poor eating habits, lack of exercise, and stressful living. Fortunately, it's never too late to shape up your act. If you start eating sensibly, exercising more, and making some healthy lifestyle changes, you'll soon find that many of your distressing symptoms have gone with the wind.

EUREKA!

TO EASE THE BLOATING that often accompanies menopause, pack in the parsley. Add the leaves to salads and sandwiches, use parsley seeds in soups and stews—and when you're dining out, eat your garnish!

Caraway Cramping Cure

Whether menstrual cramps strike like clockwork every month, or only once in a blue moon, they're sheer misery. So make 'em flee fast with this fabulous fixer.

**4 tsp. of caraway seeds
2 cups of water
Honey (optional)**

➡ Put the caraway seeds on a cutting board or a sheet of wax paper, and flatten them slightly with the back of a spoon. Bring the water to a boil, add the seeds, and simmer on low for five minutes. Remove the pan from the heat, and let the tea steep for another minute or two (but not long enough to cool off). Add honey to taste, if you like, and drink up. Just one cup should take care of the problem, but if not, sip a cup every hour or so until the pain vanishes.

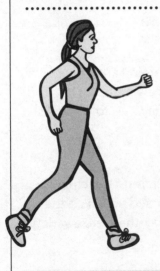

Boost Your Endorphins

■ Don't just sit around and suffer. Studies show that women who exercise regularly are less likely to have PMS, possibly because exercise increases oxygen to the muscles and boosts the amount of serotonin and other uplifting brain chemicals, called endorphins, in the blood. So what are you waiting for? All it takes is 20 minutes a day of regular exercise. And no special equipment is needed—a daily after-dinner walk can go a long way toward preventing the aggravation of PMS—and menstrual cramps, to boot.

What Would Grandma Do?

🦋 WHEN GRANDMA PUTT *had a case of premenstrual bloat, she knew just how to get relief—she'd steam some asparagus and drink the cooled cooking water. It did the trick because asparagus drippings make a great diuretic. Other diuretic foods that can aid in easing premenstrual symptoms include artichokes and watercress.*

Flower Spritz

Now, I may not know firsthand how it feels, but having a lot of ladies in my family means I've always been surrounded by people suffering from menstrual pain. So here's a DIY flower water to spritz on your skin during the day for a more fragrant life. Made from essential oils that relieve the pain and stress associated with menstruation, this elixir can be used whenever the need arises.

10 drops of clary sage oil
10 drops of lavender oil
10 drops of Roman
    chamomile oil
5 ml of rubbing alcohol
100 ml of distilled water

➤ Combine the essential oils with the alcohol, and add that mixture to the distilled water. Store the flower water in a glass sprayer bottle, and use it liberally whenever that time of the month rolls around.

Red Raspberry Relief

■ Red raspberry is a uterine tonic that may help relieve cramping and pelvic congestion. To make a tea, steep 1 heaping teaspoon of raspberry leaves in 1 cup of hot water for 10 minutes, then strain. Drink 1 to 2 cups daily. This tonic works best if it's taken every day for several weeks.

The Tummy Touch

■ Historically, women used abdominal massage to relieve cramps and bloating. Some women would sprinkle a pinch of sage, tobacco, or sacred pollen on the abdomen while singing songs to soothe away the pain. Today, there are a variety of herbal oils, such as evening primrose, that you can use.

Nifty, Thrifty Tips

Before using OTC drugs to relieve menstrual discomfort, try modifying your diet and exercising more. Cut back on the sweets, which just make you more hungry and bloated. Opt for complex carbohydrates, such as fresh fruit and vegetables. And exercise to stretch out your muscles, which, as a bonus, will lift your nasty mood.

Ladies' Tonic

There's a reason old-timers called it "the curse": Monthly woes caused by your period can literally lay you up for days without any sign of light at the end of the tunnel. Black cohosh and chasteberry have a normalizing effect on hormonal balance and may be useful when taken together for menstrual difficulties. Blend them with the two other traditional women's herbs—partridgeberry and lady's mantle—for a tea that will support you all through the month.

Dried black cohosh
Dried chasteberry
Dried lady's mantle
Dried partridgeberry
1 cup of hot water

➡ Combine equal parts of the herbs, then add 1 teaspoon of the mixture to the water and steep for 10 minutes. Strain out the solids. Drink 1 to 2 cups per day. If you drink this tea throughout the month, then when it's time for your next period to begin, you'll be in much better shape to handle the discomfort. **Caution:** If you have a history of breast cancer, take black cohosh only under a doctor's supervision.

Mind Your Minerals

■ Calcium was voted by women as one of the top treatments for PMS because it can soothe cramps, lower back pain, bloating, food cravings, and mood swings all at once. Magnesium helps, too, but you might want to go easy on the stuff because too much can cause diarrhea. The Recommended Daily Allowance (RDA) for calcium is 1,200 mg for women over 50. Good food sources are yogurt, sardines, milk, cheeses, tofu, and salmon.

✚ Certain cramps may signal a serious medical problem—such as endometriosis or fibroid tumors—that has nothing to do with menstruation. So see your doctor when your cramps do not disappear after your period ends, the pain is on one side only (rather than over the entire abdomen), or you get no relief after taking aspirin or other anti-inflammatory remedies.

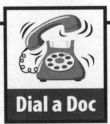

Dial a Doc

Aches and Pains Potion

Muscle aches can be a real pain in the rear, setting in and staying for days at a time. So relief can never come soon enough. To concoct a pain-relieving tea, mix up these ingredients and wave bye-bye to your woes.

2 parts dried echinacea
1 part dried lemon balm
1 part dried oat straw
1 part dried skullcap
1 part dried St. John's wort
1 cup of hot water

➡ Combine the herbs and add 1 heaping teaspoon of the mixture to the water. Cover and steep for 10 minutes, then strain. Drink 3 or 4 cups a day until the aches are gone. **Caution:** If you're taking any antidepressant or anti-anxiety medications, consult your doctor before taking St. John's wort. Don't take echinacea if you have an autoimmune disease, such as rheumatoid arthritis, lupus, or multiple sclerosis.

Ease Aches with Arnica

■ A great way to take the kinks out of sore muscles is to apply arnica cream, which relaxes muscles and helps them recover more quickly. You can also make your own muscle soother by chopping up fresh or dried arnica, adding enough water to make a paste, and spreading the mixture over the sore spots. Wrap the areas loosely with gauze and keep them covered for about 20 minutes. **Caution:** Don't use arnica on broken skin.

EUREKA!

SURE, IT FEELS GOOD, but a nice massage does more than just make you close your eyes in dreamy relaxation. It also stimulates blood flow, which can push pain-causing lactic acid out of your muscles and bring in healing nutrients. Whether you do it yourself or have someone else do it for you, it's best to use gentle pressure, always stroking toward the center of your body. To make massage even more soothing and effective, try adding a little herbal essential oil to your regular massage oil.

Aching-Muscle Magic

Muscles are very touchy and can be strained or cramped by an activity that would normally have no ill effect on them. But every so often, you'll wake up in the morning or end your day with a muscle that certainly wasn't bothering you a few hours earlier. Ease your aching muscles with a little of this minty mixer.

**1 tbsp. of petroleum jelly
6 drops of peppermint oil
Warm water**

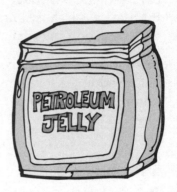

➡ Mix the petroleum jelly and peppermint oil in a small bowl, then put the bowl in a larger bowl of warm water. Soak a towel in warm (not hot!) tap water, wring it out, and drape it over the troubled area. Leave it in place for three to four minutes. Remove the towel and then massage the jelly/oil mixture into your skin for soothing relief.

Make the Right Moves

■ Sometimes a sore muscle feels like it never wants to move again—but gently stretching and moving it will speed recovery and keep it from getting tight. Try to move the affected muscle through its normal range of motion, stretching it slowly and carefully. This may mean flexing and extending your arm, arching your back, or taking a slow walk to stretch your legs. It's okay if you feel the muscle pulling and stretching, but the pain shouldn't get worse.

Snappy Solutions

You're much less likely to feel sore and strained if you ease your muscles into a workout and bring them to a gradual stop when you're done. So if you're exercising for a half hour, you should spend at least five minutes warming up and five minutes cooling down to avoid dealing with sore muscles later on.

Alfalfa Axes Aches

Some mornings we wake up and know right away that we had a bad night's sleep. How? Because our bodies just ache all over. There's no telling what you did while you were out cold to cause the pain, either. So if you're feeling a little achy in the a.m., work those knots out of your muscles with this soothing elixir.

1 tsp. of dried red clover
   blossoms
1 tsp. of alfalfa
1 cup of boiling water
1 tsp. of honey (optional)

➡ Crush the red clover blossoms, and combine them with the alfalfa before adding 1 teaspoon of the mixture to the water. Let it steep for five minutes, then strain out the herbs and sip. Add the honey, if you want, to sweeten it up a bit.

Straighten Up

■ A painful muscle cramp will eventually relax on its own, but the sooner you encourage it to do so, the sooner you'll get relief. Since the cramped muscle can't move itself, you'll need to use a free hand to straighten the affected leg, arm, or foot. Gently pull the muscle in the opposite direction of the cramp. Doing this a few times will usually relax the muscle and ease the pain.

What Would Grandma Do?

🦋 *My* GRANDMA PUTT *knew a lot about muscle injuries and how to treat them. But what she understood most (and I didn't) was that they take time to heal, and the last thing you want to do is overuse the affected muscles before the healing process is complete. As a general rule, calf pain that's only mildly irritating will probably take about 10 days to heal completely. Injuries that are slightly more serious may take 10 to 20 days, and really bad ones may take months. So when you start to feel better, don't try to pick up right where you left off, or there's a good chance you'll hurt yourself all over again.*

Apple Cider Liniment

When muscle aches and pains have you reaching for aspirin again and again, it may be time to consider a new approach to your discomfort. Here's how to make your own liniment to relieve painful muscles and get yourself back in business quickly.

½ oz. of powdered cramp bark
1 cup of apple cider vinegar
A pinch of cayenne pepper

➡ Combine the powdered cramp bark with the vinegar in a bottle. Add the cayenne pepper, put the cap on the bottle, and let the mixture stand for one week in a cool, dark place. Shake well every day, then decant and store in another clean glass bottle. Apply the elixir to sore muscles as a rub, or soak a clean cloth in the liniment and place it on the aching area. **Caution:** If you are pregnant or nursing, check with your doctor before using cramp bark.

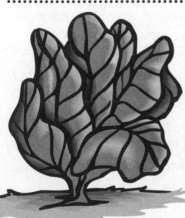

Greens for Relief

◼ The greener your midnight snack is, the less likely you are to be rudely awakened by middle-of-the-night cramps. Leafy green vegetables, such as spinach, chard, kale, and turnip and beet greens, are chock-full of cramp-stopping electrolytes—especially magnesium, potassium, and calcium. A daily salad or stir-fry that includes these ingredients should keep cramps at bay.

✚ If you're taking cholesterol-lowering medication, report any muscle aches, pains, or cramps to your doctor immediately. They can indicate a rare, life-threatening condition in which muscle—including heart muscle—is being destroyed as a side effect of your medication.

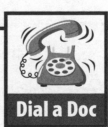

Dial a Doc

Back-in-Balance Bath

Muscle aches, cramps, and spasms could be a sign that you had something more than just a great workout yesterday. Sometimes, they could be trying to let you know that your internal electrolytes are out of balance. To make things right, reach for this recipe at night, and you'll be good to go in the morning.

2 cups of Epsom salts
2 cups of kosher or sea salt
2 tbsp. of potassium crystals

➡ Pour the salts and crystals into a tub of hot water. Slip in, and soak your aches and pains away. Potassium crystals are available in health-food stores.

The Salad Dressing Solution

■ Hot vinegar is great for relaxing cramped muscles. To use it, mix equal parts of water and vinegar in a saucepan, heat it until it's comfortably hot, and soak a small towel in the solution. Wring the towel out and hold it against the painful area for five minutes, then replace it with another towel that's been soaked in cold water. Repeat the cycle three times, keeping the hot towel in place for five minutes and the cold towel in place for one minute, always ending with the cold treatment. By the time you're done, the cramps should be gone.

Go with the Flow

■ When your body isn't well hydrated, muscle aches feel worse. Filling your water tank helps your body get rid of toxins that contribute to muscle pain. So when you're exercising or working hard, keep a bottle of water or sports drink handy and take frequent sips to stay hydrated.

Snappy Solutions

Sports drinks like Gatorade® contain minerals that your muscles need to function properly. So if your cramps are caused by a lack of nutrients, a good healthy swig of an athletic beverage before and during exercise could prevent them from occurring (or recurring).

Bath Cure-All

If you're feeling achy all over (whether it's from your daily work-out or just a bad day at the office), then you're going to need some serious pain-busting relief to get back to feeling 100 percent. For general pain, try this marvelous mixer in a soothing soak.

⅓ cup of dried chamomile
⅓ cup of dried lavender
⅓ cup of dried lemon balm
2 cups of Epsom salts

➡ First, mix together the chamomile, lavender, and lemon balm. Scoop out ⅓ cup of the mixture, wrap it up in a muslin bag, and place the bag in your tub while you run the hot water. Then pour in the Epsom salts and swirl the water to dissolve the salts. Soak in the tub for 10 to 15 minutes, or until you break into a nice healthy sweat.

Herbal Joint Remedy

■ To relieve sore joints, add 3 or 4 drops of arnica oil to ½ teaspoon of a warming wintergreen, lavender, or rosemary salve. Apply this soothing potion to sore joints three or four times a day to help increase circulation to the area. **Caution:** Don't use arnica on broken skin.

Get in the Swim

■ A great way to take the kinks out of an aching back is to go for a dip in the pool. Submerging yourself in water helps reduce muscle tension, and the water supports your weight, allowing you to exercise without putting additional strain on your back.

EUREKA!

THERE ARE MANY FOODS that can help sore joints. Nuts and beans, along with raisins, pears, apples, and other fruits, all contain the trace element boron, which can relieve pain and joint stiffness and protect against arthritis. So be sure to work these healthy foods into your daily diet.

Berry Good Tonic

Hawthorn berries are widely used for their gentle hypotensive effects. Combining them with other anti-spasmodic herbs and relaxants can really boost their benefits. So try this herbal mixer to help get your muscles back into proper working order whenever they start feeling out of whack.

Dried hawthorn
Dried motherwort
Dried passionflower
Dried skullcap
1 cup of hot water

➥ Combine equal parts of the herbs, and add 1 heaping teaspoon of the mixture to the water. Let steep for 15 minutes, then strain out the solids. Drink 2 to 3 cups daily, and you'll soon say "so long!" to aches and pains.

Stand Up for Yourself

■ The next time you get one of those awful leg, foot, or toe cramps in the middle of the night, relax—relief is just a step away. All you have to do is stand up and put weight on the leg that's got the cramp. This action stretches the muscles and almost instantly stops the pain.

Q: *I have to do the same thing day in and day out, and I always end up with painful cramps in my muscles. Is there anything I can do to prevent this from happening?*

Take My Advice

A: Some cramps happen because a muscle group becomes fatigued after being held in the same position for long periods of time. If you can schedule your day so that long tasks are broken up with shorter ones, your muscles will appreciate the break and the chance to switch gears. Get up from your desk a few times an hour, and rake leaves after working on your knees in the garden. The more frequently you change position, the less likely you are to have cramps.

Calf-Pain Reliever

Calf pain in the middle of the night can rouse you out of a deep sleep. And who knows if you'll be able to fall back to sleep? If you don't, you worry that your day will be ruined before it even starts. So if calf pain is making it difficult to get a good night's sleep, try this natural pain reliever.

Ground ginger
Dried Jamaican dogwood
Dried meadowsweet
Dried passionflower
1 cup of hot water

➡ Combine equal parts of the herbs, then steep 1 teaspoon of the mixture in the water for about 10 minutes. Strain out the herbs and let the tea cool slightly. Sip 2 or 3 cups throughout the day and have an extra cup just before you go to bed to help ensure a good night's sleep.

Bark at Your Pain

■ Cramp bark releases pain-causing spasms and promotes relaxation. To make a tea, simmer 1 heaping teaspoon of crumbled dried cramp bark in 1 cup of water for 10 minutes, then strain. Sip 1 or 2 cups daily, and you'll block any pain that comes your way. **Caution:** If you are pregnant or nursing, check with your doctor before taking cramp bark.

Play a Little Night Music

■ If you are taking medication for pain, try turning on the radio or dropping in your favorite Mozart CD. Studies show that people who are taking pain medicine experienced even more relief when they listened to music and relaxed.

EUREKA!

IT'S A FACT: Women are more likely than men to experience daily pain. And one in three women cites the trials of balancing work and family life as a significant cause of pain, which can be both physical and emotional. Stress makes you tighten your muscles for hours on end, and the result is pain. So try to eliminate some of the stress, and hopefully, you can eliminate the pain.

Comfrey Comfort Rub

The most soothing remedy for aching muscles is a nice restorative rubdown, and you'll get a lot of comfort if you use comfrey. Follow this recipe to make your own massage oil containing comfrey leaves—it's guaranteed to take the ache out of your body.

12 oz. of chopped fresh comfrey leaves
Castor oil
1 vitamin E capsule
15 drops of juniper oil
15 drops of wintergreen oil

➡ Fill a 12-ounce glass jar with the chopped comfrey leaves, and cover them completely with castor oil and the contents of the vitamin E capsule. Cap the jar tightly and steep the contents in a sunny window for one week. Shake the jar once or twice daily. Strain, then add the essential oils of juniper and wintergreen to the resulting liquid, and store the mixture in a clean glass bottle with a cap. Rub the massage oil into sore muscles as needed. To prolong the life of your oils, always store them in a cool, dark place or in the fridge.

Raise Your Heel

■ For quick relief for aching calf muscles, buy little wedge-shaped pads that slip inside your shoe and elevate and ease the muscles. The pads shorten the distance your calves have to stretch on their own, and they can be extremely effective in preventing the hyper-stretch that causes the pain in the first place. You'll find them at your local drugstore.

While you may be able to defuse your calf pain just by stretching the muscle, this doesn't help if you've injured the muscle. In fact, if the pain gets worse when you stretch, that's probably the case—and the best thing you can do is relax for a while. You certainly don't want to force the muscle to move when it doesn't want to. But if the pain does get worse, get to a doctor immediately because you may have done some real damage to it.

Dial a Doc

Herbal Healer

We all know the feeling: Some sort of pain creeps into your body, then you wait and wait and wait anxiously for it to leave. Well, the tension that often accompanies prolonged pain only creates more pain. To help you relax, use these herbs to make an elixir that will allow all of the discomfort to flow right out of your body.

Dried black cohosh
Dried chamomile
Dried Jamaican dogwood
Dried meadowsweet
Dried passionflower
1 cup of hot water

➡ Combine equal parts of any three of the herbs that you prefer (or until you find a taste that is to your liking). Steep 1 teaspoon of the mixture in the water for 10 minutes, then strain. Drink 2 to 4 cups daily. **Caution:** If you have ragweed allergies, you may be sensitive to chamomile. If you have a history of breast cancer, take black cohosh only under a doctor's supervision.

Say Ohmm!

■ Just as women in childbirth have learned that focused breathing can help get them through labor pain, that same kind of focused breathing may also help with other kinds of pain. Deep breathing relaxes your muscles, increases oxygen to the cells, and encourages your body to produce endorphins, which are natural painkillers. So inhale slowly and deeply, then exhale slowly and deeply. Be aware of your body relaxing, and feel the tension melt away. Use a mantra to help you breathe rhythmically if you so desire.

Nifty, Thrifty Tips

A cheap and easy way to get rid of pain while you sleep is to go to bed wet. When you get out of the tub or shower, don't dry off. Instead, wrap yourself up in an old sheet that's been saturated with cold water and wrung out. Then wrap up in one or two outer layers of wool blankets, and go to sleep. The sheet should feel cold for only a few minutes and will then dry out. This can be repeated once a week for deep relaxation and pain relief.

Homemade Ice Pack

An ice-cold pack can ease sore muscles, and the best part is that the effects of cold last longer than those of heat because it takes longer for your body to warm up than to cool off. To make an ice pack that will mold to your contours, follow these easy instructions. Make it now, so you'll have it on hand.

4 parts water
1 part rubbing alcohol
2 ziplock plastic freezer bags

➡ Fill one plastic bag with the water and alcohol. Put that bag into a second bag to prevent leakage, and store the pack in the freezer. The next time you're in pain, apply the pack to the injured area for no longer than 20 minutes at a time. Since the alcohol won't freeze, the pack will easily mold to your curves.

Soothe the Swelling

■ It's normal for muscles to swell after injuries, but swelling is your worst enemy because it increases both the pain and the time it takes the damage to heal. So the more you can minimize swelling, the faster your muscles will heal. If you injure your leg, start by resting the leg and putting something cold on the aching area. It's also helpful to keep your leg elevated above the level of your heart, which allows fluids to drain away from the injured tissue. In addition, wrap the muscle with an elastic bandage; it should be snug, but still loose enough so you can slip a finger underneath it.

Snappy Solutions

Good shoes with slightly raised heels are a worthwhile investment if you're prone to leg pain because they'll keep your muscles from overstretching. If you can't remember the last time you bought new sneakers, do yourself a favor and buy a pair now. Why? Because athletic shoes lose their cushioning ability over time, even when they look fine on the outside. As a general rule, you should replace them at least once a year.

Joint Remedy

As we get older, the cartilage in our joints begins to wear down, and can even disappear altogether! When this happens, you can feel a clicking as the bones rub against each other. This condition can be extremely painful and even lead to more serious consequences, like broken bones. So if you have joint pain, try soaking the aches away with this mixer.

1 cup of apple cider vinegar
1 cup of Epsom salts
Tub of hot water

➡ Add the vinegar and Epsom salts to the water. Slip into the tub and let the water wash over your entire body. The aches in your joints will soon start to dull, and before long, they'll be all gone!

Apple Away Pain

■ The next time your joints are hurting—or better yet, before the pain starts— eat a few apples. They contain the trace element boron, which can relieve joint pain and stiffness. In addition, studies indicate that they may actually protect against arthritis. Leave the skins on so you get the most out of these tasty treats.

Relief for Gym Rats

■ If joint pain tends to flare after you exercise, heat treatment can help cut down on swelling and relieve pain. Simply apply a heating pad set on "low" to aching joints before your workouts, or place a hot, moist towel on the area. Then immediately follow your workout with a cool-to-cold compress.

What Would Grandma Do?

🦋 THE NEXT TIME you have a sore shoulder, do what my Grandma Putt always did and apply heat to it. She knew that this simple remedy is just as good as over-the-counter pain relievers. Heat will relax the muscle, loosen the joint, and help prevent painful spasms. Whenever your shoulder starts feeling stiff, just hold a heating pad set on "low" or a warm compress against the area for 15 to 20 minutes at a time.

Lavender Bath Blend

My Grandma Putt used to hand-make nearly all of the Christmas and birthday presents she gave to her family and friends. With the ingredients she had around the house and the great tricks she had up her sleeve, who could blame her? The all-time favorite gift she gave to the ladies in her life was this fabulous fixer.

1 part comfrey leaves (fresh or dried)
1 part Epsom salts
1 part lavender blossoms (fresh or dried)
Lavender oil

➧ Mix the leaves, salts, and blossoms in a bowl. Add a few drops of the oil (let your nose be your guide), and blend the ingredients well with your hands or a wooden spoon. Store the mixture in a decorative jar or other lidded container. Use a handful in your bath to soothe your tired, achy muscles.

Raise Your Toes

■ One reason a muscle cramp in your leg is so painful is that the muscle is shortening more than it should. So the obvious solution is to make the muscle longer by stretching your calf, but that can be excruciating. You just have to try it to see if it makes things better or worse. The best calf stretch is to lift your toes and the ball of your foot while standing, keeping your heel on the ground. Hold the stretch for 10 to 15 seconds, then relax.

Dial a Doc

✚ If you ache all over and your muscles are always stiff, you may have a mysterious condition known as fibromyalgia. Although it's difficult to diagnose, this condition causes a deep aching pain and a burning sensation that may overtake your entire body, especially in your arms and legs. Fibromyalgia can also make you sensitive to weather changes. Although it can feel like arthritis, it has no known cause or cure. So if you've got this kind of pain, talk to your doctor immediately. You may be able to relieve your symptoms with medication.

Leapin' Liniment!

Liniments are among the best choices for relieving muscle aches and joint pains because you can use them to target the injured area to help work out the built-up tension. A gentle rubdown with this old-time elixir will bring quick relief to arthritis pain and muscle aches, and keep you rarin' to go about your day.

2 egg whites
½ cup of apple cider
vinegar
¼ cup of olive oil

➡ Mix the ingredients together, and massage the lotion into any painful body part. (Be careful not to get any of the lotion on your sheets or furniture!) Wipe off the excess with a soft cotton cloth. After a good rubdown, your body should be back to feeling normal.

Give It a Rest

■ If your muscles ache because you played six hours of softball after spending a winter on the couch, the best remedy is to head back to the sofa's soft embrace for a day or two. Rest, followed by gradual and regular exercise, will improve most muscle aches. Then as the spring and summer progress, you'll get to a point where you can play all the softball you want—pain-free.

EUREKA!

IF YOU WAKE UP in the middle of the night with leg cramps, and can't figure out what the problem is, you may be looking in the wrong places. A lack of stretching undoubtedly contributes to the problem, but it's possible that the real culprit is your sheets. If they're tucked too tight, they restrict your leg movement, which can cause cramping. So before dozing off, make sure the sheets are loose enough to give your legs plenty of room to roam. And if you tend to get cramps in bed frequently, take the time to do some slow, gentle stretches before going to sleep. That, combined with looser linens, should go a long way toward putting a stop to nighttime leg cramps.

Magical Marigold Oil

If you grow pot marigolds (a.k.a. calendulas), you've got the makings of a marvelous mixer for massaging into tired, achy muscles. (If you don't grow calendulas, check out your local farmers' market or pick up a few pots of them at the garden center.)

5 cups of wilted calendula blossoms*
Extra-virgin olive oil

➡ Put the blossoms in a 3-quart pan, and add enough olive oil to reach 2 inches above the flowers. Heat the mixture on low until the oil *almost* simmers. Let it steep over low heat, uncovered, for six to eight hours, or until the oil has turned a deep, golden-orange color and has a strong herbal aroma. (Test for "doneness" every hour or so, and make sure the oil doesn't start to simmer.) Remove the pan from the heat, and let the brew cool to room temperature. Strain it, and store the oil in a tightly capped bottle in the refrigerator between muscle massages. It will keep for a year.

* Pluck the blossoms from the plant, and let them sit in the shade for a few days.

Start with Ice

◾ As soon as muscle pain starts and for 24 to 48 hours afterward, put ice to work. Wrap some ice cubes in a washcloth or small towel, then put the cold right where it hurts for no longer than 20 minutes at a time. Cold numbs muscle pain and eases swelling.

Nifty, Thrifty Tips

Give your body—and your wallet—a break. Forget the chips, pretzels, and other salty foods when you're coping with muscle pain. Salt makes your body retain water, which can increase painful swelling inside your muscles. If you need a quick snack, fill up on vegetables or grapes, orange slices, or other fruits, all of which are naturally low in salt. They also contain a lot of water, which will help sore muscles stay hydrated and heal more quickly.

Muscle-Cooling Treatment

Sunny days make you want to get outside to play or do yard work. But believe it or not, the sun is as big a culprit in causing muscle soreness as actual work or exercise is. So when you've been working or playing hard in the hot sun, give your aching muscles this nice cooling treatment.

2 cups of witch hazel
2 tsp. of light corn syrup
1½ tsp. of castor oil
Scented oil (optional)

➡ Mix the witch hazel, corn syrup, and castor oil in a jar with a tight-fitting lid, and add a few drops of your favorite scented oil if you like. Shake the mixture well, and massage it into your sore body for almost-instant relief. There's simply no way you can go wrong with this formula.

Drink Up

■ Physical exertion depletes fluids and minerals from your body, which can create cramps, especially if you're overheated. To avoid heat cramps (and, later on, heat exhaustion or heatstroke) in the first place, drink at least one cup of water before you exercise and another cup every 15 minutes during the activity.

Q: *I know a lot of things can relieve muscle pain once it sets in, but can I do anything before I begin exercising to help me prevent it from happening in the first place?*

Take My Advice

A: Try eating the proper foods, by which I mean those that are rich in certain beneficial enzymes. Tuna, salmon, and other cold-water fish provide the CoQ10 compound that your heart, liver, muscles, and brain need to produce energy. Eating more fish will keep your entire body going and help prevent your muscles from cramping up. And don't forget to stretch before you start your exercise routine.

Oil Away Aches

Herbal oils are nearly perfect for treating muscles in your legs, shoulders, or any other area that happens to be giving you trouble. While any oil softens the skin, herb-infused oils stimulate circulation and help keep your limbs healthy and pain-free. And this doesn't just apply to your muscles: They can also be used on aching corns and calluses. Try this blend of oils (found at most health-food stores) for remarkable relief.

2 drops of carrot seed oil
2 drops of peppermint oil
1 oz. of calendula oil
5 drops of geranium oil
5 drops of lavender oil

➡ Add the carrot seed and peppermint oils to the calendula oil. Then mix in the geranium and lavender oils. Store the mixture in a small bottle and massage it into your aching muscles once a day. And if corns or calluses on your feet are also causing you problems, use this soothing blend more often to relieve the pain.

Hot Oil for Quick Relief

■ A castor oil pack is a traditional remedy to soothe and heal injured muscles, and it's easy to use. Just apply some castor oil to the area and cover it with plastic wrap, then top it off with a heating pad set on "low." The heat will help the oil penetrate your skin, where it will ease pain and any stiffness. Leave the pack on for 30 minutes, then wash the oil off. You can repeat the treatment twice a day until your muscles heal. **Caution:** Don't use this treatment for acute injuries.

Snappy Solutions

One of the best ways to relieve muscle aches is to eat some pumpkin seeds. They're loaded with fatty acids that lower the levels of the body chemicals that are responsible for muscle aches. So just chew some seeds during the day, and you should be able to say good-bye to your muscle aches.

Root for Relaxation

Most body pain is caused by inflammation that occurs after something is injured or strained past its natural range of motion. If you tame the inflammation, you can get at the root of the problem and heal yourself more quickly. These anti-inflammatory herbs help relieve pain throughout the body and may be combined with anti-spasmodic herbs to increase relaxation.

Dried calendula
Ground ginger
Dried lemon balm
Dried meadowsweet
Dried prickly ash
1 cup of hot water

➡ Combine equal parts of the herbs and add 1 heaping teaspoon of the mixture to the water. Steep, covered, for 15 minutes, then strain out the solids. Drink 2 to 3 cups daily. This herbal combination will reduce the inflammation in no time, as well as the pain that went along with it.

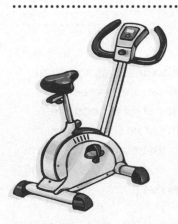

Feel the Burn, Not the Pain

■ No doubt about it—exercise is a great pain reliever. And aerobic exercise tames pain the best. In fact, people with chronic back pain felt relief after 25 minutes on a stationary bike. Even a brisk walk around the block can make you feel better—provided the walk lasts at least 10 minutes. Just be sure to start out slowly, then work up the intensity. If you feel increased pain, slow down your pace again.

Why won't the chicken cross the road? Because that's where the doctor's office is! Men are less likely to see a doctor and will do so only when they are urged by others. In fact, 38 percent of men will wait to consult a doctor until someone encourages them to get treatment for pain. Women, on the other hand, just do it. So break the trend. If you have some pain, guys, do the right thing and get help if it's persistent or really intense.

Dial a Doc

Spasm Stopper

To tone, relieve inflammation, and release spasms in the liver and biliary tract (those internal muscles that help keep your insides functioning properly), try this herbal mixer. It'll set your body straight in no time at all.

Dried artichoke
Dried butterbur
Dried dandelion root
Dried greater celandine
Dried milk thistle
Dried peppermint
1 cup of hot water

➡ Pick at least three of the herbs to use for the best effect. Combine equal parts of your choices and add 1 teaspoon of the mixture to the water. Steep for 15 minutes, then strain out the solids. Drink 1 cup, warm, between meals. **Caution:** If you take diuretics or potassium supplements, talk to your doctor before taking dandelion. Avoid dandelion if you have gallstones or active liver or gallbladder disease.

Try Turmeric

■ The same spice that gives curry its distinctive flavor also makes an excellent pain reliever, in part because it breaks down bits of pain-causing protein that circulate in damaged tissue. For best results, mix ½ teaspoon of turmeric with enough water to make a paste, and apply it to the painful area. Or mix turmeric oil with 1 teaspoon of flaxseed oil, an anti-inflammatory that may boost absorption. You can also get tumeric in capsule form at health-food stores. Take 250 mg three times daily with food to ease inflammation and relieve pain.

Nifty, Thrifty Tips

When you're in the supermarket looking for a cure for muscle pain, bypass the pricey medicine aisle and head straight to the produce section instead. Studies show that an enzyme in pineapple (bromelain) has anti-inflammatory properties, promotes circulation, cleans up the cellular debris in inflamed tissue, and may help you heal twice as fast.

A Soothing Brew

Whatever the cause of that sickening feeling, whether it's a wild ride, something you ate, the flu, or even stress, try this magical mixer. I've relied on its tummy-soothing results for years for good reason.

1 tbsp. of dried
    avocado leaves
Honey
1 cup of boiling water

➡ Steep the avocado leaves (available online) in the water for 10 to 15 minutes, strain out the leaves, and add a little drizzle of honey. Sip to ease minor stomach pain.

Olives, Anyone?

■ Does sailing make you queasy and flying turn you green? Then the next time you launch yourself into major motion, take along some olives. At the first sign of motion sickness, eat a couple. Olives contain tannins that dry your mouth, which reduces the excess saliva that can trigger nausea.

Good Morning Grapes

■ If morning sickness has you feeling so nauseated that even a glass of water sends you rushing for the bathroom, eat a bunch of grapes first thing in the morning. They're great fluid replacers, but they don't bring about that miserable queasy feeling other foods and beverages can cause.

Q: *For years I've heard the old-timers in my family say they used to keep Coke® syrup on hand for upset stomachs. Is this stuff really effective?*

A: It sure is! Just a couple of teaspoons will usually cure anything from a tiny tummy ache to a full-blown case of vomiting. Just keep some cola on hand (any brand will do). When trouble strikes, open up the can or bottle, and let it go flat. Then sip your way back to comfort.

Take My
Advice

Bet on Barley

Pearl barley
1 qt. of water
½ cup of warm milk

Ever get the urge to dine at a local dive that's said to have "the best burgers in town," if for no other reason than to see what all the hype is about? Well, oftentimes these excursions end with your stomach paying the price. So if dining out on hamburgers at the local greasy spoon gets your gut a-grumblin', here's the ideal "dessert."

➡ Boil a small handful of pearl barley (which you can find in supermarkets) in the water for an hour. Strain the liquid, then add ½ cup of it to the warm milk. Sip this concoction slowly until your stomach settles down. Try to eat the cooked barley, too, since it may help counter any lingering indigestion and diarrhea.

A Dilly of a Cure

■ A homemade infusion of dill seeds can help calm an upset stomach and ease nausea real quick. Steep 1 teaspoon of dill seeds in 1 cup of hot water, covered, for 15 minutes. Strain, and then sip.

Let It Be

■ For the first 12 hours after a bout of nausea, you should drink only clear liquids like ginger ale, plain water, or soothing teas. You need to stay hydrated because vomiting and diarrhea make your body lose a lot of liquid.

Nifty, Thrifty Tips

There are plenty of over-the-counter remedies for nausea and upset stomachs. But why waste your hard-earned dollars on pricey drugs? If you're feeling queasy, head to your fridge instead. Grab an uncut lemon, and scratch right into the peel. Now take a sniff of the clean, fresh citrus scent. That's how they handle nausea in India, and it's how you should handle it, too!

Old-Time Tummy Tamer

When nausea strikes, your stomach can feel like it's on a roller coaster ride—your insides slosh around and feel all mixed up. It seems that all you can do is just hope for the feeling to pass. Well, instead of just hoping, take action and reach for this classic remedy.

½ cup of fresh-squeezed
    orange juice
2 tbsp. of clear corn syrup
Pinch of salt
½ cup of water

➥ Mix all of the ingredients together, and store the elixir in a covered jar in your refrigerator. Take 1 tablespoon of it every half hour or so until your queasiness has flown the coop and you're good to go.

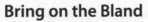

Stomach Settler

■ For nausea that's caused by stress and anxiety, try a cup of meadowsweet tea to settle your stomach. To make the tea, steep 1 heaping teaspoon of dried meadowsweet in 1 cup of hot water, covered, for 10 minutes. Strain, and sip slowly until your stomach feels better.

Bring on the Bland

■ When your appetite finally returns after a bout of nausea, scout around the kitchen for the blandest food you can find. To help you along, think of baby food. Consider eating easy-to-digest applesauce, a little plain rice, dry toast, or even a mild cooked vegetable.

✚ If your nausea is accompanied by chest pain, sweating, or shortness of breath, call your doctor immediately. These symptoms can indicate that you're having a heart attack, so you'll need immediate medical attention.

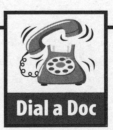

Dial a Doc

Queasiness Quencher

Spices are the most important part of traditional Indian cooking, and they also play an important role in Indian medicine. Plenty of natural cures rely on spices to heal whatever ails you. In fact, this little tonic is pretty terrific to quiet a roiling stomach.

½ tsp. of honey
½ cup of plain yogurt
2 pinches of cardamom

➡ Mix the honey thoroughly into the yogurt, then add the cardamom. Stir the entire mixture and eat it all up. This marvelous mixer will coat your stomach to make sure that the rocking and rolling soon go away.

Snap Up Some Ginger

■ Ginger is widely used to cure upset stomachs and nausea. The best part is that you don't even have to chew on the root; simply make a tea by boiling a quarter-size piece of fresh ginger in 1 cup of water for five minutes. If you're pregnant, talk to your doctor before you try this remedy.

Peppermint Stomach Settler

■ For a queasy stomach, peppermint can't be beat. The fact is, volatile oils in peppermint can help counteract nausea. So try sucking on a peppermint candy, or uncap a vial of peppermint oil and inhale the vapors for a few seconds. And if you're feeling up to a bath, add 4 to 6 drops of the oil to your tub and slide in. Just remember to breathe deeply while you're soaking your troubles away.

What Would Grandma Do?

🦋 WHENEVER WE'D TAKE A RIDE in the car, Grandma Putt made sure that I didn't suffer from motion sickness along the way. Her rules? Face forward when you ride; carefully select your seat so that you sit somewhere stable; and don't do things like read (which can cause queasiness while you're in motion). These little precautions helped me, and they can help you, too!

No, No Nosebleed Tonic

Whether you stuck something in your nose, bumped it, got hit, or you're just plain prone to nosebleeds, they're never any fun. Whenever I got a nosebleed as a youngster, Grandma Putt would sit me down and administer this tried-and-true fixer.

2 tbsp. of witch hazel
6 drops of cypress oil
Cotton balls

➡ Pour the witch hazel into a clean bottle with a tight-fitting lid and add the cypress oil. Label the bottle with the contents, and store it in your medicine chest. Then when the need arises, shake the bottle well, moisten a cotton ball with the potion, and gently insert it into the bleeding nostril. Sit up straight with your head tilted just slightly forward. Within two or three minutes, the blood should stop flowing. To speed up the process, squeeze the soft tissue of your nose firmly but gently between your thumb and forefinger.

Tilt and Pinch

■ When a nosebleed strikes from out of nowhere, sit or stand so that your head is above your heart, then tilt your head slightly forward and pinch your nostrils together just below the bony center part of your nose. Applying pressure helps halt the blood flow. In most cases, it will stop within 10 minutes.

Don't Blow!

■ Whatever you do, don't blow your nose when it's bleeding—you'll only make the blood flow harder. And ignore the common advice to tilt your head back. This will cause the blood to run down your throat, which will make you cough or choke and, if you swallow enough blood, vomit.

✚ If you've tried any of these remedies twice, and the bleeding hasn't stopped after 10 minutes or so, or is increasing at any time, call your doctor. The blood flow could be a sign of something serious.

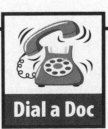

Dial a Doc

Sniff and Stop Solution

At the first sign of blood flowing from your nose, whip up this sniffable elixir. I have no idea why it stems the flood—but it does!

**Salt
Vinegar
Lemon juice**

➡ Put about a tablespoon of salt into a small, shallow bowl, and add just enough vinegar to dissolve the salt. Pour in 2 teaspoons or so of fresh lemon juice (or a few squirts of the bottled kind) and stir. Hold the bowl up close to your nose, and inhale deeply. After a few sniffs, the bleeding should stop.

Ice It

■ Usually, simply applying a cold compress to your schnozolla will dry up the flood. Wrap an ice pack, a bag of frozen vegetables, or a few ice cubes in a washcloth and hold it to your nose until the bleeding stops.

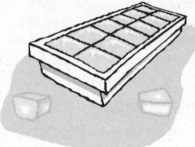

The Aftermath

■ Once you've stopped the bleeding, take things slow and easy for a day or so. Don't lift heavy objects or do anything else that might cause you to strain, and don't blow your nose for at least 24 hours. Also, keep your head elevated above your heart as much as possible. (You might want to sleep with two pillows the first night after the episode.)

Snappy Solutions

Here's a quick and easy cure for a bloody nose: Soak a cotton ball in apple cider vinegar, and gently insert it into the dripping nostril. Hold your nose closed with your fingers, and breathe through your mouth for about five minutes. Then slowly remove the cotton. If the bleeding hasn't stopped, repeat the procedure.

Bone Soup

You've heard of stone soup? Well, bone soup is a whole lot better for the health and well-being of your own bones. So pick up some soup bones at the meat counter and make a big pot of homemade soup using this simple recipe.

Soup bones (beef, chicken, ham, or whatever kind you prefer)
Vegetables of your choice
Your favorite herbs and spices
½ cup of vinegar
Water

➡ Fill a large pot with water. Add the bones, vegetables, herbs and spices, and—the magic ingredient—vinegar. Bring the soup to a boil, then lower the heat and simmer, partially covered, for 30 minutes, or until the vegetables are soft. The vinegar will dissolve a significant amount of calcium from the bones into the soup. Just 1 pint of this soup can give you as much as 1,000 milligrams of calcium!

Dig for Density

■ Moderate physical activity, such as gardening, reduces the risk of hip fracture anywhere from 20 to 60 percent. In fact, one study showed that women who did some form of activity for more than three hours a week had about half as much chance of fracturing a hip as those who were sedentary.

Chew on Some Bones

■ No, not like a puppy. But try this: Eat a can of sardines or salmon with bones once or twice a week for a quick calcium boost. Just 3 ounces of cooked salmon with bones has about 200 milligrams of calcium.

EUREKA!

SINCE LONG BEFORE anyone had heard of the word *osteoporosis*, Native Americans have been using chicory juice to heal bones. Elders, who drink lots of juice from both cooked and raw chicory, say their bone fractures due to osteoporosis heal faster. So why not give it a try?

Wild About Tea

With age come changes to our bodies that we could frankly do without. One of the most dangerous, osteoporosis, occurs as your bones lose calcium; at its worst, it can result in a bone (or bones) cracking under the weight of the rest of your body. But you can ward off this unpleasant possibility with some help from these herbs that have bone-boosting effects.

Alfalfa
Bladder wrack
Chicory
Dandelion
Horsetail
Kelp
Nettles
Oat straw
1 qt. of hot water

➡ Combine equal parts of three or more fresh herbs; then steep 1 heaping tablespoon of the mixture in the water for 10 minutes. Strain and sip. Try different combinations of these herbs until you find one that tastes best to you. Then stick with it to give your bones the boost they need to stay strong. **Caution:** If you take diuretics or potassium supplements, talk to your doctor before taking dandelion. Also, be sure to wear gloves when you're handling fresh nettles to avoid their stinging hairs.

Hit the Wall

■ Wall push-ups are a quick and easy way to strengthen the bones in your upper body. Start by putting your hands flat against a wall, level with and about as far apart as your shoulders. Take a step away from the wall, then lean in and push your body back away from the wall. Repeat several times, and do them at least three times a week to stay strong.

Nifty, Thrifty Tips

You can save yourself a lot of time, money, and worry later in life if you start dealing with your bones now. Just 60 seconds of running during a brisk walk is enough to shift your bones into a strengthening mode. Performing 30 to 45 minutes of weight-bearing exercise three times a week will help you walk or run your way to better bones.

Enjoyable Herbal Bath

The last thing you need in your love life is painful intercourse. Try a warm sitz bath using this infusion of comfrey and horsetail. It can help soothe inflamed tissues and, over time, make them less susceptible to irritation.

1 cup of comfrey root
1 pint of water
1 tbsp. of horsetail

➡ Simmer the comfrey root in the water for 20 minutes. Remove from the heat, add in the horsetail, and steep for an additional 10 minutes. Strain, and pour into your bathtub. Then fill the tub with enough warm water to come up to the top of your pelvic bone. Soak for 20 minutes. Ease into a sitz bath three times weekly for soothing relief.

Banish Yeast Infections

■ If you feel a burning sensation during intercourse—and notice a discharge like cottage cheese—you may have a yeast infection. Try an over-the-counter remedy for yeast infections, available as pills, gels, and suppositories. **Note:** If your infection doesn't clear up after taking the recommended course, see your doctor.

A Mighty Fine Tea

■ Studies show that echinacea tea can help prevent yeast infections, but you need to drink it regularly for it to be effective. Make a cup by putting ½ teaspoon of the herb in 1 cup of boiling water. Let it steep for about 10 minutes, strain, and then sip. The tea loses its effect after eight weeks. So stop the treatment for one month; then start again. **Caution**: Don't take echinacea if you have an autoimmune disease, such as rheumatoid arthritis, lupus, or multiple sclerosis.

Snappy Solutions

For some women, the uterine contractions from an orgasm can cause pain that puts a damper on the pleasure of sex. According to doctors, a simple way to prevent this and hours of pain later on is to take ibuprofen prior to intercourse.

Vaginal Wash

Even if intercourse feels great while it's happening, it can come with some pain afterward. This can be caused by a whole slew of different things, but for pain that occurs *after* intercourse, ladies should use a vaginal wash made from these soothing, antimicrobial herbs.

**Echinacea
Goldenseal
Lavender
1 cup of hot water**

➥ Combine equal parts of the herbs, and steep 1 heaping teaspoon of the mixture in the water for 20 minutes. Strain, and pour into a peri bottle (available at drugstores). Keep the bottle by your toilet, and after intercourse, wash your labia and vaginal entrance with this solution. If the irritation persists, use this wash throughout the day after every time you urinate. If the pain continues for more than a few days or worsens at any time, see your doctor.

Become the Dominant Force

■ Many women sometimes feel discomfort or pain with deep penetration. This may be a normal response to the pressure on sensitive internal parts. The most obvious solution is to avoid deep penetration. One easy—and pleasurable—way women can circumvent painful intercourse is to take control. Pin your partner to the mattress, and stay on top. If the woman sits astride the man during intercourse, she can control the rhythm and the angle of penetration for a much more enjoyable experience.

Snappy Solutions

If you regularly suffer through painful intercourse, your problem may be due to an allergy to semen. You can tell if you're allergic if your pelvic area becomes red, and you experience a very intense burning sensation after your partner ejaculates. But you don't have to give up on love. Simply ask your partner to use condoms to protect your sensitive membranes.

Body-Boosting Brew

Adults are just as susceptible to pinkeye (a.k.a. conjunctivitis) as kids are. And believe me—you don't want to know how pinkeye happens. Just know that when it is a recurrent complaint or particularly severe, you should support your whole body with these infection-fighting herbs.

Calendula
Cleavers
Echinacea
Eyebright
1 cup of hot water

➡ Combine equal parts of the herbs, steep 1 teaspoon of the mixture in the water for 10 minutes, and strain out the solids. Drink 2 to 3 cups daily until your eye clears up and your symptoms subside. **Caution**: Don't take echinacea if you have an autoimmune disease, such as rheumatoid arthritis, lupus, or multiple sclerosis.

Strawberry Soother

■ Strawberry tea can help soothe inflamed eyes and fight infection. To make the tea, steep 1 teaspoon of strawberry leaves in 1 cup of hot water for 10 minutes. Strain and cool. Use the tea in a compress, or place it in an eyecup, and rinse your eyes with it once or twice daily.

Chill Out

■ Ice-cold compresses can soothe your irritated eyes. Simply place a damp washcloth that's been chilled in the freezer or a cool, wet paper towel over your closed eyes for about 20 minutes. Stop for 30 to 60 minutes, then do it again. Chill your peepers as often as you feel the need, using a clean compress every time.

EUREKA!

WHEN YOU HAVE pinkeye, you shouldn't put anything in or near your eyes. Common eye irritants are those things we use every day: mascara, eyeliner, eye shadow, and contact lenses. So keep these items out of your daily routine until your eyes heal. And whatever you do, don't rub your eyes! You'll be rewarded with a much shorter recovery time.

The Chamomile Cure

This simple, soothing eyewash is one of the most effective remedies I've found to relieve the pain and burning of pinkeye. My Grandma Putt swore by it, and I still do, too!

> 2 to 3 tsp. of dried chamomile or 1 chamomile tea bag
> 1 pint of water

➡ Bring the water to a boil, add the dried chamomile or tea bag, and steep for 10 minutes. Let the mixture cool and strain it through a sterile cloth. Use an eyecup to rinse your eye with the solution two or three times daily until the problem is resolved. **Caution:** People with ragweed allergies may be sensitive to chamomile.

Stay Out of the Pool

■ Until your eyes have cleared up, don't go swimming! Not only can you spread conjunctivitis germs to others in the pool, but the chlorinated water can also increase your eye irritation.

Keep Your Hands to Yourself

■ For as long as your infection remains, avoid shaking hands; dispose of any tissues that you use; and be sure to disinfect doorknobs, countertops, and telephones that you come in contact with. Also, don't share towels or pillows.

Pull Down the Shades

■ Whenever you go outdoors, even on cloudy days, wear sunglasses to protect your eyes from glare and irritation. (Remember, even when you can't see the sun, its rays are still potent enough to burn.) Besides increasing your comfort level, you'll look classy, and you'll feel less self-conscious about your pink peepers.

✚ Once in a great while, a case of conjunctivitis can do some real damage. If your pinkeye doesn't clear up within a week, or if you have a fever or changes in vision along with it, call your doctor.

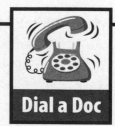

Dial a Doc

Drip-Stopper Tonic

The causes of postnasal drip include the usual suspects: colds and flu, allergies, cold weather, and chronic sinus problems. Attack that drip with this herb combo that reduces congestion, strengthens mucous membranes, and supports immunity.

Calendula
Elder
Eyebright
Goldenrod
1 cup of hot water

➡ Combine equal parts of the herbs, and steep 1 teaspoon of the mixture in the water for 10 to 15 minutes, then strain. Sip 1 to 3 cups daily for as long as your drip continues (which shouldn't be long after you try this drip-stoppin' solution).

Bathe Your Nose

■ You can simply wash away that irritating, thickened mucus with a nasal douche or a Waterpik® that's got a nasal nozzle. Start by making a solution of 1 teaspoon of baking soda or salt in 1 pint of warm water. Use it to irrigate your nose two to four times a day. If this treatment seems like too much trouble, try using a simple saline nasal spray to moisten your nasal passages instead.

Steam-Sniffing Solution

■ Sniffing steam is a great way to clear out nasal passages, and if the steam is infused with a healing herb, it works even better! Fill a basin with steaming water, then add a few drops of eucalyptus oil to it. Grab a big towel, and use it as a tent to contain the healing vapors. Pop your head under the towel, and breathe in deeply. Just be careful not to burn your cheeks!

What Would Grandma Do?

🦋 *WHENEVER I WOULD GET A RUNNY NOSE, I didn't want to drink anything. I was already leaking, so why worsen it with water or juice? Well, Grandma Putt knew better, and she would make me drink lots of water. You see, mucus thins out when you have a lot of fluid in you, and at least eight glasses of water a day will help thin the gunk.*

Natural Nasal Balm

Dripping up a storm? Well, don't let it get you down. Just whip up a batch of this simple mixer. You'll think it's the best friend your nose ever had.

¼ cup of petroleum jelly
Eucalyptus oil
Peppermint oil
Thyme oil

➡ Put the petroleum jelly in a small saucepan, and warm it until it melts. Remove it from the heat, and stir in 10 drops *each* of the eucalyptus, peppermint, and thyme essential oils. When the balm has reached room temperature, pour it into a clean, lidded jar for storage. Apply a small amount to your nostrils one to three times daily. The petroleum jelly prevents the essential oils from being absorbed into your skin, so you can inhale the volatile oils for a prolonged period. Aaah . . . now you're breathing easy!

Humidify Your Home

■ Dry indoor air can thicken mucus. Install a humidifier, or do what I do—put pans of water on top of your radiators. Worried about spillage? Check your local hardware store for little trays that hang from radiators.

Cut the Caffeine

■ Even though drinking plenty of fluids will help stop your postnasal drip, avoid coffee, tea, cola, and anything else that contains caffeine. These drinks act as diuretics and actually deplete your body's water supply.

✚ Sometimes polyps develop from chronic sinusitis, and these can cause an irritating, persistent postnasal drip. If you suspect a polyp may be behind your particular drip, consult an otolaryngologist, who will examine the interior of your nose. A fiber-optic scope, a computed tomography (CT) scan, or X-rays can pinpoint the offending polyp, which can then be treated with medication or surgically removed if necessary.

Dial a Doc

Corn Silk Tea

For thousands of years, folk healers have used corn silk to treat dozens of ailments. One of its most well-known roles is as a first-class remedy for prostate problems. When corn is in season, head out to a farmers' market (or your own garden), grab some ears, and proceed as follows.

6 ears of fresh corn
1 qt. of water

➡ Cut the silk from the corn, and put it in a pot with the water. Bring it to a boil, then reduce the heat and simmer for 10 minutes. Strain and pour the tea into a jar. Drink a cup three times a week.

A Toast to Tomatoes

■ As little as two servings a week of foods made with cooked tomato sauce, such as pizza, pasta with marinara sauce, chicken Parmesan—or even tomato soup or tortilla chips and salsa—can help cut your risk of developing prostate cancer in half. That's because cooked tomatoes contain an antioxidant called lycopene that fights off cancer cells.

Make Whoopee

■ Doctors say that regular ejaculation can help keep your prostate from getting stagnant and inflamed. So the fact of the matter is that you'll just have to grin and bear it, guys!

EUREKA!

FOR A HEALTHY SEX LIFE, men need to get plenty of zinc. The prostate must have this mineral to produce semen. And true to its legend, the good old oyster really is just "shuck-full" of zinc. Try this quick recipe to restore the roar: Heat 2 cups of peanut oil in a heavy frying pan. One by one, dip six oysters into ½ cup of flour, then into a dish with two beaten eggs, and finally roll them in 1 cup of bread crumbs. Fry the oysters in the oil until golden brown, serve, and enjoy.

Manly Tonic

There's so much information about prostate health and the dangers that an enlarging prostate can pose to men that it's hard to know what to do. But remedies for just such a problem have been around for many years. This elixir, for example, was specially created for us guys, and drinking a cup or two a day may keep prostate problems at bay.

1 tsp. of fennel seeds
1 tsp. of hawthorn berries
1 tsp. of marshmallow root
1 tsp. of saw palmetto berries
½ tsp. of licorice root
6 cups of water

➥ Combine all of the herbs, then put them in a pan filled with the water. Bring the mixture to a boil and let it simmer for 25 minutes. Allow the tea to cool, strain out the herbs, and then bottoms up—here's to a better man (both inside and out)!

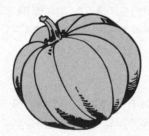

Pick Some Pumpkin Seeds

■ Pumpkin seeds are particularly good for men because zinc, one of their major nutrients, is crucial for prostate health. Try adding them to your salad instead of croutons, or simply pick up a package and crunch them throughout the day. You'll be glad you did.

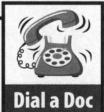

Dial a Doc

After age 60—and earlier if your doctor recommends it—get a prostate-specific antigen (PSA) blood screening as part of your regular physical exam. And call your doctor if you develop any of these symptoms: You need to urinate more frequently than usual, especially at night; you have trouble starting your urine flow or the flow is weak; blood appears in your urine; no matter how recently you've urinated, your bladder doesn't feel empty; you feel a burning sensation during urination; you feel pain behind the scrotum; or ejaculation is painful.

Ease the Pain Oil

Your sciatic nerve is not only your body's biggest nerve, but it can also produce one of its biggest pains. If you've ever had sciatic pain, you'll understand why it hurts where it does. If you currently have sciatic pain, try this oil mixer to ease that nerve back into place as well as whatever is pressing against it to cause the pain.

Arnica oil
Castor oil
St. John's wort oil

➡ Combine equal parts of the oils and gently massage the mixture onto the nerve track, starting at your buttocks and proceeding down the back of your leg. Do this once or twice a day for a week. If your symptoms persist, or if the pain seems unusually severe, see your doctor right away because sciatica can lead to permanent nerve damage.

Take C for Sciatica

■ Vitamin C has been shown to help repair muscle damage that can lead to tightness as well as nerve pain. You'll want to take up to 3,000 milligrams of vitamin C a day if you have sciatica caused by a back injury. That's a lot more than the usual daily dose, so it's a good idea to take it in several smaller doses throughout the day.

Q: *I've noticed that my sciatica seems to be worse in the morning. Why is that?*

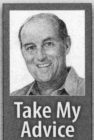

Take My Advice

A: If your sciatica is caused by a herniated disk, the pain may be more intense in the morning because your spinal disks absorb water during the night, while you are lying flat. As a result, they press harder on the surrounding nerves and you really feel it. During the day, gravity pushes the water out, making the disks flatter—and less likely to pinch any nearby nerves.

So Long, Sciatica Smoothie

Legions of sciatica sufferers have found blessed relief from this sweet-and-tangy mixer. The secret lies in the interaction of the ingredients, which reduces the inflammation that causes the pain and also helps rid your body of toxins.

➡ Put all the ingredients in a blender or food processor, and liquefy the contents until they are smooth and thick. Then pour the smoothie into a glass, sip slowly, and savor the flavor.

½ cup of milk
½ apple
¼ avocado
Juice of 1 orange
Juice of ½ lemon
1 heaping tbsp. of shelled hemp seeds (available at health-food stores)
1 tsp. of honey
1½- to 2-inch piece of fresh ginger, peeled

T Is for Turmeric

■ People with sciatica who like spicy foods should definitely seek out recipes that contain turmeric, since this fragrant herb has powerful anti-inflammatory effects that help counteract sciatic flare-ups. You'd have to eat a lot of turmeric to get enough of the active ingredient, though, so supplement your menu with turmeric capsules. Check with your doctor first, then start with about 250 milligrams three times daily, preferably with food.

EUREKA!

BECAUSE NERVE INFLAMMATION is behind the excruciating pain of sciatica, taking a couple of good old-fashioned aspirins can bring welcome relief—and it will work even better if you take those two tablets with a cup and a half or so of coffee. The caffeine in the java helps your body absorb the medication more efficiently. You'll feel the full effects in 30 minutes, and they'll last for three to five hours. **Caution:** Aspirin and caffeine can worsen reflux, gastritis, and ulcers and may increase inflammation in some folks.

Herbal Peri Wash

Hopefully, you've never had an STI. But, if you have, then you probably know how painful and dangerous one can be. While STIs should be treated with conventional medications, you can relieve burning and itching symptoms with this cooling peri wash.

Comfrey root
Echinacea
Goldenseal
1 cup of hot water

➡ Combine equal part of the herbs, and steep 1 heaping teaspoon of the mixture in the water for 15 minutes. Cool and strain into a peri bottle (available in drugstores and online). Leave it by the toilet, and rinse yourself two or three times daily. If symptoms don't go away in a couple of days, then use it every time you urinate, and see your doctor immediately.

Get Tested Routinely

■ If you are sexually active and not monogamous, get tested at least once a year—and when you have a new partner—for any sexually transmitted infection. Most women get an annual gynecological checkup and Pap smear. Let your doctor know you want to be routinely checked for infections, too. Then ask your partner if he or she has ever had an STI, or has been tested for one.

There are a number of infections that cause different degrees of discomfort and risk. Among the most common are chlamydia, herpes, gonorrhea, trichomoniasis, and human papillomavirus. Be aware of the symptoms—including an unusual discharge or odor, genital or anal itching, a burning sensation when urinating, sores, swollen glands in the groin, pain in the groin, vaginal bleeding, and testicular swelling. If you have any of these symptoms, you should get to your doctor immediately to get tested and properly treated. Some STIs have mild symptoms that may go unnoticed. However, if your partner has any symptoms, you both should be tested and treated.

Dial a Doc

Herpes Helper

Neem has long been known as one of the best natural antiseptics in the world. And that makes it ideal for treating the pain of herpes with this soothing wash.

3 or 4 handfuls of neem leaves
Water

➡ Put the leaves in a pot with enough water to cover them by 2 to 3 inches. Boil until the water turns a greenish shade, then strain out the leaves and pour the water into a bowl or basin. Treat the infected area twice a day with the liquid, allowing it to dry naturally. You should begin to notice relief within a couple of days.

The Double-L Remedy

■ To help cut the healing time for genital herpes, reach for two antiviral herbs—lemon balm, also known as Melissa, and licorice. Check your health-food store for an ointment containing lemon balm and apply it two to four times a day. Or apply a gel containing glycyrrhetinic acid, also available in health-food stores, three times a day.

Get Cultured

■ If you're taking an antibiotic for chlamydia or gonorrhea, you can offset the side effects—namely an overgrowth of yeast—by eating a cup of yogurt that contains live cultures of the "good" bacteria acidophilus daily. Check your supermarket or health-food store for live-culture yogurt.

Nifty, Thrifty Tips

When you first feel the burning that signals a herpes outbreak on the horizon, get out the ice tray. Wrap some cubes in a small towel and apply it to the area for 10 minutes at a time several times a day. Not only will the burning subside, but you may even keep lesions from appearing—without spending a penny on medications or other commercial treatments.

Immune System Strengthener

The bad news is that you've contracted an STI. So get your doctor to put you on medication. The good news is that you can help strengthen your body's immune system from the inside out with this elixir.

Echinacea
Goldenseal
Licorice root
1 cup of hot water

➥ Combine equal parts of the herbs, steep 1 heaping teaspoon of the mixture in the water for 15 minutes, and strain. Drink 2 to 3 cups daily. While it won't get rid of your STI, you'll certainly be giving your body a better than fighting chance of getting rid of the infection quickly. **Caution:** If you have high blood pressure or kidney disease, don't take licorice root. Don't take echinacea if you have an autoimmune disease, such as rheumatoid arthritis, lupus, or multiple sclerosis.

Eat Well

■ Support your healing with nature's pharmacy of immune-boosting, nutrient-dense foods. Make sure your diet includes plenty of garlic, dark leafy greens, orange and yellow vegetables, and seasoning herbs each day.

Get Shot

■ If you are sexually active, have had multiple partners, and do not use adequate protection (i.e., latex condoms), you're also at risk for the hepatitis B virus, which can result in liver failure. Ask your doctor if you should be vaccinated.

Snappy Solutions

To *save yourself from potential problems down the road, until your test results are in and you are certain you and your partner are not infected with an STI of any kind, use latex condoms— for at least six months. Most doctors say that if you have been mutually exclusive in your sexual relationship for at least six months, and you both have tested negative for STIs, it is probably safe to have sex without using a condom.*

Pain Be Gone Paste

The agonizing pain of shingles can have you all but climbing the walls. Fortunately, this marvelous—and marvelously simple—mixer can help you stay grounded.

2 aspirin tablets
2 tbsp. of rubbing alcohol

➡ Crush the aspirin tablets into a powder, and combine it with the rubbing alcohol to make a paste. Apply the mixture to the affected areas three times daily and heave a sigh of relief. **Caution:** Do not apply over broken skin.

Keep 'Em Clean

■ Wash shingles blisters twice a day with regular soap and water. Resist the urge to cover them with bandages. And hang in there—the rash will usually run its course in three weeks or so.

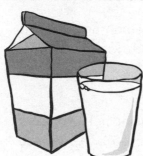

Look to Lysine

■ This amino acid, which prevents viruses from growing and spreading, may bring your bout with shingles to a quicker end. You can easily boost your lysine intake simply by drinking milk and eating potatoes and chicken.

Snappy Solutions

Doctors say the best way to prevent the pain of—and time-consuming treatment for—shingles is to maintain a healthy lifestyle and strong immune system. Because poor nutrition contributes to weakened immunity, make sure you eat at least five vegetables and fruits daily, along with a variety of whole grains, dairy products, lean meat and fish, and moderate amounts of healthy monounsaturated and polyunsaturated fats.

Shingles Remedy

Shingles is a booby-trap disease; it's completely hidden, patiently waiting for something to spring the trap. If you have shingles, you're probably too busy hurting and itching to care where it came from. But to reduce residual nerve pain after a shingles outbreak, try this herbal fixer.

30 drops of astragalus
30 drops of Jamaican dogwood
30 drops of licorice
30 drops of St. John's wort

➡ Add each of the extracts to a glass of water, then drink three glasses a day for up to 20 days. Astragalus (an immune booster), Jamaican dogwood (a nerve sedative), licorice (an antiviral), and St. John's wort (a wound healer) work together to keep things under control. **Caution:** If you have high blood pressure or kidney disease, don't take licorice. Avoid St. John's wort if you're taking antidepressant or anti-anxiety medication.

Take It to the Tub

■ A leisurely soak in a tub of lukewarm water can help ease the discomfort of shingles. And if you add either colloidal oatmeal or baking soda to your bathwater, you'll get even more soothing relief.

Be Pretty in Pink

■ After you dry off from your shower or bath, apply some calamine lotion to your skin. The pink salve works wonders for soothing the itch and pain of shingles.

EUREKA!

ALTHOUGH SHINGLES CAN RUN ITS COURSE without treatment, see your doctor early to head off any possible infection. Starting treatment with antiviral drugs within three days of an outbreak can shorten the duration of the rash and lessen the severity of the outbreak. These medications also help prevent the pain that can follow shingles.

Shingles Tonic

There are many possible triggers for the virus that causes shingles: age, illness, medication, and stress are some of the most common. To concoct an immune-stimulating and pain-relieving tea, use these herbs to knock out every shingle pain.

2 parts echinacea
1 part lemon balm
1 part oat straw
1 part skullcap
1 part St. John's wort
1 cup of hot water

➡ Combine all of the herbs, then steep 1 heaping teaspoon of the mixture in the water, covered, for 10 minutes. Strain out the solids. Drink 3 to 4 cups a day. Your whole body will benefit from having the shingles knocked out. **Caution:** Consult your doctor before using this tea if you're taking antidepressant or anti-anxiety medication. Don't take echinacea if you have an autoimmune disease, such as rheumatoid arthritis, lupus, or multiple sclerosis.

Take Valerian Tea

■ Valerian sedates the nervous system and helps put a damper on the pain of shingles. This is especially useful when you are having difficulty sleeping because of the pain. To make a soothing nighttime tea, steep 1 heaping teaspoon of valerian in 1 cup of hot water for 10 minutes. Drink 1 cup after dinner and before bed. **Caution:** Do not take this herb with any other pain relievers or with anti-anxiety or antidepressant medication.

Nifty, Thrifty Tips

A cheap and easy way to handle shingles pain is by rubbing hot-pepper ointment on the sores. While this remedy may not sound as though it would put out the fire, ointments that contain capsaicin, the element that provides the heat in hot peppers, help some people with shingles. Substance P is the active ingredient, and it works on pain close to the surface of the skin. Apply the ointment three or four times a day, and within one or two weeks, the pain should gradually ease.

Dream Spirits Pillow

There's nothing more comforting or soothing than the idea of a restful night's sleep. But it doesn't have to stop there. How about a restful night's sleep filled with wonderful dreams? The better your dreams are, the better you'll feel in the morning. Here's how to create your own dream machine for a great night's sleep.

½ cup of dried hops
½ cup of dried lavender
½ cup of dried lemon balm

➡ Combine all of the herbs, and dump the mixture into a muslin bag. Pull the drawstring closed and slip the bag into your pillowcase or under your pillow. Lay your head down, and then it's sweet dreams, baby!

Set Your Brain Clock

■ Sleep is malleable like a muscle and, with some limits, it can be trained and refined. Try to repeat the same sleep pattern every day so your brain clock gets set to a good schedule. Your body will adapt to the regularity and get ready for sleep, with glands and hormones functioning and by-products breaking down. Stay consistent and don't skimp on sleep, and you'll feel great in the morning.

Q: *I sleep eight hours every night, which is more than a lot of people can say. But what's the big deal? Why do I need a specific amount of sleep time each night?*

Take My Advice

A: Sleep restores energy to the brain's nerve cells. So while you're asleep, your brain is recharging. This is why you feel so much brighter and smarter in the morning, even without a jolt of java. Eight hours of sleep is the amount your body and mind need to recover completely, and get you ready for the next day.

Dreamy Dream Maker

Sometimes the best way to forget your troubles is with a good night's sleep. But if you find that you're unable to get proper rest because life's little (or big) stresses are weighing heavily on your mind, try this helpful herbal nightcap.

1 oz. of catnip tincture
1 oz. of hops tincture
1 oz. of passionflower tincture
1 oz. of skullcap tincture
1 oz. of wood betony tincture

➡ Put all of the tinctures together in a glass container, cap it with a lid, and give it a few good shakes to blend. Then take an eyedropper and fill it with the liquid. Put 20 drops of this mixture into a glass of water and drink it right before you go to bed. Reseal the bottle and store it in a cool, dry place in your house—like maybe your nightstand.

Catnip Promotes Catnaps

■ Catnip may turn your lazy feline into a rowdy cat, but believe it or not, it has just the opposite effect on us humans. In fact, a little catnip tea after dinner might be just the ticket for winding down after a long day, so why not give it a try? To make it, steep 1 teaspoon of dried catnip in 1 cup of hot water for 10 minutes. Strain, then drink and enjoy. Just be sure to keep your stash of catnip out of reach of your curious kitties!

What Would Grandma Do?

🦋 WHENEVER I HAD a bad case of insomnia and woke up feeling like I had gotten only an hour of sleep, Grandma Putt would march upstairs and help me start cleaning out my room. We put everything where it belonged, cleaned the room from top to bottom, and even rearranged some of the furniture so the area was restful and serene. She listened to how I wanted the room to feel, and we'd have the room looking much better in no time at all. And, sure enough, that night I would sleep like a baby. Try de-cluttering your bedroom and see for yourself.

Jet Lag Dip

Some jobs require a lot of traveling, which is exhausting on its own. But when you travel across time zones, your body ends up conflicted between your natural sleep cycle and the time of day that it actually is wherever you happen to be. This pick-me-up bathtub formula will douse your jet lag blues and give you the boost you need to get through the days until your internal clock is reset. **Caution**: Don't use this treatment on raw, irritated, or broken skin.

½ cup of lemon juice
½ cup of lime juice
5 to 6 drops of lemon extract
½ cup of baking soda (see note)

➤ Mix all of the ingredients together in a bowl, and pour the solution into tepid bathwater. Ease into the tub and soak your sleepy-time woes away. When you get out, you'll be ready for action! **Note:** Don't add the baking soda unless you have hard water.

Fake It

■ No, not the orgasm, the sleep. You can use guided imagery, a form of self-hypnosis, to help you get to sleep. Listen to a meditation tape or use a progressive muscle relaxation exercise to get deeply relaxed; then picture yourself comfortably asleep. Imagine you're in a more comfortable bed, maybe in a luxury hotel, on a mountaintop, or in a gently rocking sailboat. If you visualize every detail of the scene, it will increase the power of suggestion.

Snappy Solutions

If you just can't sleep no matter what, save yourself all the tossing and turning and just stop. Trying to sleep only makes the problem worse, so if you haven't fallen asleep after a little while, get up and distract yourself. Sit in another room and pick up a good book or do some paperwork—anything to get your body out of bed and your mind off your predicament.

Sleepy-Time Tea

Ever had one of those restless nights of tossing and turning, acutely aware of each passing hour? The terrific herbal trio in this elixir blends nicely into a sleeping remedy that'll put an end to that restlessness. Try this easy recipe, and you can't lose—you'll snooze!

20 drops of valerian root tincture (or 1 tsp. of dried valerian root)
1 tsp. of dried chamomile flowers
Pinch of cinnamon
1 cup of boiling water

➥ Mix the first three ingredients together in a bowl. Put 1 teaspoon of the mixture into the water and steep for 10 minutes. Strain out the chamomile flowers, and your bedtime drink is ready and waiting for you. Before you know it, you'll be waking up the next morning feeling refreshed!

Darken Your Room

■ Your body needs darkness to trigger its sleep cycle. So if you have a big street-light shining in the window, or if you have to sleep during the day because you're working the night shift, close the blinds or pull opaque drapes across your window so the light won't get through.

Block Out Night Noises

■ Music soothes the savage beast, and it can help the rest of us sleep better, too. So make a tape of whatever sounds relax your body and calm your mind, and play it as you turn out the lights. Sweet dreams!

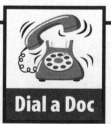

Dial a Doc

✚ As you age, you need to pay attention to your aches and pains. The real reason older people sometimes sleep less is that they have more medical conditions, like arthritis, that keep them awake. So don't be a stiff-upper-lipper when it comes to pain. Talk to your doctor and do something about it. You don't want to wait until it's too late!

Sweet Dream Tea

There are plenty of "tips" and over-the-counter remedies for insomnia, but they can be as much of a sham as they sound. If you don't want to count sheep or take a sleeping pill, you can easily fall into a peaceful slumber with this special soothing solution.

1 tsp. of dried catnip leaves
1 tsp. of dried chamomile leaves
1 tsp. of dried marjoram leaves
1 tsp. of dried mint leaves
1 cup of boiling water

➡ Blend all of the herbs together, scoop out 1 to 2 teaspoons of the mixture, and stir it into the water. Let it steep for about 10 minutes. Strain out the herbs, and then sip yourself into dreamland. **Caution:** People with ragweed allergies may also be sensitive to chamomile.

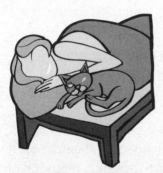

Get a Purring Security Blanket

■ Many people sleep with their pets, and some say their furry friend is just like a security blanket. They know that should anything go wrong during the night, their dog or cat will wake them up. This reassuring thought helps them relax when they go to bed and primes them for sleep.

EUREKA!

IF YOU'RE SUFFERING from a bout of insomnia, you can save yourself many restless nights simply by deciding which type of sleeper you normally are. You'll have to decide if you're a morning person and are most effective in the morning, or an evening person who is most effective in the evening. Insomnia usually comes from fighting your natural sleep type. So figure it out sooner, rather than later, and you'll be back on track in no time at all.

Four-Alarm Fire Reducer

A sore throat is usually the first sign that something is wrong and you've contracted a virus. Once it sets in, your throat will get very scratchy and raw. But when you feel like you've got a four-alarm fire blazing in your throat, put out the flames with this old-time magical mixer.

1 crushed garlic clove
1 tsp. of salt
A tiny pinch of
**   cayenne pepper**

➡ Mix the garlic, salt, and cayenne pepper in a glass, fill it with warm water, and stir. Gargle with the solution, and repeat as needed. (But if your throat doesn't feel better in a day or so, or if it's accompanied by a high fever, call your doctor.) This same potion can also be used as a rub to speed the healing of a chest cold or bronchitis. Apply it with olive oil and massage it onto your chest several times a day.

Pucker Up

■ No cough drops or candy handy? Soak half a lemon in salt water, and suck on it for a while. This treatment will moisten your throat and relieve soreness.

G-g-gargle

■ Gargling with salty water helps dissolve mucus, cleanse your throat, and add some astringency to your body chemistry to reduce swelling and inflammation. It also helps minimize postnasal drip. Here's what you need to do: Put 1 teaspoon of salt in 8 ounces of hot water, and gargle four or five times a day. Don't be heavy-handed with the salt because too much will irritate your throat. The gargle should taste a little salty, but not overwhelmingly so.

✚ If your sore throat is accompanied by difficulty swallowing, you may be having a life-threatening allergic reaction to something. So call your community's emergency response team, or have someone get you to a hospital immediately.

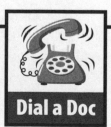

Dial a Doc

Pain-Away Spray

Lots of things can leave your throat sore—allergies, infections, a physical injury, or too much smoking or talking. Whatever the cause, however, you can count on there being inflammation, pain, and an itchy or scratchy feeling. Here's a nifty, natural way to get the lumps and irritation in your throat to beat a hasty retreat.

3 tsp. of dried echinacea
3 tsp. of dried licorice
3 tsp. of dried slippery elm
3 cups of water

➡ First, get yourself a small sprayer bottle or mister and set it aside. Next, combine the herbs in a saucepan, then add the water. Stir well, bring the tea to a full boil, reduce the heat, and let simmer for 10 to 15 minutes. Strain out the herbs and pour the brew into the sprayer bottle. Open your mouth, stick out your tongue, and spray the back of your throat as needed during the day. **Caution:** Don't use echinacea if you have an autoimmune disease, such as rheumatoid arthritis, lupus, or multiple sclerosis. If you have high blood pressure or kidney disease, don't use licorice.

Sore Throat, Be Gone!

■ For those unfortunate times when you get a sore throat on top of a lingering cold or the flu, licorice can help soothe the scratchiness and make it easier for you to swallow. Try this easy-to-make gargle. Boil 1 teaspoon of licorice root (fresh, dried, or powdered) in 1 cup of water. Simmer for 10 to 15 minutes. Let it cool down enough so you can swish it around in your mouth and gargle. Or simply sip it to soothe your sore throat. **Caution:** If you have high blood pressure or kidney disease, don't use licorice root.

Nifty, Thrifty Tips

The fastest (and cheapest) way that I've ever come across to get rid of a lingering sore throat is to wrap up your throat. Soak a clean washcloth in warm water, wring it out, and place it around your neck. The warmth will help relieve soreness and loosen up any mucus.

Scratchy Throat Solution

Have you ever woken up with your throat hurting so much that when you swallowed you'd swear your tonsils were made by Gillette®? And if that weren't enough, your morning orange juice stings like hydrochloric acid? To relieve that kind of intense sore throat pain, you need this elixir to stimulate your immune system.

Dried agrimony
Dried cleavers
Dried echinacea
Dried sage
1 cup of hot water

➤ Combine equal parts of the herbs, then steep 1 heaping teaspoon of the mixture in the water for 10 minutes. Strain. Sip the hot tea slowly three or four times a day to give your throat the chance it needs to heal quickly and pain-free. **Caution**: Don't take echinacea if you have an autoimmune disease, such as rheumatoid arthritis, lupus, or multiple sclerosis.

Violet Flower Tea

■ Violets are not only beautiful, but they're medicinal, too, helping ease the pain of a sore throat. To make a tea, steep 1 heaping teaspoon of violet flowers in 1 cup of hot water for 10 minutes. Sip slowly, and drink 2 to 3 cups per day.

The Calendula Cure

■ For a speedy ending to a sore throat, ask a friend to paint your throat with fresh calendula juice or tincture. Dip a long cotton swab in the juice, and thoroughly apply it to the back of your throat, paying particular attention to the sides. Too unpleasant? Then make a strong infusion of calendula by steeping 1 heaping teaspoon of the dried herb in ½ cup of hot water and gargle with it as needed.

EUREKA!

WHEN YOUR THROAT IS SORE, the less work your throat muscles and membranes have to do, the better you will feel. So save the speeches until your throat has healed. In fact, don't say a word and your throat will have plenty of time to heal quickly. You'll be good as new in no time at all.

Sweet-and-Spicy Sore Throat Cure

Sometimes your sore throat just needs a little boost to get it back on the healing track. So give it some TLC with this double-dip gargle. It will send your sore throat packin', pronto, and leave you rarin' to go!

⅛ tsp. of cayenne pepper
⅛ tsp. of powdered cloves
⅛ tsp. of powdered ginger
1 cup of hot water
1 cup of ice-cold pineapple juice

➡ Mix the spices in the water. Pour the pineapple juice into a glass, and set it aside. First, gargle with a swig of the spicy water mixture. Then follow up by gargling with the pineapple juice. Switch back and forth between the hot and cold liquids one or two more times, and repeat the routine several times a day. The combination of hot and cold liquids will ease the burning sensation, and the dual action of the spices and bromelain (an enzyme in the pineapple) will loosen the irritating mucus in your throat.

Wear a Carrot

■ Some naturopaths suggest wrapping a sore throat in a carrot poultice. To make one, grate a large carrot and spread it on a clean cloth. Wrap this cloth around your throat for 20 minutes, covering it with a scarf to keep it in place. You also have the choice of placing either an ice pack or a hot compress over the poultice to make it even more effective.

Snappy Solutions

If you're out and about during the day with no time to properly care for your sore throat, suck on some lozenges or hard candies to keep your throat moist. Look for cherry lozenges with benzocaine to numb your throat temporarily and help with swallowing. Slippery elm lozenges are a good choice, too.

Anti-Stress Spray

The skin allows a lot of things to soak into your body. Because it's very permeable, it's easy for different enzymes and minerals to be absorbed right through it. But the same goes for a host of toxins that can cause your body to feel stress. To help ease the tension, try misting your skin with this herbal anti-stress spray.

1 tsp. of salt
5 drops of bergamot oil
5 drops of chamomile oil
5 drops of clary sage oil
5 drops of geranium oil
5 drops of lemon balm oil
5 drops of lavender oil
5 drops of rose oil

➡ Combine the salt and all of the essential oils in a 2-ounce sprayer bottle, and top it off with water (preferably distilled water). Gently mist your skin to feel refreshed, or mist the air and take a big, deep breath. Inhaling the aroma of these calming and stimulating herbs will ease your troubled mind, too.

Play at Your Desk

■ Experts say that the major source of stress for adults is workplace pressure, and we may do well to revive certain kindergarten pastimes. Stock your pencil holder with colored pens, for instance, and when you're jotting down notes or thoughts, do it in a fun color like purple—and keep scribbling, doodling, and coloring if you have the time and the privacy. This little throwback to childhood can help release tension and have a deeply calming effect.

EUREKA!

LOTS OF PEOPLE CLENCH THEIR TEETH when they're uptight and under stress. Here's an easy exercise to relax your jaw, face, and neck muscles. Take a deep breath, and drop your jaw right now. Next, open your mouth and exhale with a long *haaaaaaa* sound. Finally, gently close your lips. Since it only takes five seconds to do, repeat this exercise throughout the day. You'll soon become aware of how often your jaw clenches—and how that tightness moves tension down into your neck and shoulders.

Bath Salts, Over Easy

While a little stress can improve productivity, the hormones generated by extreme or chronic stress can be damaging to your physical and emotional health. But as easy as it is to get stressed, a nice soothing bath can be all it takes to get rid of it. And luxury bath treats don't come any easier than this fixer!

1 cup of baking soda
1 cup of Epsom salts
1 cup of table salt

➡ Combine the baking soda and salts, and store them in an airtight container at room temperature. At bath time, pour about 2 tablespoons of the mixture into warm running water. For an aromatic bath, add a few drops of your favorite essential oil as the tub fills. Then slip into the water, and your stress will just melt away.

Switch Gears

■ If you are strumming your fingers on your desk as you pore over a report that is already late and not as good as you'd like it to be, get up and walk away from it. Take a break, and shift to something mindless—even if you're on deadline. You'll come back less stressed and better able to concentrate on what you're doing.

Move That Bod!

■ Studies have consistently found that even a single exercise session can make you feel calmer. A simple morning walk at a brisk pace enhances the flow of brain chemicals that block the effects of stress. And in a pinch, even a dash up and down the nearest staircase will help.

Snappy Solutions

After a long, hard day, don't take time whipping up a bath mixer to soothe your spirit and soften your skin. Instead, reach for some brewskies. Just pour three bottles of beer into a tub of water, settle in, and think lovely thoughts!

Be Calm Spritzer

Here's one stress-relieving fixer you can carry with you wherever you go. Just mix up a batch of this aromatic spritzer, and tuck a bottle of it into your pocket or purse. Then, whenever you're feeling stressed and out of sorts, pull out the bottle and give yourself a fragrant lift.

1 tsp. of rubbing alcohol
10 drops of chamomile oil
10 drops of clary sage oil
10 drops of lavender oil
3½ oz. of distilled water

➡ Mix the ingredients together, and store the elixir in a glass sprayer bottle. Keep it close at hand, so that whenever you're feeling tense, you can spray your skin liberally. The fragrance of the essential oils will help ease your stress and lift your spirits.

Munch on Schisandra

■ Ongoing stress can wear out your adrenal glands, but schisandra, an herb available at health-food stores, can help perk them up like a jolt of java—without the jittery side effects. How you take schisandra is up to you: You can either chew 1 teaspoon of berries twice daily, sip 2 cups of tea per day, or add 15 to 25 drops of tincture to a glass of water and drink it once a day. No matter which form of schisandra you use, you can be sure it will counteract the stress effect. **Caution:** Don't take schisandra if you're pregnant.

What Would Grandma Do?

🦋 YOU COULDN'T ASK for a more effective calming bath than this fabulous fixer from Grandma Putt's day. It's just the ticket to relaxing at the end of a long, tough day. First, cut an orange into thin slices. Then wrap a few chamomile tea bags or a handful of dried chamomile in a cheesecloth pouch or an old panty hose leg. Hang the pouch from the bathtub spigot and let warm water flow over it as the tub fills. Toss the orange slices into the water, climb in, and let your troubles float away.

Bring on the Bubbles Mix

It's difficult to think of any disorder in which stress does not play an aggravating role. In fact, studies show that your risk of a heart attack triples within two hours of an extremely stressful incident or major meltdown. But there are plenty of relaxing ways to keep stress out of your life. And if your idea of relaxation is sinking into a tub full of bubbles, this mixer's for you!

1 gal. of water
2 cups of soap flakes
½ cup of glycerin
2 cups of shampoo
Scented oil (optional)

➡ Mix the water, soap, and 2 tablespoons of the glycerin in a pot over low heat, stirring until the soap flakes have dissolved. In a large bowl, add this mixture to the rest of the glycerin, the shampoo, and, if you'd like, the scented oil. Store in quart containers at room temperature. To use, add 1 cup of the mixture to the water as your tub is filling.

Have a Girls' Night Out

■ If you're a woman, head to the park with your best pals or join the local bowling league. Women "tend and befriend"; in many species of mammals, females respond to stress by seeking social contact with others, especially other females, or by nurturing their young. Both seem to be big stress reducers.

Snappy Solutions

Get out the Godiva®! The good news is that research has shown that chocolate—yes, chocolate!—helps release endorphins, which are those brainy chemicals that control your mood. As it turns out, some people may crave chocolate to compensate for a magnesium deficiency. Stress stimulates the body to excrete magnesium, which, in turn, causes a depletion of endorphins.

Foaming Bath Crystals

When you're feeling stressed to the limit, down in the dumps, or just plain tired and achy all over, it's good to have a big, beautiful jar of these colorful crystals on hand. (They make great gifts, too!)

6 cups of rock salt
½ cup of liquid hand soap or mild dishwashing liquid
1 tbsp. of vegetable oil
4 to 5 drops of food coloring

➡ Put the rock salt in a bowl. In another bowl, mix the liquid soap, vegetable oil, and food coloring together, and pour the solution over the salt. Stir to coat the crystals, and spread them out on wax paper. When they're completely dry (usually in about 24 hours), put them in a jar. At bath time, pour ¼ cup of the crystals into the tub under running water for a soothing soak.

Five Minutes to Heaven!

■ Prayer is an invaluable tool for stressful times. But don't wait until your world falls apart before you make prayer a regular part of your day. Instead, start by spending 20 minutes or so each morning and evening centering yourself and reconnecting with your Maker (whoever it happens to be).

Q: *I have a friend who swears by massage as a cure-all for stress. I'm sure it works, but I have a hard time justifying the expense. Is massage worth the price?*

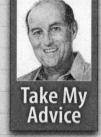

Take My Advice

A: It may seem like a big splurge, but besides making you feel more relaxed, professional massage can help head off a lot of serious—and expensive—problems. Massages can cut cortisol levels, lower blood pressure, and boost immunity. To find a licensed therapist near you, contact the American Massage Therapy Association at www.amtamassage.org.

Lemon Belly Balm

Do you ever have a feeling in your gut that something is eating at you, but you can't quite figure out what it is—or how to get rid of it? An abdominal massage with this fixer can help release nervous tension and emotional stress, both of which are often held in the belly.

4 drops of chamomile oil
4 drops of lemon balm oil
1 tbsp. of massage oil

➥ Add both essential oils to the massage oil. Lie down on your bed and, using gentle pressure, smooth the oil over your abdomen in nice wide circles. Begin at your belly button and, making small circles with your fingertips, slowly massage in a clockwise direction in gradually bigger circles, until the circle is going from one side of your abdomen to the other. By the time you're there, you should feel the tension melting away, and you should be really, really relaxed.

Get Ease with Teas

■ Choose one of the following herbs to make your own tension-tamer tea: lemon balm, chamomile, passionflower, vervain, wood betony, or skullcap. Try each one for a week at a time until you find your favorite. Then every time you feel stressed, steep 1 teaspoon of your preferred herb in 1 cup of hot water, covered, for 10 minutes, then strain out the solids. Drink 1 to 3 cups a day. **Caution:** If you have ragweed allergies, steer clear of chamomile.

EUREKA!

IF YOU CAN'T MEDITATE WITH THE DALAI LAMA, being in the room with your golden retriever may be the next best thing. Studies have shown that pets serve as a buffer against acute stress and make you feel less hassled—even more so than being in the presence of a spouse or close friend. One reason for this: Pets neither judge nor evaluate you.

Make Mine Minty Bath Powder

A bath can be the most soothing way to end a day, especially if the day was full of mind-numbing stress. So how can you make an ordinary bath even better? Combine it with a sweet smell that we're all familiar with—mint. If you love the fresh aroma of mint, here's a bath powder that's just for you.

5 tbsp. of slippery elm powder
1 tbsp. of cornstarch
2 drops of peppermint oil

➡ Combine all of the ingredients in a bowl, and mix them well with a wooden spoon. Pour the mixture into a shaker (like a large salt shaker) or a container that's got a lid and a big powder puff. After your bath, dust yourself with this powder, and you'll feel as good as new! **Note:** Talcum powder is loosely associated with increased ovarian cancer risk. That's why this recipe calls for slippery elm powder. You can substitute calendula powder if you prefer.

Visualize Relief

■ When you feel your stress level rising, close your eyes. Breathe deeply, and visualize a peaceful scene from nature. Try to keep the scene in your mind for 15 to 20 minutes. If you do, you'll find that you feel a lot more relaxed afterward. If nature isn't your thing, then picture anything that makes you feel completely carefree. Stay focused and your cares should soon subside.

Snappy Solutions

Believe it or not, keeping stress under control can help you avoid the time and hassle of dealing with bad hair days. That's because stress can boost your output of sebum, the fatty oil produced by the skin to keep your scalp from drying out. When there's too much sebum, your hair becomes flat, greasy, and sprinkled with dandruff. In other words, when you're weighted down with worry, your hair may become weighted down with oil.

Soothing Soaker

A hot bath is a super stress buster, and when the right scents are added, the bath becomes an instant stress reliever. Here's how to make your own heavenly fragrant soak that'll soothe you when you're tired and irritated.

2 cups of nonfat dry milk
1 cup of cornstarch
1 tbsp. of your favorite scented oil

➡ Combine all of the ingredients in an old blender. Add ½ cup of the mixture to your bathwater, sink into the tub, and relax. You'll be amazed at how quickly your stress disappears. The remaining mixture can be stored in an airtight container at room temperature until you need it.

Commune with Nature

■ As we gardeners know, being outdoors is both enjoyable and calming. Now we know why: Researchers believe that biochemical pathways in the brain may respond positively to contact with nature. The interesting part is that you don't even have to be outside! Strolling through a warm, aromatic greenhouse or simply admiring your neighbor's lawn or the park across the street can also do the trick.

Pinch Yourself

■ Once or twice a day, press firmly on the fibrous spot between your thumb and index finger, about an inch from the edge of the web. This acupressure point corresponds to the large intestine, and pinching it may help tone your exhausted adrenals and improve your ability to handle stress.

Nifty, Thrifty Tips

You can spend a lot of money on different remedies for stress, but sometimes your own emotions are all you need to kick the nasty stress right out of you. Try hugging someone—studies have shown that this can help you remain calm during a chaotic day. Just be sure to ask permission first. Or, go ahead and be a crybaby. Believe it or not, having a good cry can reduce your body's levels of stress hormones.

Triple-Treat Bath Blend

Soaking in a soothing, great-smelling bath is a classic way to relax. The next time you feel your stress level rising, reach for three of nature's most potent relaxing aids: baking soda, milk, and salt.

1 cup of baking soda
1 cup of nonfat dry milk
1 cup of salt
10 drops of vanilla or lemon extract

➥ Combine the ingredients, and store the mixer in a moisture-proof container with a tight lid (a clamp-lidded glass canning jar is perfect). Add about ¼ cup to your bathwater, and soak away your stress-filled day. You'll come out of the tub relaxed and refreshed, and your skin will be soft and smooth.

Catch the Catastrophic Thoughts

■ It's a proven fact that what you tell yourself can absolutely add to your stress level. So the next time you hear yourself saying, "I can't handle this," take a deep, calming breath and swiftly replace that thought with this one: "I am strong, I am in control, and I am handling this."

Q: *I find myself unbelievably stressed every day, from the time I wake up until the time I go to bed. I know this can't be good, but nothing I try seems to get rid of it. Is there anything else I can do before I go crazy?*

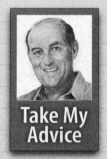

Take My Advice

A: Sometimes the easiest thing you can do is decide whether this stress is really worth it. Try asking yourself these questions: Is this really important to me? Would a reasonably prudent person be this upset? Can I do anything to fix the situation? Would fixing it be worth the cost? If you answered "yes" to all the questions, take action. But if you answered "no" one or more times, then just ride out the stressful situation.

Ultra-Simple Stress Soother

If you're anything like me, when you're feeling tired and irritated, the last thing you want to do is mix up some complicated formula. So don't do it. Instead, stroll into your kitchen and grab the ingredients for this simple mixer. It'll help you kick back and let your cares flow away.

½ **cup of nonfat dry milk**
¼ **cup of cornstarch**
1 **tsp. of vanilla extract**

➡ Combine the ingredients, then pour the mixture into running bathwater. Sink into the milky bath, and soften your skin while you're soothing your mind with the wonderful vanilla aroma.

Get Your B's

■ If your life is in overdrive, it's vital to include plenty of fish, milk, beans, peas, whole grains, broccoli, cauliflower, and kale in your diet. These foods all provide a bushel of pantothenic acid, which is critical for keeping your adrenal glands up to snuff when they may be maxed out. To be on the safe side, supplement daily with a B-complex vitamin that contains 50 milligrams of pantothenic acid.

EUREKA!

IF YOU'RE A SURVIVOR of a traumatic event like an auto accident, sexual abuse, or a physical attack, it's all but guaranteed that you are less stress-hardy than folks who have not suffered similar mishaps. But here's good news: A simple method called EMDR (eye movement desensitization and reprocessing) seems to help lower stress and anxiety in just two or three sessions. In a nutshell, the patient recalls the stressful event while following a therapist's finger moving rapidly back and forth in front of her eyes. To find out more, call the EMDR International Association toll-free at 866-451-5200 or visit the organization's Web site at www.emdria.org.

Fresh and Fruity Smoothie

Whether you're recovering from a stroke or simply aiming to prevent one, this fresh-fruit fixer is just what the doctor ordered. It's chock-full of anti-stroke superstars, including vitamin B, vitamin C, and potassium. What's more, it's just about as delicious as a drink can get.

➤ Combine the apple, banana, juice, and milk in a blender, and blend until smooth. Pour into a chilled glass, and drink up.

1 apple, peeled, cored, and chopped
1 frozen banana, peeled and chopped
½ cup of freshly squeezed orange juice
¼ cup of milk

Keep Your Spuds Covered

■ A baked potato in its skin packs 903 milligrams of stroke-lowering potassium—tons more than any other food. But take away the skin, and you'll get only 641 milligrams. So buy organic potatoes (or grow your own), scrub them well, bake them in their jackets, and gobble up each and every bite.

Snappy Solutions

Calling all couch potatoes! There are few events in life that will cost you more recovery time than a stroke. So get up, already—and get moving. The more you move your body, the stronger your cardiovascular system gets, and the less likely you are to have a stroke. If you can't even remember the last time you did anything more strenuous than stroll to the kitchen to make a sandwich, start by getting a clean bill of health from your doctor. Then take off by going for a walk every day. It doesn't have to be fast or far—a moderately brisk walk to the corner and back will do for starters. Gradually increase your time, speed, and distance until you're really exercising—walking, running, biking, swimming, even dancing—for 15 to 20 minutes each and every day.

Lovely Liniment

Thanks to medical advances, people who suffer strokes these days are frequently able to recover, but it's typically a long road back. A warming herbal liniment may help increase circulation to paralyzed muscles.

2 oz. of powdered rosemary leaves
1 oz. of powdered lavender flowers
½ oz. of cayenne pepper
1 qt. of rubbing alcohol

➥ Mix all the ingredients and pour them into a capped bottle. Let the mixture stand for seven days, but shake it well each day. Strain through a coffee filter into another clean bottle with a cap. Then use once or twice daily.

Stroke-Preventing Tea

■ A number of studies associate good ol' black tea with reduced risk of heart disease and stroke. Scientists believe it works because the tea's antioxidants maintain the health of the circulatory system and reduce the risk of blood clots.

Raise a Stink!

■ This is one folk remedy backed by solid science! Garlic stimulates circulation, reduces high cholesterol, and decreases the stickiness of platelets—all of which may help prevent stroke. So chop some garlic and sprinkle it onto your favorite foods. For best results, eat one to three raw cloves a day.

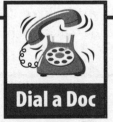

Dial a Doc

If you suddenly experience weakness or numbness in your face, arm, or leg on one side of your body—all hallmarks of a stroke—head to an emergency room right away. Also, get help if you have difficulty speaking or understanding others, dimness or impaired vision in one eye, an unexplained dizzy spell, or a severe headache with no apparent cause. Even if the symptoms pass, get immediate help because you may have had a mini stroke, which is a sign that another such incident could occur.

Capsule Cure

Did you spend more time out in the yard than you were expecting to on that first day of spring? Or maybe you went to the beach and forgot to put some sunscreen on right away? Whatever the reason, if you find yourself with a sunburn, take care of it immediately. If left unchecked, it can create a lot of problems. Here's a nice soothing oil for a case of mild sunburn.

6 capsules of vitamin A oil
6 capsules of vitamin E oil
¼ cup of flaxseed oil
¼ cup of aloe vera juice (optional)

➡ Add the contents of the vitamin A and vitamin E capsules to the flaxseed oil. Apply frequently to the sunburned areas. If that alone doesn't work, try adding the combination to the aloe vera juice, and smooth it over your skin. **Caution:** Don't use this remedy on blistered skin.

A Cooling Lavender Spray

■ Lavender is an antiseptic, cooling herb that can relieve burning and protect against secondary infections. To make a healing preparation, fill an 8-ounce sprayer bottle with cold water, and add 6 drops of essential oil of lavender to it. Shake the contents well, and spray on sunburned areas for an instant cool-off.

Chug-a-Lug

■ When you're sunburned, drink plenty of water to help heal your overheated skin. Avoid drinking alcohol or caffeinated beverages because they are diuretics that will steal much-needed moisture from your skin.

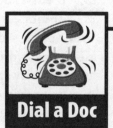

Dial a Doc

✚ Call your doctor if you experience chills, fever, nausea, swelling, or blisters along with a sunburn. You could have second-degree burns or sunstroke, both of which require medical care. And never ever use any ointments, antiseptics, sprays, or home remedies on a severe burn.

Cool-Aid for Burns

Once those warm summer days come around, we all like to sit out in the sun and shake off what's left of the winter blues. But when you linger too long and your skin turns a painful shade of way-too-hot pink, reach for this cooling— and healing—sunburn fixer.

2 capsules of vitamin E oil
½ cup of aloe vera gel
1 tsp. of cider vinegar
½ tsp. of lavender oil

➡ Using sharp scissors, open the tip of each vitamin E capsule and squeeze out the oil into a bowl. Then mix in the other ingredients. Gently smooth the cool mixture directly onto your ailin' skin until the pain goes away. And by the way, even though Grandma Putt took her aloe straight from the plants on her windowsill, you can easily buy a tube at the drugstore and keep it stashed in your medicine chest.

Try Some Mallow Aloe

■ Ointments made with the fresh gel of aloe or a paste from the Indian herb country mallow are Ayurvedic remedies for sunburn. Rub one of these on your sunburned skin—but only if your skin is unbroken and there is no chance of infection. Another remedy involves the paste or oil of sandalwood. Just put some on your forehead, and—it's reported—it will cool down your entire body.

Nifty, Thrifty Tips

You can save your money on sunburn remedies if you buy the proper sunscreen protection from the very start. Choose a sunscreen with a sun protection factor (SPF) of 30 or higher. Use a waterproof brand if you'll be swimming or if you perspire heavily. And apply it at least 20 minutes before going outside—it takes that long for the protective ingredients to "kick in"—and reapply it frequently throughout the day. All of these little things can keep big bucks in your wallet and sunburn out of your life.

Soothing Sunburn Bath

Kids seem to get sunburned pretty easily. The problem is that they don't always take too kindly to being smeared up with lotions and gels. So try this alternative—kids love the foam, even when they don't have sunburned skin. (Plenty of grown-ups go for it, too!)

1 cup of vegetable oil
½ cup of honey
½ cup of liquid hand soap
1 tbsp. of pure vanilla
    extract (not artificial)

➥ Mix all of the ingredients together, and pour the mixture into a bottle that's got a tight stopper. At bath time, shake the bottle, then pour ¼ cup or so of the mixture under lukewarm running water. The oil can make the tub slippery, so use caution helping the kids into the water. Rinse them thoroughly with fresh water after bathing.

Be Cool as a Cucumber

■ Soothe the burn by placing chilled slices of cucumber on your simmering skin. A dab of cold plain yogurt or a splash of vinegar will do the job, too.

The Morning-After Sunburn Remedy

■ An enzyme called photolyase, which is made from ocean algae, is said to be the magic elixir for a painful sunburn. It even reverses some of the critical DNA damage that is caused by soaking up too much ultraviolet light. In fact, studies have shown that photolyase reduced redness and DNA effects by as much as 45 percent! It's scheduled to be in sunburn remedies soon. Check labels for details.

EUREKA!

ONE OF THE BEST THINGS you can do right away when you get sunburned is to crack open the medicine chest. There you'll probably find some aspirin, ibuprofen, or other pain reliever. The drugs won't help the burn heal, but they're very effective at reducing pain while nature takes its course. So follow the package directions and take a dose.

Sore Face Soother

Spring has sprung, and you were so eager to start planting that you rushed out to the garden without applying any sunscreen—and you stayed outdoors way too long. Now your face is feeling the results. Instead of chewing yourself out, treat your face to this intensive treatment.

5 capsules of vitamin E oil
2 tsp. of plain yogurt
½ tsp. of honey
½ tsp. of lemon juice

➡ Drain the contents of the vitamin E capsules into a bowl, and add the yogurt, honey, and lemon juice. Stir well, and apply the mixture to your face with a cotton ball. Wait about 10 minutes, and rinse with tepid water.

Cool It Down
■ To ease a painful sunburn, fill your tub with cool to lukewarm water. Add some baking soda or colloidal oatmeal, and soak long enough for your skin to chill out. Or you can place cold, damp cloths on your skin (but don't rub!). If your sunburn is severe, submerge your burned skin under cool water instead of lukewarm water, and stay under until it stops the pain.

Let the Soap Slide
■ For the first day or two after getting sunburned, don't use soap on the painful areas. It dries the skin and only makes the pain worse. Of course, you may have to use soap if the area is dirtier than usual. But it's better to have a little irritation than risk a more serious infection.

Snappy Solutions

You can save yourself hours or even days of discomfort after your sunburn starts healing if you follow this simple rule. When your skin starts to peel or the blisters break, gently remove any dried fragments, and apply an antiseptic ointment or hydrocortisone cream to the raw skin below.

Sunburn Cooler

Here's a variation on the old-time cucumber cure for sunburn: It's a fresh, cooling lotion that eases the pain while helping the skin to heal. It's worked so well for me and my family that we keep a bottle of it handy year-round.

1 cup of witch hazel
3 tbsp. of coarsely chopped cucumber
Juice of 1 lemon

➡ Mix the ingredients in a clean glass jar that's got a lid. Let the mixture sit for two days, strain out the cucumber, and pour the liquid into another clean bottle with a cap. Keep it in the refrigerator, and dab it on with a cotton ball whenever the need arises.

Go Green

■ When green tea is applied topically to skin, it may help prevent sunburn damage and skin cancer. And if you're already burned, it may stave off cellular damage. So brew a pot of green tea, let it cool, then pour it into a sprayer bottle. Gently spritz it on the burned areas daily, and the green may help stop the red.

Cure It with Calendula

■ Herbalists are quick to sing the praises of calendula when it comes to repairing damaged skin. Make an infusion by adding 1 heaping tablespoon of the dried herb to 1 cup of boiling water. Steep 15 minutes, strain, and cool. Apply it to the burn and cover the area with a light bandage or gauze. You can reapply it a few times a day until your skin has healed.

What Would Grandma Do?

🦋 WHEN I WOULD GET A NASTY SUNBURN *from being outside all day in the garden with Grandma, she would try to cure me with food. To help skin heal itself and to protect it from the free-radical damage that can cause skin cancer, Grandma would have me eat berries, citrus, mango, papaya, dark leafy greens, broccoli, Brussels sprouts, and other healthy foods until my skin went back to its natural shade.*

Douse the Denture Pain Rinse

Attention, denture wearers! At the first sign of denture pain—whether your choppers are brand new or you've had them for years—treat your aching gums to this antibacterial mouthwash. It will not only ease the soreness, but will also help head off infection.

2 tbsp. of rosemary
1 tbsp. of cloves
2 cups of boiling water

➥ Put the rosemary and cloves in a heat-proof glass bowl or measuring cup, pour the water over them, and let them steep overnight. Strain out the solids, and store the fluid in a tightly capped bottle or jar. Rinse your sore mouth three times a day with ½ cup of the elixir.

Brush Often

■ Plaque and tartar, the same nasty substances that promote tooth and gum disease, can also adhere to dentures. Once plaque and tartar build up, they can push your dentures out of alignment. To prevent trouble, brush your chops every night at bedtime, using denture cleanser or paste. Don't use regular toothpaste, because it's too abrasive. Some formulas can actually damage the material to the point where the dentures don't fit properly.

The Clove Cure

■ Clove oil—a traditional toothache remedy that you can buy at any health-food store—works just as well for sore gums, and it takes effect almost instantly. Simply dip a cotton swab in the oil, and dab it directly onto the sore area.

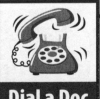

Dial a Doc

✚ Ill-fitting dentures can be more than just a pain in the mouth. They can also contribute to poor nutrition (because you won't feel like eating) and lead to severe gum infection. See your dentist immediately if you notice red inflammation on your gums; you have soft, white, slightly raised sores on your gums, cheeks, or tongue; or your dentures simply don't fit as well as they once did.

Homemade Toothpaste

If you like the taste, texture, and ease of commercial toothpastes, but you'd rather not pay supermarket prices, this tooth-pleasing mixer is for you. It's easy to make, and it does an excellent job of keeping those pearly whites pearly *and* white.

3 parts baking soda
1 part salt
3 tsp. of vegetable glycerin
10 to 20 drops of flavored oil or extract
1 drop of food coloring (optional)
Water

➡ Mix the first five ingredients thoroughly in a bowl, and add just enough water to give the mixer the consistency of toothpaste. Spoon the concoction into a small plastic squeeze bottle, then use the paste to brush away to your heart's content.

Be Gentle

■ Don't brush your teeth as though you're trying to scrub shellac off the floor. Hard scrubbing damages your teeth and won't remove any more plaque than gentle brushing. A good rule of thumb is if your brush bristles are worn down after a month, you're brushing way too hard. Brush gently, but thoroughly.

Buy the Right Brush

■ Look for a brush that has soft bristles with rounded ends (if the bristles are hard, they can wear away tooth enamel and damage your gums). Replace the brush every three to four months, or sooner if the bristles fray.

EUREKA!

KEEP YOUR TEETH HEALTHY by doing what Mom always told you to do—drink your milk! And while you're at it, eat plenty of cheese, walnuts, rice, and oats. These and other calcium-rich foods keep your jawbone strong so your teeth don't loosen up. Calcium also helps prevent gum inflammation and bleeding.

Perfect Peppermint Toothpaste

 Aside from getting the occasional tooth snapped off in the throes of a ferocious ice hockey game, most of us lose teeth in a much more predictable—and preventable—way: from decay, cavities, and the resulting extractions. So do yourself and your teeth a favor by brushing twice a day with this mouth-pleasing mixer. It'll leave your teeth sparklin' clean and make your breath kissin' sweet.

1 tbsp. of baking soda
¼ tsp. of peppermint extract
Dash of salt

➤ Combine the ingredients until you get a toothpaste-like consistency. Then brush and enjoy. Your mouth will feel refreshed, and you'll feel even better when you realize how much money you saved making this homemade paste.

Go for Green Tea

■ Green tea contains tooth-loving tannin, which kills decay-causing bacteria and stops them from producing a sticky substance that helps acid-generating bacteria adhere to your teeth. So take a trip to your local market and pick up some green tea; it's widely available in tea bags and as loose tea. Drink it hot or cold after every meal to keep your teeth in tip-top shape. **Caution:** If you have clotting disorders or take heart medications, check with your doctor before drinking green tea.

Nifty, Thrifty Tips

Save yourself a lot of time and money on costly tooth repair by following one simple rule: Brush at least twice a day. Although saliva is a natural cleanser, your body doesn't produce much while you're sleeping and that's when plaque typically does its dirty work. So brush in the morning *before* you eat breakfast to remove plaque that formed overnight, then brush again before you go to bed. Plaque takes 16 to 24 hours to develop, so brushing twice a day helps keep it away.

Strawberry-Leaf Mouthwash

Strawberry leaves (and the fruits, too) contain plaque- and germ-fighting chemicals that keep your teeth and gums strong and healthy. If you don't grow your own strawberries, venture out to a pick-your-own berry farm, harvest a good supply of the tasty fruits, and make several batches of this easy elixir.

1 cup of fresh strawberry leaves
1 cup of boiling water
2 tsp. of vodka or lemon juice

➡ Put the strawberry leaves into a heat-proof glass or ceramic bowl, and cover them with the water. Let the brew steep until the water has reached room temperature, strain it into another bowl, and mix in either the vodka or lemon juice (not both). Store it in a capped bottle in the refrigerator, and use it as you would any other mouthwash.

Look, Ma—No Toothpaste!

■ To make strawberries part of your dental hygiene plan, simply mash a berry in a bowl or saucer, dip your toothbrush in the pulp, and brush as you would with your regular toothpaste. Hold off rinsing as long as you can (half an hour or so if possible) because the longer the berry juice remains on your teeth, the more effective it will be at removing tartar.

Snappy Solutions

We all know that an apple a day keeps the doctor away. Well, guess what? It can help keep the dentist away, too! Apples contain compounds that fight tooth decay and inhibit the gum-destroying enzymes secreted by oral bacteria. So if you can think of more pleasant ways to spend your time than leaning back in a chair having your teeth drilled and/or gums fixed, be sure to munch a slice or two of apple after every meal or snack to help keep your mouth clean between brushings.

Guardian Angel Elixir

Angelica (*Angelica archangelica*) is a slightly sweet, slightly bitter carminative herb with a long history of use in nausea medications. This tasty elixir helps halt vomiting in a hurry by relieving stomach spasms.

1 tbsp. of angelica
stems and root
2 cups of water
1 tsp. of aniseeds

➡ Make a decoction by simmering the angelica in the water for 20 minutes. Add the aniseeds, then remove the brew from the heat, and strain. Take 1 tablespoon every 30 minutes until your stomach settles, or no more than 2 cups a day.

Go for the Gatorade®

■ Keep a few bottles of sports drinks on hand in case you need to restore electrolytes—the sodium, potassium, and other chemicals that keep body fluids in balance—lost via vomiting. If you don't care for sports drinks, get an over-the-counter oral rehydrating solution or mix, such as Kaolectrolyte®. These powders are available without prescription, they come in several flavors, and quickly dissolve in water. Just be sure to follow package directions.

Excuse Yourself

■ From the dinner table, that is. If you're feeling ill, let your stomach rest from its usual work of digestion. Don't eat anything or even spend time around the aromas of food until the vomiting has passed completely. Your belly will let you know when it's safe to eat again. Start with bland foods, like plain toast, rice, and applesauce, to ease your stomach back to work.

Nifty, Thrifty Tips

Don't waste your pricey prescriptions by taking your usual medications while you're vomiting. You won't be able to keep them down. But if your stomach upset is causing you to miss rather than delay doses, ask your doctor for guidance on what to do.

Mint Magic

The most common causes of vomiting are viral infections, motion sickness, migraines, morning sickness (in pregnancy), food poisoning, food allergies, and side effects from medication. But the volatile oil contained in these minty herbs can help relieve spasms and may help allay bouts of vomiting.

Calamint
Catnip
Lemon balm
Peppermint
Spearmint
1 cup of hot water

➡ Mix together your choice of at least three of the herbs. Try different combinations until you find the one that works best (and tastes best) to you. Make a tea by steeping 1 teaspoon of the dried leaves of your mixture of choice in the water for 10 minutes. Strain, then take small sips while it's still warm. Your ailing tummy will thank you very much!

Make It Salty, Sweetie!

■ When you've been vomiting, avoid water or fluids that don't have any salt or sugar because they'll usually come right back up. Instead, sip clear, sweetened liquids like flat ginger ale. And clear liquids and broth will stay down better than juices and cola-based sodas.

Q: *As a kid, if I felt like I was going to throw up, I was always told to get up and walk around, and breathe deeply. But this has never worked and I blame it on not being able to control the vomiting. Why doesn't this old remedy work for me?*

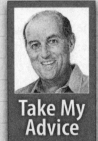

Take My Advice

A: Moving about actually makes you feel worse. Try to rest quietly in one place until the need to vomit passes. Just sitting in a calm spot with a small plastic trash can in your lap and some baby wipes at your elbow can absolutely soothe your psyche—and maybe even your belly.

Part Two

A More Beautiful You!

You don't have to be a supermodel or a TV celebrity to care about your appearance. Even my Grandma Putt, who was the most down-to-earth person I've ever met, knew that when we look our best we tend to feel and perform better, too. But Grandma also knew that putting your best face forward doesn't have to mean shelling out a lot of money for fancy cosmetics and elaborate treatments. In fact, she'd have a fit if she could see some of the overpriced products—and often downright dangerous procedures—people fall for these days.

Well, friends, this section is right up Grandma's alley. I've filled these pages with about a gazillion fixers, mixers, and elixirs that will keep you and your family looking terrific—including a boatload of Grandma's own commonsense grooming secrets and homemade (and often home-*grown*) beauty potions.

So whether you're looking for relief from a chronic concern like dandruff, dry skin, or brittle fingernails, or you're simply suffering from a bad hair day, help is close at hand. You'll find lots of bright ideas and fabulous formulas that will give you shiny, full-bodied hair; sweet-smelling breath; and soft, smooth skin.

And for those of you who have small children or grandchildren around the old homestead, I'll also share some timely tips, tricks, and tonics that will help you deliver extra-special TLC to the tiny tykes.

A Honey of a Cleaner

Honey has been used since ancient Egyptian times as a beauty aid because it retains moisture and can be applied to the face or added to bathwater for smoother skin. Add a couple of extra ingredients and keep acne away with this daily skin cleanser.

1 tbsp. of plain yogurt
2 tsp. of honey
½ tsp. of milk

➤ Combine all of the ingredients, and apply the mixture to your skin. Leave it on for a few minutes, then rinse it off and watch your face glow.

No Digging Allowed!

■ Don't even think about excavating blemishes with a mechanical or electric pore extractor. They can force bacteria deep into your skin tissues, causing deep-rooted inflammation and infection. The result: acne that's so angry it may leave scars that only lasers can remove. And that's the last thing you want.

Be a Soft Touch

■ All the scrubbing in the world won't make those zits disappear—in fact, it might just cause them to spread. So when it comes to cleaning, be gentle.

Q: *I seem to have a lot more acne than my sister ever had. Does it have something to do with being a boy?*

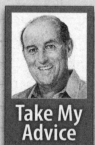

Take My Advice

A: Actually, it does. Most girls start noticing pimples around age 11, and most boys by age 13, when the adolescent body begins producing large amounts of androgen, which seems to cause an overproduction of the oils that trigger acne. Boys produce about 10 times as much androgen as girls, which is why we see many more pimply-faced boys than girls in high school.

Blackheads Be Gone Facial Paste

Pimples are a pain in the fanny no matter how old you are. But blackheads can be even more annoying—they're just as unsightly, but more of them can congregate in a single area. Plus, they're even harder to get rid of. So banish blackheads with this simple, but highly effective, fixer.

1 egg white
1 part dry oatmeal
1 part honey

➡ Mix the ingredients together to make a paste, adding more oatmeal or honey as necessary. Smooth the mixture onto your face, and wait 10 minutes or so. Rinse with warm water, and pat dry.

Try Tea Tree Oil

■ This herbal oil, which you can find at health-food stores, battles acne just as well as over-the-counter medicines do, but with much less skin irritation. The only drawback: It works more slowly, has an unpleasant odor, and may sting a bit if your skin is irritated. If you're willing to give it a try, use a cotton ball to apply the oil directly to pimples.

Grab Some Goldenseal

■ If you've got acne, don't leave your health-food store without picking up some powdered goldenseal root, which is a mild, but effective, disinfectant. Add ½ teaspoon of powdered goldenseal to 12 drops of tea tree oil, and dab the resulting paste onto your blemishes. Rinse after about 20 minutes. Apply the paste twice a day, and your pimples will vanish into thin air!

EUREKA!

TAKING 2 TABLESPOONS OF FLAXSEED OIL or evening primrose oil daily could make up for a deficiency of essential fatty acids in your diet. Both oils are excellent sources of the acids that spur production of an anti-inflammatory prostaglandin known to promote healing. That means they'll help clear things up—including acne—a whole lot quicker.

Clean and Soft Facial Scrub

As teens, we could cover up the angry bumps—those on our foreheads, anyway—with a fringe of bangs. Adult acne, which typically crops up on the chin, isn't so easily hidden. And it's possibly even more vexing than the teenage variety because it's so unexpected—and so totally unfair. But you can fight back! For skin that's squeaky clean *and* as soft as silk, reach for this marvelous mixer.

2 tbsp. of shelled almonds
2 tsp. of milk
½ tsp. of flour
½ tsp. of honey

➤ Grind the almonds to a fine powder in an old blender or coffee grinder. Then mix all of the ingredients together to make a thick paste. (If it's too thick or too thin, add more milk or flour as necessary.) Rub the mixture into your skin and rinse with warm water.

Wine Away

■ Here's a skin-care solution that even teetotalers will love: You can control facial breakouts by dabbing a little wine on your skin. Do it once or twice a day after washing your face and you'll have things under control in no time at all.

Defeat Dull Skin

■ For a super-simple skin cleanser, you can't beat this fixer: Grind shelled almonds to a fine powder in an old blender or coffee grinder. Then wet your face and rub the almond powder gently into your skin and rinse with warm water. It will keep your skin soft and smooth.

Nifty, Thrifty Tips

Here's a cheap, easy cleanser to deal with oily skin: Combine ½ cup of buttermilk with 2 tablespoons of fennel seeds and heat in the top part of a double boiler for 30 minutes. Turn off the heat and let the mixture steep for three hours. Strain, cool, and pour into a bottle. Apply to skin once a day with a cotton ball and keep it refrigerated between uses.

Happy Hour for Skin Freshener

Here's a skin freshener that your face will love, and you can make it at home whenever you feel like you need a little pick-me-up. And as delicious as it sounds, just keep telling yourself, "It's for my face, and not my . . ."

1 cup of white wine
1 lemon, sliced
1 tbsp. of sugar

➤ Put the wine and lemon slices in a glass or enamel pot, and bring to a boil over medium heat (or put them in a microwave-safe bowl and bring to a boil—about 1½ minutes on "high"). Boil for another full minute, remove the pan from the heat, and stir in the sugar. Let the mixture cool, strain it, and store it in a tightly capped bottle. Be sure to label the bottle so no one accidentally drinks the contents. Then whenever you need facial refreshment, just dab the lotion onto your skin with a cotton ball.

Heirloom Acne Stopper

■ Have you (or your favorite teenager) broken out in pimples? Then reach for this heirloom helper: Mix 1 teaspoon of onion juice with 2 tablespoons of honey, and apply it to your face. Wait 10 to 15 minutes, and rinse twice—first with warm water, then follow up with cool water.

Sweeten Away Pimples

■ Got pimples that you're not pleased with? Dissolve a little sugar in a few drops of water, then dab it onto the spots with a cotton ball. Repeat every couple of days, and the pimples should disappear—fast!

What Would Grandma Do?

🦋 WHENEVER I WOULD GET A PIMPLE, *Grandma Putt would go straight to her medicine cabinet. She grabbed something that I would never have guessed would help me get through puberty: toothpaste. That's right—you can give pimples the brush-off by dabbing them with a tiny glob of toothpaste. Let it dry, and rinse with cool water. You'll be amazed by how quickly those blemishes vanish.*

Milky Lime Maneuver

If you (or other members of your family) are perturbed by pimples and bothered by blackheads, try this simple money-saving mixer. The all-natural ingredients will make your face feel great!

1 cup of whole milk
Juice of 1 lime
1 tsp. of glycerin (optional)

➡ Boil the milk and stir in the lime juice. Let the liquid cool, then wash your face with it. If your skin is dry, add the glycerin to the mixture.

Garlic Peel

■ To make blemishes vanish, peel and mash six garlic cloves, and apply the mash to the affected areas, avoiding your eyes. Leave it in place for about 10 minutes, rinse with warm water, and pat dry. Your face may smell a little, but it'll feel great and the odor will disappear fairly quickly.

Attack with Acid

■ If your chest or back looks like a connect-the-dots game, check your local health-food store for SalAc®, a commercial shower rinse that contains salicylic acid. It is a gentle de-oiler and a mild peel that helps open clogged pores.

Q: *Can't I eliminate my pimples a whole lot easier by simply squeezing out the pus and letting my skin dry out?*

Take My Advice

A: Unfortunately, the answer is no. I realize that it is oh-so-tempting to squeeze those zits, but curb the urge. It'll only make matters worse because when you press on a pimple, you push pus and bacteria farther into the pore, causing deeper, more serious inflammation. Instead, apply a warm washcloth to the blemish once or twice a day. This will coax the bacteria to the surface so the pimple bursts naturally.

Anti-Aging Lotion

The only reason we develop age spots is because we've lived long enough to soak up a lot more sun than the neighborhood six-year-olds. If age and too much time in the sun have left you with spotty skin, lighten those splotches with this mixer.

4 tbsp. of plain yogurt
2 tbsp. of honey
Juice of 1 lemon
Juice of 1 lime

➡ Mix all of the ingredients together, and gently massage the lotion into each spot at least once a week. Store the mixture in a covered container in the refrigerator. Within a couple of weeks, your spots will not only lighten up, but your skin will feel much smoother and softer, too!

Cover and Camouflage

■ You can hide age spots with smart makeup application. Many of today's foundations are made to even out skin tone over time. Make sure you choose the proper shade, however, or you'll wind up with a mask-like look. And take advantage of in-store experts—ask a cosmetics pro how to best blend your makeup for the most natural look.

Make a Fashion Statement

■ A wide-brimmed hat or visor can actually eliminate half the sunlight that would otherwise reach parts of your face. So slap on a chapeau—you'll be stylish and skin savvy, too!

Nifty, Thrifty Tips

You can save yourself a lot of time, trouble, and money when dealing with age spots by getting serious about sunscreen. Make sure to slather sunscreen on any exposed skin, including legs, arms, and hands. And if you have a sassy short haircut, don't forget your ears! Most women fail to reapply sunscreen every time they wash their hands. It really does make a difference, so find a brand of sunscreen you like, and keep a small bottle in your purse.

On-the-Spot Bleach

I've always had freckles on my arms, but when I noticed a few larger, darker ones cropping up on the backs of my hands, I absolutely refused to admit they were "age spots." I didn't want to look "old," and, well, they're called age spots for a reason. Here's a fixer that'll bleach tell-tale spots and help you look younger a little longer.

1 tsp. of grated horseradish
1 tsp. of lemon juice
1 tsp. of vinegar
3 drops of rosemary oil

➡ Combine the ingredients in a bowl. The lemon juice and vinegar are natural bleaches and are safe to use on skin. Rub this concoction onto your age spots, and they'll fade away.

First, Pass the Test

■ As women who color their hair know, it's important to do a test patch first to be sure that any product (including natural ones) won't irritate your skin. Here's how: Smear a drop of the solution on a small patch of skin under your jaw. Check it the next day. If there is no sign of redness or irritation, then it should be safe to use on your face.

Q: *I know that exposure to sunlight causes age spots over time, so I stay in the shade or only go outside when it's kind of cloudy. But I still get sunburned. What's going on?*

Take My Advice

A: Remember—light reflects. Reflected light that bounces off the parking lot, the deck of your boat, or snow on the slopes is actually more harmful than overhead sunlight beaming down on you. Snow reflects 88 percent of light, which can hit your skin on the way back up. So don't think you're safe just because you try to avoid intense sunlight.

Spot Fader

Spots can pop up anywhere your skin has been overexposed to the sun's destructive rays. Some people develop more of these "freckles" than others, getting them on the face, chest, or hands. Traditional herbal blood purifiers are said to clear the skin of blemishes and spots. To try one, make a batch of this terrific tea.

Dried burdock
Dried dandelion root
Dried yellow dock
Honey
Lemon
1 cup of boiling water

➡ Mix equal parts of the herbs, and steep 1 tablespoon of the mixture in the water for 20 minutes. Strain and then drink, adding honey and lemon to taste. Drink a cup or two every day, and you'll soon say good-bye to age spots.

Flower Face Wash

■ Elderflowers, known for keeping complexions free and clear of unsightly blemishes, have their origins in folk medicine and are still used today in many commercial skin creams. Make your own elderflower water by steeping 1 ounce of fresh elderflowers in 1 pint of distilled water overnight. Strain, and use the mixture as a wash following your daily cleansing regimen. Refrigerated, the solution will keep for four to five days. Then whip up a fresh batch so you can keep up the age-defying routine.

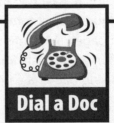

Dial a Doc

Most age spots are harmless, but always examine them carefully to be sure they're not skin cancer. If a spot enlarges, changes color or shape, bleeds, itches, or thickens, have your doctor check it out right away. Remember the easy ABCD test of melanoma: A is for asymmetry (both halves of the spot should match), B is for border (the spot should not have irregular edges), C is for color (they should be the same color all over), and D is for diameter (it shouldn't be larger than the head of a pencil eraser). If any of these don't seem right, see your doctor immediately!

Halitosis Helper

Got dinosaur breath? Does your bed partner stuff his or her head under the pillow when you lean over for a good morning smooch? In either case, you need help! Good old peroxide is great for curing bad breath, and this recipe couldn't be any easier.

Hydrogen peroxide
Water
Flavored oil (optional)

➥ Mix equal parts of hydrogen peroxide and water in a cup, and swish it in your mouth. Do not swallow it! Spit it out and rinse your mouth again with cool water. If the taste of hydrogen peroxide doesn't suit you, add a drop or two of your favorite flavored oil, like peppermint.

An Apple a Day

■ An apple a day not only will keep the doctor away, but it will keep bad breath at bay as well. In fact, an apple is a great remedy for garlic breath. In a healthy mouth, garlic odor usually goes away after a while, but you'll speed up the process if you dilute the pungent aroma by eating an apple, and then brushing your teeth.

Brush Up on Your Oral Hygiene

■ Are you brushing your teeth twice a day with a soft brush? And are you brushing for at least two minutes each time? The bedtime brushing is important, so plaque doesn't form during the night (when saliva production is off-duty). Massage your gums with the brush, too, and gently brush your tongue. And before you brush, floss. Flossing every day helps remove plaque—and odor-causing bacteria—from between your teeth.

Nifty, Thrifty Tips

Here's a cheap and easy way to make mouthwash at home to help handle your bad breath. Stir 1 teaspoon of myrrh tincture into ¼ cup of water. Gargle, swish it around, spit, and you're good to go!

Myrrhvelously Sage Mouthwash

While you're sleeping, your saliva production factory is off-line. Busy little bacteria take over, multiply, and form plaque. A few hours later, you wake up with real roadkill breath. Try this herbal mixture to fight the bacteria, protect tissues, and prevent infection.

5 drops of calendula tincture
5 drops of myrrh tincture
5 drops of sage tincture

➡ Add the tinctures to a small amount of warm water, and swish the mixture in your mouth for several minutes two to three times a day. Then when you're sleeping, you'll be armed with a serious bacteria buster!

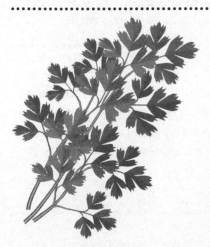

Chew on a Few Leaves

■ Some Native American traditions use spearmint or bergamot leaves as a quick and easy digestive aid and breath freshener. If you want to try it, chew a leaf or two slowly. Then make a cup of mild mint rinse by steeping three leaves in a cup of hot water, letting it cool, and using it as a gargle, rinse, or spray. You can also carry a sandwich bag of mint or parsley leaves to chew on throughout the day.

EUREKA!

MOST BAD BREATH comes from the wet, boggy areas in the back of your mouth, where bacteria like to breed a sulfur-smelling plaque on your tongue. To clear it out, reach into your mouth as far as you can go without gagging, before brushing, and scrape away the plaque. Plastic tongue scrapers are available at most pharmacies, or you can simply use your toothbrush. You should also brush your tongue whenever you brush your teeth.

Red Pepper Mouthwash

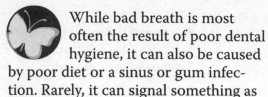 While bad breath is most often the result of poor dental hygiene, it can also be caused by poor diet or a sinus or gum infection. Rarely, it can signal something as serious as kidney failure, liver disease, or diabetes. But if you know that it's just bacteria, then kill your dragon breath with cayenne's fire power. Cayenne not only kills germs, but it leaves your breath feeling spicy fresh, too!

5 to 10 drops of cayenne tincture
5 to 10 drops of myrrh tincture
½ glass of warm water

➡ Dilute both tinctures in the water. Take a swig of this fiery drink, swish it around your mouth (or gargle if you'd like), and spit it out. Your mouth will feel great, and be in fine fettle to keep bacteria at bay for a while.

Wash Out Your Mouth . . .

■ But unless you deserve it, not with soap! Instead, use an antiseptic mouthwash that kills bacteria. Other mouthwashes just mask odor with a minty solution, but some can be quite pleasant and long lasting. Try making your own odor-masking mouthwash by steeping a couple of whole or ground cloves in hot water. Let it cool, then swish the mouth odor away.

Snappy Solutions

You can cut off bad breath problems long before they start by eating your veggies. Vegetables and fruits not only are valuable sources of vitamins and antioxidants, but they also contain chlorophyll, a natural deodorant that sweetens your breath. If you can, eat five to nine servings a day for a healthy body and healthy breath, too. And while you're at it, throw in some sour foods, like pickles and lemons. They will jump-start the flow of saliva, which helps flush away those nasty halitosis-causing bacteria in your mouth.

Spicy Breath Spray

The power of hot spice is extremely potent for killing bad breath because many bacteria (including those that cause halitosis) can't handle heat. So try this spicy mixer to kick those bacteria to the curb and keep your breath smelling sweet and fresh.

¼ cup of vodka
5 drops of cinnamon oil
5 drops of clove oil
5 drops of orange oil
¼ cup of water

➡ Mix all of the ingredients together, and pour the solution into a dark-colored glass bottle that's got a sprayer top. Shake well before using. When you feel as though your breath could use a little extra jolt (or you just feel like refreshing it), spritz a couple of sprays into the back of your mouth and you'll feel the spice kick into action.

Don't Suck on Lemon Drops

■ Lemon-flavored drops may seem like they'd be good breath fresheners, but they're actually highly acidic and create a haven for halitosis. So stick with mint, which is always a safe (and best) bet as a halitosis helper.

But Do Suck on Lemons

■ Lemons, on the other hand, are a great remedy for bad breath because they boost the flow of saliva and help flush away odor-causing germs. Simply squeeze the juice of half a lemon into ½ cup of water, swish it around, and spit it out.

EUREKA!

REGULAR SPRITZING WITH a saline nasal spray helps thin out mucus from postnasal drip and keeps it from collecting on the back of your tongue. If you don't thin it out, bacteria use this protein-rich gunk to make smelly sulfur molecules that leave a sour taste in your mouth. Make your own nasal spray by dissolving ½ teaspoon of table salt in a glass of warm water, placing it in a bulb syringe, and spraying it into each nostril.

Splendid Spice Mix

Here's a cleansing and refreshing mixture that will clear up bad breath while brightening teeth, and it makes a fine gargle and mouthwash. You can use this tooth powder daily, or alternate it with your favorite commercial brand.

1 tbsp. of baking soda
½ tsp. of powdered allspice
½ tsp. of ground sage
½ tsp. of sea salt or kosher salt

➡ In a small dish, combine all of these ingredients. Then sprinkle this well-blended mixture onto your toothbrush and brush, or stir 1 teaspoon of the combo into 1 cup of warm water and gargle with it. Whichever method you choose to use, your mouth will certainly feel cleaner and smell much better in no time flat.

Drink Lots of Water

■ Keeping yourself well hydrated is a good health practice in general, and especially important to help prevent bad breath. So drink eight glasses of water a day to keep saliva production going, which will reduce bacteria buildup.

Seedy Relief

■ Chewing fennel or dill seeds after meals will help freshen your breath and promote healthy digestion. So munch a bunch of either when your dinner is done, and your bad breath worries will be history.

What Would Grandma Do?

I USED TO GO THROUGH TOOTHPASTE like it was candy when I was little. Of course, most of it ended up in the sink. Grandma couldn't always get to the store to buy some more, so she'd whip up some of her own at home. All you do is add a few drops of hydrogen peroxide to baking soda to make an effective toothpaste. Just don't expect it to taste good while you brush, although afterward your mouth will be wonderfully fresh and clean.

Hurry the Healing Paste

Big blisters sometimes take a long time to heal, but there are ways you can help speed up the process. Using this potent but gentle fixer is one of the best. The key ingredient, yarrow, naturally draws out the fluid, allowing the blister to decrease in size more quickly.

Yarrow (either fresh or dried)
Water
Adhesive or gauze bandage

➡ Chop the yarrow (available at health-food stores) as finely as you can, then add water to make a paste. Apply the paste to the blister, and cover with an adhesive or gauze bandage. Replace it daily until the blister is gone.

Let It Breathe

■ Even though it's good to protect a blister with a bandage, you want to expose it to the air for at least 20 minutes a day. A little air circulation will help protect the area from infection-causing bacteria, which thrive in dark, moist places.

Comfrey Comfort

■ Ointments that contain comfrey root promote speedy healing. If you're going to try it on open, inflamed blisters, add a pinch of powdered goldenseal or echinacea to the ointment to prevent infection and soothe irritated tissues.

Snappy Solutions

Like most problems in life, blisters can be a lot easier—and less time-consuming—to head off than to cope with after they've appeared. They're most likely to develop if your feet are too sweaty or your skin is too dry. If your socks are often soggy, the origin of your blister problem may be that sweaty skin. So try sprinkling a little cornstarch into your socks before you put them on, and dust some between your toes, too. On the other hand, if the skin on your feet is very dry, apply a thin film of petroleum jelly to it before you pull on your socks and sneakers.

Infection Fighter

If you're worried about a blister becoming infected, you can reduce that risk with these two herbs, which are probably the strongest antiseptic herbs in your kitchen. Try this fantastic fixer on your next blister; you'll be glad you did!

1 tbsp. of dried rosemary
1 tbsp. of dried thyme
1 cup of hot water

➡ Add each herb to the water, and steep for about 10 minutes. Let the liquid cool to room temperature, pour some on a cloth, and hold it against your blister for about 20 minutes. You can repeat the treatment once or twice a day until the blister is gone.

Catch 'Em Quick

■ Before a blister appears, you'll usually notice a hot spot—a red, tender area on your skin. Fast action at this stage may prevent a blister from forming. If you've had a burn, quickly apply ice to the area and keep it there for about 20 minutes. If the hot spot was caused by friction, cushion the area with moleskin, gauze, or other padding. Replace the padding frequently, before it thins out and stops doing its job.

Wash Away the Germs

■ The best way to keep infection-causing germs out of blisters is to clean them (and the surrounding skin) once or twice a day. Wash the area well, but gently, with soap and water, then dry it thoroughly. This step is important because too much moisture will soften the blister and make it more likely to break open before it's ready.

✚ The persistence of one or more blisters, swelling, inflammation, or bleeding can be a sign of infection, and you should see a doctor. And if a blister is accompanied by fever or other symptoms of infection, call your doctor immediately.

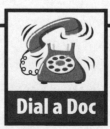

Dial a Doc

Tan Your Hide

Tannins are compounds that are present in many plants and trees. They are especially good at strengthening skin. To make your skin stronger and prevent blisters, soak your hands and/or feet in this tannin-rich infusion.

Black tea
Oak bark
Pine twigs

➡ Soak a handful of the tea, bark, and twigs in a basin of boiling water. When the water cools down, strain the infusion, and soak your hands and/or feet for 10 to 15 minutes. Repeat this treatment weekly to keep your skin in tip-top shape. **Caution:** If you have diabetes, check with your doctor before soaking your feet in anything.

Lace Up Right

■ When putting on running or other sports shoes, be sure to lace them up properly so your foot is held firmly in place. Otherwise, your foot will rub around against the inside of the shoe, and soon enough, you'll have a painful blister or two.

Lose the Shoes

■ Some athletes, especially runners, like to toughen up their feet by going barefoot as often as possible. If this sounds appealing to you, try running barefoot on the beach or in a grassy field for 10 to 15 minutes after your regularly scheduled workout. That should do the trick.

EUREKA!

ONE OF THE BIGGEST CAUSES OF BLISTERS is friction against your feet. To reduce the rubbing, try this two-part friction fighter. First, apply a commercial friction-reducing gel, such as Hydropel®, to your feet. Then wear silk or fine-cotton sock liners under your regular socks for smoother movement. You can find sock liners at most sporting goods stores.

Calendula Cream

Native Americans have long relied on calendula to freshen skin because of its mild, pleasing fragrance and skin-soothing minerals. A cream made from the flower's essential oil absorbs well into the skin, and keeps you smelling great all day long.

½ oz. of beeswax
½ oz. of cocoa butter
1 tbsp. of glycerin
1 tbsp. of rose water
3 to 4 drops of calendula oil

➡ Melt the beeswax and cocoa butter together in a double boiler, stirring occasionally. Add the glycerin, rose water, and calendula oil, and stir to blend completely. Store the cream in a glass jar with a lid. The cream may separate between uses, but that doesn't affect its potency. Just mix it around in the jar before applying it to your underarms.

De-Stink the Sweat

■ Normally, sweat is odor-free because it's composed primarily of electrolytes and salts. The odor comes when perspiration mixes with the bacteria, yeast, and fungi that thrive in the damper, hairier regions of your body. If you've washed these areas with a mild antibacterial soap and you still smell funky, you may have excess protein in your diet. Try limiting foods such as fish, garlic, cumin, and curry, which contain protein oils that linger in the body's secretions.

✚ Like fatty, sugary, low-fiber foods, antibiotics can upset the pH balance in your intestines, inhibit your digestion, and increase body odor. But they aren't the only pharmaceutical offenders. Betaine (Cystadane), which removes excess homocysteine from the blood; bupropion (Wellbutrin) and venlafaxine (Effexor), which are prescribed for depression; and pilocarpine (Salagen), which is used to treat dry mouth, can all raise a stink. If you suspect that medications you're taking may be the root of your trouble, talk to your doctor.

Dial a Doc

Chlorophyll Cleansing Tonic

Aren't you glad we're not living back when people bathed once a week—or less frequently—and masked their body odor with heavy perfumes, powdered wigs, and lots of rarely washed clothes? I sure am. Whee-ew! If you're having a problem with odor, try taking chlorophyll, which is a potent odor eliminator.

> **Juice of 1 lemon**
> **1 tsp. of chlorophyll**
> **1 glass of water**

➡ First thing each morning, drink a glass of water with the lemon juice and chlorophyll stirred into it. This will help cleanse your system from the inside out. While you may not start smelling like a rose, you'll certainly stop smelling like sweat and dirt (or whatever your own personal odor is).

Natural Neutralizers

■ If foot odor is your particular stinkeroo, then the next time you buy deodorant, pick up one of these natural odor neutralizers, too: sage, tea tree, or green clay. Sprinkle your choice in your shoes, and you'll say *sayonara* to smelly dogs.

Eat Sweet

■ Some body odor is caused by what you eat. The infamous smells of garlic and onions can come right through your pores. But there's no need to boycott these favorites. Just neutralize their potent aromas by also eating parsley and other leafy green vegetables that contain chlorophyll. If you keep it up, you'll notice a difference in just a few short days.

What Would Grandma Do?

🦋 As I started to hit puberty, *my pits got up and running like nobody's business, so Grandma Putt had to get a remedy ready in a hurry before she let me back in the house! She made me drink a lot of water to flush the bacteria out of my system—eight glasses to be exact. And she'd always squeeze some fresh lemon in there because the juice helped clear the bad stuff out of my system more quickly.*

Cream Deodorant

 Our bodies need to sweat to regulate temperature, but perspiration's not the problem—it's nearly odorless water. The odor comes from the presence of bacteria and fungi in the sweaty areas. If you're noticing an odor of your very own, this simple mixer will keep you feeling as fresh and dry as any store-bought brand.

2 tbsp. of baby powder
2 tbsp. of baking soda
2 tbsp. of petroleum jelly

➡ Combine all of the ingredients in a pan, and place them over low heat until the mixture is smooth and creamy. Store it in an airtight container. Dab some under your arms before you go out each morning.

Add Some Alfalfa

■ To deodorize your body along with your breath, drink up to 3 cups of alfalfa tea daily. Steep 1 heaping teaspoon of dried alfalfa in 1 cup of hot water for 10 minutes. Or take alfalfa tablets, which are available at health-food stores. **Caution:** Don't take alfalfa if you are pregnant, nursing, or on blood-thinning therapy (e.g., warfarin).

Clean Up Your Digestion

■ Just as old garbage can stink up your whole house, the odor from decaying matter in your intestines can radiate throughout your body. For starters, cut back on red meat, which can sometimes create a foul odor. Beef protein is harder for your gut to break down, and the more food hangs around, the more smelly bacterial by-products will hang around, too.

EUREKA!

SPLASHING SOME RUBBING ALCOHOL under your arms may reduce the bacteria population and eliminate a smelly situation. For a persistent odor problem, try using alcohol in place of deodorant—just not after shaving or if you have any nicks or cuts in your skin. That'll sting like crazy!

Dust-Well Dusting Powder

Those busy little odor-causing bacteria love to get between your toes, into your armpits, and on your private parts. Clothes can also get pretty smelly from the stale perspiration they absorb if they're not washed often enough. Here's a dusting powder that'll help keep odors at bay and your feet feeling fresh.

➡ Combine all of the ingredients in a bowl. Then sprinkle the mixture on your feet before slipping them into your socks and shoes, rub some under your arms, or dust you know where. It'll help keep you dry all day long while you go about your business.

2 parts dried calendula flowers
1 part aluminum-free baking soda
1 part dried lavender flowers
1 part dried slippery elm

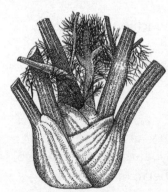

Feel Fresh with Fennel

■ Fennel tea makes a sweet post-meal drink, especially if you've had garlic, onions, or other smelly foods that not only cause bad breath, but may also cause odor to pour from your pores. Make the tea by steeping 1 heaping teaspoon of fennel seeds in 1 cup of hot water for 10 minutes. Fennel is such an excellent natural deodorizer that Indian restaurants often offer fennel seeds instead of after-dinner mints.

Nifty, Thrifty Tips

Here's one of the best ways to eliminate body odor and eliminate a big hurt on your wallet. Just cut back on coffee. You probably already know that odorous oils in garlic, onions, fish, and exotic spices can linger in your body, but coffee and tea are also bad news because they increase the activity of the sweat glands. Try doing without these offenders and see if the foul funk doesn't fade fast.

Flower Powder

We've all had occasions when no matter how frequently or ferociously we've scrubbed, we still smell more foul than fresh, and the lingering odor has turned our favorite sweaters into instant castoffs. This powdered flower fixer can help absorb even the toughest odors.

Powdered calendula flowers
Powdered lavender flowers
Slippery elm powder

➡ Mix together equal parts of the powdered flowers, and add them to an equal part of slippery elm powder. Dust under your arms once or twice daily, and your odor will be gone. You'll smell fresh and clean, and everyone (yourself included) will thank you for it!

Carve That Jack-o'-Lantern

■ A deficiency of zinc can prompt body odor, so start munching on pumpkin seeds, which provide a good, concentrated source of the mineral. If you're not keen on the seeds, take a zinc supplement daily to help reduce body and foot odor—but not without your doctor's guidance.

Load Up on Yogurt

■ The best way to control odor-causing "bad" bacteria in your gut is to fill it with "good" bacteria. You can accomplish this by eating yogurt that contains live, active cultures of *Lactobacillus acidophilus*. Check the label to make sure, and remember that frozen yogurt and yogurt-covered snacks don't contain any live, active cultures.

Nifty, Thrifty Tips

The easiest thing you can do to help cure your bad body odor is to try your fridge's best friend. That's right—the handy helper in the bright orange box. Baking soda keeps your fridge odor-free, so why not you, too? You can use it as a dusting powder or body rub, or sprinkle a handful in your bath.

Inside-Out Cleaner

Your skin is your largest organ and, therefore, an important player in the elimination of toxins. Body odor can sometimes be the result of sluggish or poor elimination. If that's the case, use these gentle herbs, fresh or dried, to help clean your body on the inside.

Calendula
Cleavers
Peppermint
Red clover
Yarrow
1 qt. of warm water

➡ Combine equal parts of the herbs, and steep 1 heaping tablespoon of the mixture in the water for 15 minutes. Strain out the solids and drink the tea throughout the day. Your body will start to be cleaned quickly, and you should notice a difference in how you feel right away.

Change Deodorants Periodically

■ After years of use, your regular deodorant may no longer work as well as it used to. It may have been altered, your own body chemistry may be changing, or you may simply have developed a tolerance for the brand. If so, then try another—change is good! If you get a rash from one deodorant, try one that's designed for sensitive skin. And you may want to look for a plain deodorant because antiperspirants contain aluminum hydrochloride, which can be a skin irritant.

Q: *I feel suffocated by the things I wear. But I like my style and don't want to change it. What can I do to feel better in what I wear?*

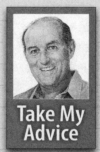

Take My Advice

A: Simple—wear clothes that breathe. Polyester and most synthetic fabrics keep odors close to your body. Cotton, silk, and some of the new wicking fabrics designed for athletes allow moisture to circulate, so it won't cling to your body or clothing. Try a sports-supply or camping store for lightweight wicking underwear.

Odor-Killing Herbal Swipe

The culprits of body odor are bacteria that thrive on skin. When they devour the fatty sweat produced by the apocrine glands in the underarms, scalp, and genitals, the result is a very pungent smell. But these ordinary cooking herbs can help solve your odor problem lickety-split. Try 'em—you'll like 'em!

1 tbsp. of ground rosemary
1 tbsp. of ground sage
1 cup of baking soda

➡ Mix the herbs with the baking soda, and swipe some of the resulting mixture under your arms. The herbs are a dynamite odor-fighting duo—the piney rosemary has natural antibacterial properties, while the tangy-smelling sage contains compounds that can fight odor-causing bacteria.

Freshen Up with Juice

■ Using a juicer is a great way to get a variety of chlorophyll-rich foods, such as kale, chard, and other dark green vegetables, all in one shot. Chlorophyll can restore the pH balance of blood that's too acidic—and therefore too friendly to bad bacteria—due to a diet that's heavy on meat and other proteins.

Sip Some Sage

■ Sage tea can help curb sweat gland activity and may be especially helpful when your perspiration is stress induced. To make the tea, steep 2 teaspoons of dried sage in 1 cup of boiling water for 10 minutes, strain, then savor it in small doses—but only during tense situations. **Caution:** Regularly ingesting sage may cause dizziness, hot flashes, and other problems. Don't drink sage tea if you're pregnant or nursing.

✚ Keep in mind that strong body odor can sometimes be a sign of a serious medical condition or skin infection. So call your doctor if an unusual odor permeates your skin, despite your best attempts to get rid of it.

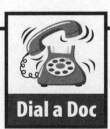

Dial a Doc

Sage Spritz

Body odor is no laughing matter. It can make you repulsive to those around you and can even get so bad that you start to smell it yourself. That's when you know it's time to make a change. To banish body odor of any kind, try this combination of essential oils that make a lovely spray.

**5 drops of coriander oil
5 drops of lavender oil
5 drops of sage oil
2 oz. of distilled witch hazel**

➡ Add each of the oils to the witch hazel in a sprayer bottle. Shake well, then spritz away. You can find the herbal oils at most health-food stores. Witch hazel is a great source of tannic acid, which helps close the pores of the sweat glands and starve odor-causing bacteria.

Get Sweaty

■ Encouraging sweating—say, by sitting in a sauna—can help detoxify your system, keep your liver and gastrointestinal tract functioning at optimal levels, and diminish body odor. So when you work out, don't be afraid to sweat.

Run Off Athlete's Foot

■ You can stamp out smelly athlete's foot fungus by soaking your feet in a basin of warm water that's been spiked with 2 to 3 teaspoons of tea tree oil. Soak them for 15 minutes twice daily. While you're doing this, go barefoot or wear open-toed shoes as often as possible. And when you have to, change into clean socks several times a day.

What Would Grandma Do?

WHENEVER MY FEET STARTED TO STINK, Grandma Putt would turn to a tried-and-true method for getting rid of the reek: vinegar. Just soak your smelly feet in a solution of 1 part vinegar and 1 part warm water for 10 minutes twice a day for three weeks. The sour vinegar soak will make your stinky feet smell good!

Spray Deodorant

Aside from general odor that makes you feel like you need to rub deodorant all over your body, your odor may be due to some sort of infection. Odds are that your natural scent has just turned somewhat sour. Here's a fast-acting spray deodorant you can use anytime you need a little body boost.

½ cup of witch hazel
2 tbsp. of vodka
1 tbsp. of glycerin
½ tsp. of liquid chlorophyll

➥ Mix the ingredients together, and pour the solution into a sprayer bottle. Take the bottle along with you anywhere you think you'll need it. You can also keep one in your desk drawer or in your car for the long day ahead. Just spritz the deodorizer under your arms morning, noon, and night.

Go for the Stone

■ If you're going through deodorants and antiperspirants like there's no tomorrow, consider trading your stick for a stone—a crystal deodorant stone, that is. Not only will one stone last a lot longer than a standard stick, it may be much kinder to your system. Standard antiperspirants contain aluminum hydrochloride, which completely plugs up the sweat glands; crystal stones contain alunogenite, a natural astringent that may only partially block the glands. You'll find deodorant stones at your local health-food store.

EUREKA!

UNCOOKED VEGGIES AND FRUITS provide roughage that helps escort smelly waste through—and out of—your intestinal tract. Cooked foods, on the other hand, are much slower moving through your intestines. And when you cook foods, you change their oxidation, which can prompt more odor during digestion. So when you take a carrot out of the fridge, wash it, peel it, and eat it as is!

Bunion Buster

A bunion is simply a protruding bump of tissue on the joint of the big toe. Wearing shoes with insufficient toe room forces the big toes to angle toward the other toes, and an unsightly bunion is the result. The next time your bunions are barking, stop at a health-food store and get these ingredients for a soothing herbal fixer.

6 parts dried comfrey root
6 parts dried oak bark
3 parts dried marshmallow root
3 parts dried mullein
3 parts dried walnut bark
2 parts dried wormwood
1 part dried lobelia
1 part dried skullcap
Olive oil
Beeswax

➥ Put the herbs in a double boiler, add enough olive oil to cover them, and cook for one to two hours. Strain out the herbs and throw them on your compost pile. Add an equal amount of beeswax to the oil and store the mixture in an ointment jar with a tight-fitting lid. Apply it daily whenever the bunions on your feet are hurting.

Ease the Pressure

■ Surround a burgeoning bunion with an OTC doughnut-shaped moleskin or a gel-filled pad to reduce pressure and friction from shoes. Check your drugstore or supermarket for protective pads impregnated with anti-inflammatory medicines. They'll deliver first aid to your bunion as they cushion it.

Snappy Solutions

The main cause of bunion pain, and the one thing that always makes it worse, is wearing shoes that don't fit. Shoving your foot into a poorly fitting shoe literally changes the shape of your foot. So to save yourself the time and hassle of dealing with bunions, always have your feet measured when you buy new shoes. And avoid narrow styles with pointy toes. You want shoes that are wide enough for your feet to slip into comfortably, preferably with a flat or low heel.

Bunion-Soothing Footbath

Comfrey contains chemical compounds that soothe away bunion pain fast. To make an excellent elixir for your tender tootsies, just follow this easy recipe. Then soak your feet for sweet relief.

1 oz. of dried comfrey leaves (available at health-food stores)
2 to 3 cups of water

➥ Heat the water until it's simmering, add the comfrey, and continue to simmer for 10 minutes. Add enough cool water to make the temperature comfortable, pour the water into a basin, and soak your sore feet for 20 minutes or so.

Rub Out Pain

■ Massage is excellent for reducing bunion pain, and you'll get even better results when you combine it with a soothing bath. The next time you're in the tub, lather your hands with soap. Slip your fingers between the toes of one foot and gently reach around to massage the bottom of your foot. Bend your ankle while you rub so your foot moves in every direction. Then do the same thing with your other foot. You may be a little sore the first few times you do it, but after that, your bunions should start feeling a whole lot better.

Head to the Shore

■ Your feet might benefit from a trip to the beach as much as you do. Walking barefoot in the sand is a great way to strengthen your feet and make them less sensitive to bunion pain.

Nifty, Thrifty Tips

If your big toe is starting to drift and a bunion is sprouting, a toe spacer, available for just a few bucks at drugstores, can encourage your big toes to maintain their proper position and relieve the pressure while you're wearing shoes. Start with a small spacer and gradually use wider ones until your toe feels comfortable.

Anti-Cellulite Wrap

You can work out every day to look and feel terrific. But some cellulite seems to linger no matter what, and it's a pain in the you know what. Here's an anti-cellulite mixer made with grapefruit juice that works just like the ones used in fancy spas.

1½ cups of fresh
    grapefruit juice
1 cup of corn oil
2 tsp. of dried thyme

➡ Combine the ingredients in a bowl, then massage the mixture into your hips, thighs, and buttocks, and cover the areas with plastic wrap. Hold a heating pad over each section for five minutes or so. Repeat this treatment every day, and you'll take care of the cellulite, and prevent any more from showing up.

Kick It with Coffee

■ If you're concerned about cellulite on your hips and thighs, wake up and smell the coffee! Then (after you've drunk a cup or two), let the grounds cool off, and rub them onto your problem areas. Believe it or not, they contain the same active ingredient—caffeine—as most commercial cellulite creams!

Work It Out

■ Some experts say that exercise will put a layer of muscle under the fat on your thighs and legs. With more exercise, eventually the muscle can replace the fat altogether. So work out every day with a brisk walk, jog, or bike ride to firm up the muscles in your hips, thighs, and buttocks.

EUREKA!

THE EASIEST WAY to get rid of that nagging cellulite is to change your diet. Try eating fruits and raw vegetables instead of sugary snacks. And stop eating foods that are high in fats or have too much salt. Also, drink lots of water to clean out your system, flush out toxins, and eventually eliminate cellulite altogether.

Farewell, Cellulite Massage Oil

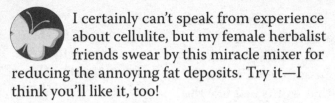 I certainly can't speak from experience about cellulite, but my female herbalist friends swear by this miracle mixer for reducing the annoying fat deposits. Try it—I think you'll like it, too!

**3 tsp. of almond oil
2 drops of fennel oil
2 drops of rosemary oil**

➡ Blend the essential oils thoroughly and massage them into the problem areas once a day. Before long, those unsightly bumps will vanish.

Brush, Brush, and Brush Some More

■ As often as you can, brush your skin using a soft brush, a massage glove, or a rough sisal mitt. It doesn't matter whether your skin is wet or dry, but always brush in long, sweeping strokes over the afflicted area, working in the direction of your heart.

Vim and Vinegar

■ My Grandma Putt never heard the word *cellulite*, but she was just about the biggest booster apple cider vinegar ever had. I know that if she would've had to battle the little bulges, she'd use this fabulous fixer: Just mix 3 parts apple cider vinegar with 1 part of your favorite massage oil, and gently knead the solution into the affected areas twice a day.

What Would Grandma Do?

🦋 MEDICAL SCIENCE *has proven what Grandma Putt always knew—that stress (or getting all hot and bothered, as she put it) is bad for your health. So do your body a favor: Don't let yourself fly into a tizzy over a few fat deposits. Just get plenty of fresh air and exercise, eat sensibly, and use whatever de-stressing techniques work best for you. Before long, you may find that while you're busy enjoying life, your cellulite melts away all by itself.*

Invincible Ivy Paste

If you've got ground ivy growing in your yard, you have an endless supply of a first-class cellulite fighter. Put your prunings to good use with this marvelous mixer.

1 handful of ground ivy leaves
20 drops of chamomile oil
Gauze bandage or soft cotton cloth

➡ Crush the ground ivy leaves, mix them with the oil to make a paste, and spread it on the bandage or cloth. Rub the affected area with hot water and a brush or massage mitt. Dry your skin, apply the bandage, secure it with tape, and leave it on for three to four hours. Repeat the treatment two or three times a week until you see the results you want.

Pick the Plant Kingdom

■ When you're shopping for commercial anti-cellulite creams, choose ones that have botanical ingredients at the top of the ingredient listings. Ground ivy, barley, sweet clover, lemon, strawberry, fennel, and coconut oil are especially effective in helping reduce the unsightly fat deposits.

Lemon Aid with a Kick

■ Looking for a drinkable fixer for cellulite? Try this: Squeeze a fresh lemon, pour the juice into a glass of water, and add a pinch of cayenne pepper. Give it a stir and drink up. Three glasses a day could make your cellulite melt away.

Snappy Solutions

No *matter what anti-cellulite preparation you use, you can double its potency—and therefore decrease the time it takes to see results—with one simple step: Massage the stuff into your skin thoroughly with your fingertips. That's because, if truth be told, the massaging action is more effective than any fixer, mixer, or elixir you can find, whether it's commercial or homemade.*

Baby Bath Formula

Babies require extra-special care, especially when it comes to washing them. Every ounce of their bodies is fragile and requires a soft, soothing touch. Whenever one of her young friends had a baby, my Grandma Putt gave her a jar or two of this extra-gentle bath mixer.

¼ cup of dry buttermilk
¼ cup of nonfat dry milk
1 tbsp. of cornstarch

➡ Combine all of the ingredients, and put the mixture in a covered glass jar. When baby's bath time rolls around, pour 1 tablespoon of the powder into a baby bathtub, or ¼ cup into a full-size tub. He or she will love it!

So Long, Stuffy Nose

■ For a toddler, a stuffy nose is pure misery. To unclog that tiny sniffer, dissolve ¼ teaspoon of salt in 8 ounces of water, and insert 2 drops of the solution into each nostril, using a medicine dropper. Then use a suction bulb to draw out the saline and mucus. Repeat as needed up to six times a day.

No More Hard Knocks

■ Help guard the toddlers in your life from bumps, bruises, and cuts by covering chair and table legs with foam pipe insulation. Just cut it to the right length, and slip it around the leg. If the stuff won't stay put, secure it with electrical tape.

Q: *My baby has just started to crawl, and he goes so fast and comes down so hard that his poor little knees take a pounding. Do have any ideas for cushioning the blow?*

A: I sure do! Just cut the tops off a pair of child's tube-type socks, and use them as knee pads for your tiny tyke.

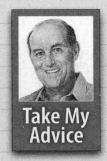

Take My Advice

Bathtub Cookies

These bath-time "cookies" are the perfect bribe for reluctant young bathers. They also make great gifts.

➡ Mix all of the ingredients together to form a dough, roll it out, and cut out shapes with cookie cutters. Bake at 350°F for 10 to 12 minutes. (Don't overbake!) Let the cookies cool completely. To use, just add one or two cookies to the bathwater, and enjoy!

2 cups of fine-grain sea salt*
½ cup of baking soda
½ cup of cornstarch
2 tbsp. of light vegetable oil
1 tsp. of vitamin E oil
1-2 eggs
6 drops of food coloring (optional)
6 drops of scented oil (optional)

* If your supermarket doesn't have fine-grain sea salt, use kosher salt instead, and run it through your blender or coffee grinder.

Hands Off!

◼ Are there small children around your house who can't tell the hot water faucets from the cold ones? You can protect those tiny fingers from burns by marking the hot faucets with red nail polish. Of course, make sure the youngsters know those marks mean "Don't touch!"

'Til the Tooth Fairy Comes

◼ It's easy for us grown-ups to forget how scary it can be to lose your first baby tooth and see the blood flow out of your mouth. But you can stop the flow and set the youngster's mind at ease the old-fashioned way. Just roll a moist tea bag into a tight cylinder, and hold it on the spot where the tooth used to be.

Snappy Solutions

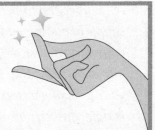

Fresh out of baby powder? Don't rush out to the store and buy some. Reach for the cornstarch instead—it makes a perfect substitute in a pinch.

Bombastic Bubble Solution

Have you ever known a baby who was not entranced by the sight of pretty bubbles floating through the air? I sure haven't! That's why, at my house, we make a never-ending supply for visiting tykes by using this simple recipe.

2 parts dishwashing liquid
1 part vegetable oil
2 parts water

➡ Mix the ingredients together in a shallow bowl or tub. Then dip your bubble blower into the fabulous fluid, and make marvelous bubbles.

Nifty Needle Relief

■ Sometimes I think that to infants and toddlers, life must seem like one round of shots after another. After your baby's next vaccination, comfort the "victim" by applying a cool, wet tea bag to the scene of the "crime."

Don't Give Boots the Boot!

■ New baby on the way? If you have a cat and are worried about allergies, you may not need to give up your precious pet, as was once widely recommended. Studies reveal that early exposure to a cat, and therefore its dander, may actually protect children from developing a feline allergy. That's because the dander works like a vaccine, helping the immune system build up resistance so it's less likely to react to the allergen.

Snappy Solutions

As any parent knows (and anyone who was once a kid remembers), summertime seems to deliver a constant supply of bumps, bug bites, and sunburn. So be prepared to supply first aid with one simple fixer: Pick up some aloe vera gel at the drugstore, squeeze it into an ice cube tray, and stash it in the freezer. Then, the next time your youngster lingers too long in the sun or winds up on the wrong end of a stinging insect, pull out a cube and deliver instant relief.

Colic Remedy

 Few babies—or parents—escape the misery of colic. Dill and savory are classic tummy-trouble tamers, and both are gentle enough for infants and toddlers.

> 1 tsp. of dill seed
> 1 tsp. of powdered savory
> 6 oz. of water or infant formula

➡ Bruise the dill seed with the back of a spoon. In a pan, heat the water or formula to about 100°F. Stir in the dill and savory. Remove the pan from the heat, and let it sit for 10 minutes. To use the remedy right away, reheat it to 100°F—no hotter; it should be warm, not hot. If you plan to serve the elixir later, put it in the refrigerator immediately, and use it (reheated) within three hours. Discard any unused portion that's older than that. For infants over 2 months old, use a dropper and give 5 to 10 drops; for toddlers, 30 drops or ½ teaspoon.

Relax Already!

■ Very often, colic is a baby's way of responding to what he perceives as a stressful environment. If that's the case with your little one, you may have a super-simple fixer for a highly annoying problem. What is it? Just make sure mealtimes are quiet and peaceful affairs. Turn off the TV or radio news and talk shows, or your favorite contemporary pop music. Then put some Mozart, Vivaldi, or other soothing classical music into the CD player, and keep the sound low. If you're nursing, drink a cup or two of warm, relaxing herbal tea before you start "serving." Chances are you'll find that you and your child will rest a whole lot easier.

What Would Grandma Do?

🦋 WHENEVER YOU BATHE AN INFANT, *do what Grandma always did: Wear cotton gloves. They'll give you a better grip than you'd have with bare hands, and they'll feel a whole lot better on the baby's tender skin than rubber gloves would.*

Homemade Baby Wipes

Why buy expensive baby wipes when you've probably got everything you need to make your own? Here's how it's done.

➡ Cut the roll of paper towels in half with a serrated knife, and remove the cardboard tube. Place half the roll, on end, in the plastic container. Mix the liquid ingredients, pour the solution into the container, and close the lid. The towels will absorb the liquid. As you need them, pull the wipes up one by one from the center of the roll.

1 roll of soft, absorbent paper towels (premium brands work best)
1 plastic container with a tight-fitting lid to hold the paper towels
2 tbsp. of baby oil
2 tbsp. of liquid baby bath soap
2 cups of water

Boost Their Brainpower

■ Recent medical research shows that the minute you begin reading to an infant or toddler—even if she can't understand the words—you "turn on" thousands of cells in her growing brain. Existing connections between brain cells grow stronger and new cells form, adding more definition and complexity (a.k.a. brainpower) that will remain largely in place for the rest of the child's life. So start early—even right after birth isn't too young. Although she won't have a clue what you're saying, your baby will enjoy hearing the sound of your voice. Recite nursery rhymes or read simple books using a pleasant, singsong delivery. Then as the baby grows, give her sturdy, colorful, drool-proof books to play with. She'll be hooked on books before she's even out of diapers!

EUREKA!

IF YOU HAVE SMALL CHILDREN or grandchildren who ride their bikes, trikes, or pedal cars in your driveway, here's a super safety tip: Lay an extension ladder across the end of the drive to keep the youngsters from riding into the street.

Classic Anti-Corn-and-Callus Concoction

In my Grandma Putt's day, medical treatment wasn't sophisticated by a long shot. But she and her pals sure had their share of simple—and effective—remedies. When it comes to bidding good-bye to annoying (and often painful) corns and calluses, you can't beat this old-time mixer Grandma used.

2 slices of white bread
2 slices of onion
1 cup of vinegar
(any kind will do)

➡ Soak the bread and onion in the vinegar for 24 hours. Place the bread over the trouble spot, top it with one of the onion slices, wrap the area with a bandage, and leave it on overnight. Repeat as needed until your corn or callus is gone—which shouldn't be too long!

Do the Ol' Soft Shoe

■ Stiff leather shoes may look great, but they don't feel so good when you have corns (small calluses on your toes). The only way to get rid of the corns is to get rid of the friction that causes them. That means wearing shoes made from cloth or soft leather for a few weeks. Sandals are also a good choice (weather permitting), as long as the straps don't rub up against tender skin areas.

Lemon Smoother

■ Lemons help soften calluses. Rub half a lemon on your feet, elbows, and heels, and those rough spots will be smoother before you know it. For corn relief, press a piece of lemon peel, inner side down, to the top of the corn and tape it in place. Leave it on overnight, and repeat the procedure each night for a week.

✚ Calluses are never a medical emergency. But if you have a callus that hurts so much you can hardly stand it, or if it starts to ache or bleed, call your doctor for some relief.

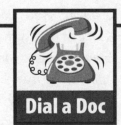

Dial a Doc

Easy Callus Remover

They're not cute, but they're clever. Calluses are your body's way of protecting delicate layers of skin from the effects of heavy pressure or friction. They're areas of thick, dead skin that are usually found on the bottom of your feet and on your fingertips or palms. This mixer will gently remove those annoying calluses wherever they build up.

1 to 2 tbsp. of cornmeal
1 tbsp. of avocado oil
Pinch of kosher salt

➤ Mix the ingredients to form a paste that's got a meal-like texture. Take the mixture in the palm of your hand, and rub both hands together, working the gritty stuff into the calluses and around your fingers. Do the same on your feet and toes. Repeat once or twice a week, and before long, your skin will be smooth and callus-free.

Go Barefootin' at the Beach

■ Those gray, gritty pumice stones we use to sand down our calluses are made of volcanic rock. And while few of us have access to volcano slopes, sand on the beach acts just like a pumice stone—only better! So if you live near a beach, walk in the sand as often as you can, and your feet will feel fabulous.

Snappy Solutions

You can take care of your calluses at home in no time at all with a soothing soak in a pan of water with 1 teaspoon of baking soda added to it. As the callused skin loosens, gently rub it away a bit at a time with a pumice stone or emery board. Follow up with a revitalizing lotion or cream to soften your feet. **Caution:** This remedy is not appropriate for people with diabetes, who may have poor circulation in their feet and thus may injure their skin. If you have diabetes, check with your doctor before soaking your feet in anything.

Fight the Flakes Formula

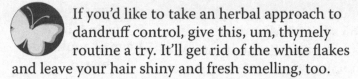

If you'd like to take an herbal approach to dandruff control, give this, um, thymely routine a try. It'll get rid of the white flakes and leave your hair shiny and fresh smelling, too.

Dried thyme leaves
1 qt. of water
Thyme oil
Olive oil

➡ Boil a handful of dried thyme leaves in the water for about five minutes. Strain out the solids and set the liquid aside to cool. Then, about an hour before washing your hair, dab thyme oil diluted in olive oil (4 drops of thyme oil per teaspoon of olive oil) onto your scalp. After shampooing, rinse your hair with the cooled thyme water, and you'll be flake free.

Wash It Daily

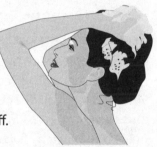

■ It's important to wash your hair every day to break up larger flakes of dandruff, making them less noticeable. Regular cleaning also prevents the buildup of hair spray, gels, and other gooey preparations—some of which can look a lot like dandruff flakes as they wear off.

Serious Medicine

■ For really stubborn dandruff, look for anti-dandruff shampoos containing zinc pyrithione and selenium sulfide—and purchase both. These two minerals scruff up the scalp, initiate cell turnover, and can break cornflake-size flakes into less noticeable ones.

Nifty, Thrifty Tips

When you're choosing a hairdo, you can save yourself a big chunk of change if you use a little common sense. Use only oil-free gels or mousses when styling your hair because greasy hair fixatives can make a dandruff problem worse. Or just skip the gels and hair sprays altogether and go "au naturel." Your wallet will be glad you did!

Homemade Dandruff Shampoo

Ever feel as though you live inside one of those little snow globes? All around you, people might be strolling through spring, summer, or fall—but for you in your dark suit, it's snowing on your shoulders all the time. There are a lot of expensive treatments for dandruff nowadays, but for my money, this easy treatment beats 'em all.

5 aspirin tablets
1 cup of apple cider
  vinegar
⅓ cup of witch hazel

➥ Mash the aspirin tablets and put them in a bottle with the vinegar and witch hazel. Cap the bottle and shake it thoroughly to mix the ingredients. After you shampoo as usual, comb the solution through your hair. Wait 10 minutes, rinse it out with warm water, and say farewell to the flakes!

Squeeze a Lemon

■ One simple way to get rid of dandruff is with a rinse. After shampooing, rinse your hair with ½ cup of lemon juice or vinegar in 1 gallon of water. (The vinegar smell will disappear quickly.) This treatment will leave your hair shiny and squeaky clean. Rinsing with or dabbing these weak acids onto your scalp helps remove itchy flakes, too.

Q: *I use different dandruff-prevention shampoos and conditioners every day to keep flaking in check. But I still find myself with some unsightly dandruff. Is there anything else I can do?*

Take My Advice

A: Depending on your situation, if you're using a hair dryer, it may be time to hang it up. That hot wind really dries out your scalp, making you more vulnerable to developing dandruff. So whenever you can, let your hair dry naturally, rather than blowing it dry. And when you must have extra volume for a special occasion, be sure to use a lower setting.

Steam Cleaner

Most folks shed a dandruff flake or two every now and then, especially in winter, when scalps tend to be drier. More serious dandruff, however, results when tiny oil glands at the base of the hair roots run amok. Steaming the scalp with these nutritive herbs will give you a deep-cleansing treatment to plow away a blizzard of flakes.

Nettles
Peppermint
Rosemary
2 cups of hot water

➡ Mix equal parts of fresh or dried leaves of the ingredients together. (If you're using fresh nettles, be sure to wear gloves while preparing the infusion to avoid getting stung.) Place 2 tablespoons of the dried mixture, or ½ cup of fresh, in the water, and steep, covered, for 10 minutes. Strain the infusion, let it cool slightly, and carefully apply it to your scalp. Cover your hair with a shower cap and wrap your head in a hot towel right out of the dryer. Leave the covering on for 30 minutes, then rinse your hair with warm water.

Flake Out

■ Getting rid of a few flakes can be as simple as changing the way you brush your hair. You should brush from the scalp outward with steady, firm strokes. This carries excess oil away from your scalp (where it can cause dandruff) to the hair strands, where it gives your hair a nice healthy shine.

Hop to It

■ Hops (one of the main ingredients in beer) is an old-time cure for dandruff. To get rid of the flakes, just add a squirt or two of beer to your regular shampoo.

What Would Grandma Do?

🦋 YOU COULDN'T FIND an easier dandruff cure than the one Grandma Putt used to use. Simply pour a tablespoon of salt onto your head, rub it into your scalp, and then shampoo as usual. Those white flakes will vanish like snow falling on warm ground!

All-Faces Mask

Unlike the woman on TV who seems to be best friends with an alligator, most of us hate dry skin. It itches, it looks dull, and living inside it is no fun at all. Here's a mask mixer that works for any skin type—just by altering one ingredient.

¼ cup of nonfat dry milk
1 egg
Juice of 1 lemon
1 tbsp. of whiskey

➡ Mix all of the ingredients together, then smooth the mixture over your face, avoiding the eye area. Let it dry, and remove it with a warm, wet washcloth. Keep the mixture in the refrigerator, and use it once a week. Now for the skin-type secret: For normal skin, use the whole egg; for dry skin, use only the yolk; and for oily skin, use only the white.

Honey, Please Pass the Milk!

■ A milk-and-honey massage is one way to start your day off right. Mix equal parts of honey and milk and, starting at your feet, massage the lotion into your thirsty skin. This treatment is best done in the shower, where you can simply rinse off when you're done.

Just the Fats, Ma'am

■ Dry skin, especially in the winter, can be the result of insufficient fats—the right kind of fats. Since skin is the place where water and oil meet, both are essential to good skin health. So make sure your diet includes one or more servings a day of omega-3 fats, found in cold-water fish, nuts, and seeds.

Snappy Solutions

While a nice long soak may feel so relaxing and soothing that you never want to leave the tub—especially if you have some music or a good book with you—don't overstay your welcome. Just remember: A bubble bath and even some bath oils can dry out your skin if you stay in too long.

Anti-Alligator-Skin Fix

Winter weather means dry indoor heat, and that makes your skin as parched as a thirsty sponge. Here's one of my favorite fixers for turning dry skin back to its healthy, moisture-filled self.

Fresh marigold blossoms
Olive oil
1 vitamin E capsule (800 IUs)

➡ Fill a glass jar with cleaned and dried marigold blossoms. Douse the flowers with olive oil, seal the jar with a lid, and stick it on a windowsill that will get plenty of sunshine. After two weeks, strain out the blossoms, leaving the oil. Refill the jar with a new batch of blossoms. You may need to add a tad more olive oil. Reseal the lid, but this time, put the jar inside a brown paper bag, and then place it back on the sunny windowsill for another two weeks. Strain out the blossoms and pour the remaining oil in a dark glass bottle. Add the contents of the vitamin E capsule and store the fixer in a dark place until you're ready to use it. You won't believe how well this concoction works!

Moisturize Slowly

■ We are often so rushed that we barely have time to apply any moisturizer after a shower, which is the best time to do so because our skin is damp and can absorb the moisturizer better. So give yourself a few more minutes in the morning for a mini massage, and rub a moisturizer all over your body. The massage will stimulate blood flow to your skin, making the moisturizer even more effective.

Nifty, Thrifty Tips

The single cheapest way to keep your skin hydrated and moisturized is to make sure your internal rain barrel is full. That's right—you need lots and lots of water for all parts of your body to work well. And the more water you drink, the more water is available for your body to pump up and out to your skin so that it stays in tip-top shape. So don't be stingy with the water—drink at least 8 to 10 8-ounce glasses of H_2O each and every day.

Berry Good Facial Mask

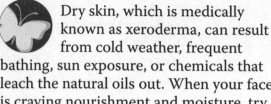

Dry skin, which is medically known as xeroderma, can result from cold weather, frequent bathing, sun exposure, or chemicals that leach the natural oils out. When your face is craving nourishment and moisture, try this mask—it's the berries!

3 to 4 ripe, medium-sized
    strawberries
1 tbsp. of evaporated milk
1 tbsp. of honey
1 tsp. of cornstarch (optional)

➡ Puree the strawberries in a blender or food processor. In a medium-sized bowl, mix the puree with the milk and honey. If it's too runny, add the cornstarch. Apply the mixture to your face and neck with your hands, gently rubbing in circles. Leave the mask on for 10 minutes, rinse with lukewarm water, and you're done.

Bathe with Bath Oil

■ To moisturize your skin, add a fragrant bath oil to your bathwater, soak, pat yourself dry, and apply a good moisturizer. Experiment with different bath oils to find ones that feel best to you. And in places that are extremely dry, like your feet, rub on additional moisturizer. Then wear cotton socks to bed so you don't get your sheets greasy.

EUREKA!

FOR YEARS, DERMATOLOGISTS have lauded petroleum jelly as the thickest emollient and, therefore, the best treatment for very dry skin. Now there's evidence that moisturizers with large amounts of glycerin may work just as well, if not better. Glycerin appears to increase space between cells, which creates a reservoir of moisture-holding ability that makes the skin more resistant to drying out. So look for a glycerin-laced moisturizer to use in place of petroleum jelly products.

Cereal Scrubber

Your skin is the largest organ in—or on—your body. So it should be treated with just as much care as any of your other organs. If you don't keep up with a moisturizing routine, your skin can dry out and feel awful. Here's a quick, easy, and gentle mixer that'll soften up rough heels, knees, elbows—your whole body, for that matter.

1 part baking soda
1 part dry oatmeal
3 parts water

➡ Mix the ingredients together in a bowl. Then use a washcloth to apply the mixture to your body in a circular motion, paying special attention to any areas that are rough, dry, or cracked. Your skin will feel better in no time, and it'll have a healthier glow, too!

Select the Right Soap
■ Check your health-food store for oil-based bars that contain super-moisturizing olive oil or coconut oil, are not labeled "soap" (which is drying), and are scented with palmarosa, rosewood, and/or sandalwood. All of these factors can help stimulate oil production to keep your skin moist.

Open Sesame
■ Women in India have long used sesame oil, which is rich in both vitamin E and linoleic acid, to moisten and soften dry, cracked hands and feet. To try it, pour ½ cup of sesame seeds and ¼ cup of warm water in a blender and process them for three minutes. Strain the lotion, apply it to your skin, and leave it on for as long as possible. Rinse with warm water, then cool water, and blot dry.

✚ If your skin is itchy and flaking, it could be an allergy or infection, or a systemic condition. Some dry skin, known as ichthyosis, is an inherited disorder that is linked to a poorly functioning thyroid or lymphoma. If your skin is rough, scaling, wrinkled, and itching, see your doctor.

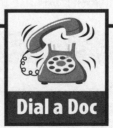

Dial a Doc

Heavenly-Scent Healer

Roses and herbs are among the most beautiful smells that Mother Nature ever dreamed up. And the good news is that these wonderful smells are quite helpful in soothing dry skin. This recipe is a great healing remedy that'll leave you feeling relaxed and moisturized.

Rose petals
Calendula
Chamomile
Comfrey
Lavender
Vegetable oil
1 vitamin E capsule
Lavender oil

➡ Put a handful of rose petals into a 1-pint glass jar with a tight-fitting lid, then add a sprinkling *each* of calendula (leaves or flowers), chamomile, comfrey, and lavender. Fill the jar nearly to the top with vegetable oil, then break open the vitamin E capsule and squeeze its contents into the oil. Twist the lid on tight, and stash the jar in a warm place, maybe near your stove. Every morning, give the jar a rousing up-and-at-'em shake. Do this for a couple of weeks, then open the jar, and strain out the herbs using a fine-mesh sieve. Finally, add a few drops of lavender essential oil to the mix. You now have your very own heavenly-scent massage oil that'll revitalize your dry skin like magic.

Soak Away Psoriasis

■ To soften scaly areas of skin on your hands and feet that are caused by psoriasis, sprinkle 1 cup of Epsom salts in your bathwater and soak. After patting the itchy areas dry, rub them gently with some warm peanut oil, and top the oil off with a paste made of baking soda and castor oil. Put on some white cotton gloves and socks, and say "Nighty-night." After a few days, your scales should disappear. **Caution:** Don't use this treatment on raw, irritated, or broken skin.

Nifty, Thrifty Tips

Dry skin is often lacking in certain acids, like lactic acid. So instead of buying fancy creams and hoping they work, reach for something that naturally has lactic acid—buttermilk. It's loaded with the stuff—and will soften and soothe even the driest skin.

Herbal Steamer

If you don't like to put creams or gels all over your face, there are other options for getting moisture back where it belongs. This herbal facial steamer can deep-six dryness—especially because the geranium oil encourages oil production in your skin. It'll also give your cheeks a healthy rosy glow.

Fennel oil
Geranium oil
Peppermint oil
Rosehip oil
Rosemary oil
3 cups of water

➤ In a saucepan, bring the water to a boil, then remove the pot from the stove. Add one drop of each oil to the water, and drape a towel over your head to capture the steam and create a kind of mini sauna. Bend over the pot and remain there for about five minutes. Just be careful not to get close enough for the steam to burn your face. Indulge in this skin-moisturizing treatment once a week and you'll soon see a noticeable improvement in your complexion.

Refresh with Rosehips

■ Alcohol-based toners can strip away much-needed oils from your skin, but rosehip oil has a high linoleic acid content, which can both tone and moisturize. Look for the oil in your local health-food store, then douse a cotton ball with it and dab it all over your face, neck, and upper chest.

Snappy Solutions

*W*hile it may not seem like it, your lips are skin, too, just a slightly different shade of pink. They can become as dry and cracked as the rest of you. You'll save a lot of discomfort if you can determine the source of your dry lips. Start by checking out the ingredients in your toothpaste. If it contains cinnamate—a flavoring agent that can be drying—you've got the culprit. Simply switch to a brand that's cinnamate-free and isn't labeled "tartar control." Like long-lasting lipsticks and mouthwashes that contain alcohol, tartar-control products can also dry out your lips.

How Sweet It Is Moisture Mask

If your skin dries out, it doesn't necessarily mean that it's simply lacking in moisture. It could also indicate that it's malnourished. Vitamins A and E are important for soft, healthy skin. And you can soften and nourish your hungry hide every day with this sweet-smelling facial fixer.

2 tbsp. of mashed strawberries
1 tbsp. of coconut oil
1 tbsp. of olive oil
2 drops of vitamin E oil
Witch hazel

➡ Combine the berries and oils in a bowl. Smooth the mixture sparingly onto your face and go about your business for a couple of hours. Then rinse it off with warm water, and use a cotton pad to pat your face with the witch hazel. Store any leftover mask in a covered container in the refrigerator, and use the whole batch within a few days.

Smooth Your Skin with E

■ As an ingredient in lotions or as an oil, topical vitamin E reduces skin roughness, the length of facial lines, and wrinkle depth. And when it's combined with vitamin C, the effects may even be enhanced. So check your health-food store for skin-care products that include both of these skin-friendly vitamins.

EUREKA!

MADE FROM THE SHEA NUT of the karite tree, shea butter is loaded with vitamins A and E and may even protect your skin from oxidative damage. Perhaps its best quality, though, is that it's a thick emollient that sinks into your skin and feels smooth, not greasy like petroleum jelly. Check your health-food store for shea butter that's either sold alone or combined with other skin-care ingredients.

Oatmeal Scrub

A nice hot bath can have a lot of healing properties, working wonders on getting rid of stress and depression. But it can also give you a chance to clear your skin of impurities and dry patches. This bath time mixer cleanses, tones, and softens your whole body. Use it and you'll start looking healthier than you have in years!

1 cup of dry oatmeal
½ cup of almonds, coarsely ground
1 ripe avocado

➡ Mix the oatmeal and almonds, and put the mixture in a bath mitt or a clean panty hose foot. Peel the avocado, and mash it up in a small bowl. When you're in the tub or shower, use the filled mitt or panty hose foot to scoop up some avocado, and rub it onto your skin. After your bath, rinse, pat dry, and follow with your regular moisturizer.

Take a Hint from Mister Ed

■ Oats will do more for you than simply provide a hearty breakfast; you can also use them to treat yourself to a whole-body oat mask. Start by making a big pot of oatmeal. Let it cool to a tolerably warm temperature, then slather it on from head to toe. Leave it on your skin for 20 minutes or until it's dry, and then rinse. Better yet, soak it off in a warm tub. For ease of removal, you might want to lightly oil your skin before applying the oatmeal.

Nifty, Thrifty Tips

When your skin starts feeling tight and itchy, it's time to say so long to hot baths and showers. Hot water washes protective oils right off, leaving your skin desert-dry. So jump into a quick, tepid shower instead, then pat yourself dry with a soft towel and slather on the moisture. Extra-virgin coconut oil (found in health-food stores) is just what your thirsty skin craves. Prefer moisturizing with lotion? Check the label for shea butter; it'll leave your skin feeling oh-so-smooth.

Satiny-Smooth Solution

The sharp, chilling winter winds can leave any exposed areas feeling as dry as twice-used sandpaper. But don't fret—make your skin feel silky smooth again with this herbal bath mixer.

½ cup of dried calendula petals
1 muslin bag or cheesecloth
   with a drawstring
Dry milk powder or oatmeal

➤ Carefully put the flower petals inside the bag or cheesecloth and tie it up, then fill your bathtub with warm (not hot) water. Pour a little dry milk powder or a few teaspoons of oatmeal under the faucet. Add the bag of calendula petals and let it float around like a rubber ducky. Hop in, and soak yourself in the bath while the herbal oils work their rejuvenating magic.

Brush Up

■ Starting at the soles of your feet and moving up your legs toward your heart, gently rub your body in a circular motion with a super-soft, dry-bristle brush. Then do the same with your hands and arms. Brushing will help stimulate your sebaceous glands to produce more sebum and will remove any dead skin that makes you look dry, dull, and old.

Q: *I hate that my skin gets super dry every time winter rolls around. But I don't think anyone has ever told me what makes it dry out. Do you know why it does?*

Take My Advice

A: As we get older, the uppermost layer of our skin naturally loses some of its ability to hold water. While aging isn't within our control, other factors contribute to dry skin, including indoor heat, prolonged sun exposure, leisurely baths, and even frequent air travel. If you can eliminate any of these causes, you can help your skin stay moist a bit longer.

All Eyes on You

The easiest way to hide dark eye bags is to cover them with makeup. But sometimes, you wind up applying too much. And then the problem is getting it all off at night, which isn't so easy. Here's a great mixer that's a gentle and soothing eye-makeup remover.

1 tbsp. of castor oil
1 tbsp. of olive oil
2 tsp. of canola oil

➡ Mix all of the ingredients together. Apply the mixture with a tissue or cotton ball to remove eye shadow, eyeliner, or mascara safely and without irritation. Discard any of the mixture that's left over. And remember: It's probably better to not use so much makeup in the first place!

Bag the Bags
■ Black tea has an astringent nature that makes an excellent remedy for baggy eyes. Simply wet two black tea bags, and place one over each eye while you rest for 20 minutes or so. Take 'em off, and admire the new you!

Potato Patties Prevail
■ You can lessen eye bags by making a potato patty compress. Simply grate a raw potato and wrap it in clean cheesecloth or gauze. Place the compress over your eyes for about 20 minutes while resting. A simpler method is to thinly slice a raw potato and apply the potato directly to your skin. Follow up with your favorite anti-aging cream, taking care not to stretch the delicate skin around your eyes.

Snappy Solutions

Save yourself from dealing with unsightly eye bags by simply minimizing them. How? By concealing them. The skin on your baggy lower lids is usually darker than the rest of your eye area. If this is the case, use a concealer there, but don't go overboard. It should be only one tone lighter than your regular foundation. Once you add foundation or powder over it, the concealer will set for a longer-lasting look.

Brighten 'Em Up!

Eye bags have two causes: Either they're a temporary result of fluid retention, or they may be fat deposits that have accumulated over the years. Unfortunately, there is no diet or exercise to diminish the latter kind. But for the former kind, eyebright is a favorite herb for any eye ailment, and a warm compress of this excellent elixir will certainly refresh your eyes.

1 tsp. of eyebright
1 tsp. of fennel seeds
1 cup of hot water

➥ Make a tea by adding the eyebright and fennel seeds to the water. Dip a clean cloth into the mixture, and let the tea steep for 10 minutes. Wring out the cloth, then sit back and lay the cloth over your eyes. Leave it on for 20 minutes. Indulge in this treatment once or twice a day, and your eyes should start to look and feel better fairly quickly.

Fabulous Fennel

■ A cold compress made with fennel tea can reduce the swelling around puffy eyes. Just pour 1 cup of boiling water over 2 teaspoons of fennel seeds. Cover the mixture, and allow it to steep for 10 minutes before storing it in the refrigerator overnight. In the morning, strain out the seeds and your eye-pleasing medicine is ready to use. Just dip a paper towel into it, lie down, and put the moistened paper towel over your eyes for 10 minutes or so for soothing relief.

EUREKA!

THE NEXT TIME you want fast relief from puffy, swollen eyes, reach into your cutlery drawer and pull out two metal spoons (either silver or stainless steel will do fine). Run cold water over them until they're good and chilly. Then lie down, lay one spoon (curved side down) over each eye, and relax for a minute or two. Then get ready for peepers that will feel—and look—a whole lot better!

Almond Face Cleanser

Your face is the first thing people see when they meet you, so make sure it's healthy and glowing every day. Here's a facial fixer that's perfect for all skin types, and that can be made in a flash.

1 cup of almonds
1 cup of uncooked oatmeal
1 cup of dried orange peel

➡ Put all of the ingredients in a blender or food processor, and grind them to a fine powder. Scoop some into the palm of your hand, add a few drops of water, and rub the mixture onto your face. (Be careful not to get any in your eyes.) Rinse with warm water, and pat dry. Store the powder in an airtight container at room temperature for future use.

Lemony Skin Care

■ For a great facial cleanser, try this tangy recipe. First, grind some lemon peels in a blender or food processor, then mix about 1 tablespoon of the ground peels with enough plain yogurt to make a paste. Wash your face with this mixture, rinse with cool water, and pat dry. If your skin is on the dry side, substitute vegetable oil for the yogurt.

Calendula Wash

■ Calendula's bright orange flowers can be made into a refreshing facial wash. Just steep 1 teaspoon of calendula flowers in 1 cup of hot water for 10 minutes. Cool and strain. After cleansing your face as usual, rinse it with the calendula wash, then pat it dry with a soft towel.

Snappy Solutions

If you've got dry skin—and not much time to fuss with elaborate cleansing routines—try this simple scrub. Apply a little sesame oil to your face and neck, and scrub gently with a warm, damp washcloth. Rinse with warm water, and pat dry. That's all there is to it!

Apple and Wine Mask

When a lot of gunk starts clogging up the pores on your face, it can feel like you're carrying around a couple extra pounds that you really don't want (or need). Here's a super solution that will slough off dead skin cells, refine your pores, and gradually even out your skin tone.

2 tbsp. of dry oatmeal
2 tsp. of apple juice
2 tsp. of red wine

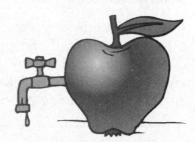

➡ Grind the oatmeal into a powder in a coffee grinder or blender. Then mix it with the other ingredients in a small bowl until it forms a spreadable paste (add more liquid if you need to). Smooth the mixture onto your face and neck, and leave it in place for 20 to 30 minutes, or until it's dry. Then rinse with warm water and pat dry.

Super Skin Smoother

■ If you've got dry skin, this soother's for you. After every bath or shower, apply mineral oil to your wet skin. Then towel dry. The towel will remove excess oil, but a thin layer will stay on your skin, providing much-needed moisture.

Soap Away Oily Skin

■ Here's a great way to clean oily skin: Pour a little liquid castile soap into the palm of your hand, and add about 1 teaspoon of cornmeal to it. Gently massage the mixture into your face until it lathers, being careful to avoid your eyes. Rinse it off with warm water, and pat dry.

Nifty, Thrifty Tips

If your skin is extra-oily, keep plenty of witch hazel on hand. It's the perfect balancing agent—and it's a whole lot cheaper than commercial skin balancers. Just dab it onto your face with a clean cotton ball in the morning and before bed—or whenever you get that oily feeling.

Apple Astringent

Some days, it can look and feel like your entire face is sagging. You can't even imagine going out into the world and letting friends and family see you like that. Well, if that's the case, then try this magical mixer. The acids in the apple juice tone your skin and help keep it clear—and they're mild enough for even sensitive skin.

½ cup of fresh apple juice
4 tbsp. of vodka (100 proof)
1 tbsp. of honey
1 tsp. of sea salt

➡ Pour all of the ingredients into a bottle, cap it tightly, and shake it well. Apply the solution to your face and neck twice a day with a cotton pad. Just be careful around any areas that have cuts or nicks—100 proof vodka will make them sting something fierce!

Cleanse with Calendula

■ Many folks just assume that if their skin is oily and prone to pimples, they should be scrubbing it like crazy. Not true! The key to keeping outbreaks under control is to wash with a gentle touch. Using your fingers (not a washcloth), cleanse your skin with warm water and a mild herbal soap like calendula, which you can find at health-food stores. The herb is a gentle but potent natural astringent that will safely strip your skin of oils. Finish up with a splash of cold water to close the pores and you're done.

Snappy Solutions

*W*hy go to the salon for a facial and wait 45 minutes before anyone even has the time to see you? Here's how to get the same soothing results right at home. Just puree half a cucumber in a blender. Stir in 1 tablespoon of plain yogurt, apply the mixture to your face, and leave it on for about 30 minutes. Rinse it off with warm water and pat dry. Then say "Aaahhh!"

Citrusy Smooth Face Cream

At the end of a long day, there can be a buildup of bad stuff on your face. Between makeup, dirt, dust, and other pollutants that are always doing damage to your skin, it can be hard to keep looking beautiful. So try whipping up this fabulous face cream to remove makeup and clean and soften your skin.

Juice of 1 lime
1½ cups of mayonnaise
1 tbsp. of melted butter (not margarine)

➡ Combine the lime juice, mayonnaise (the real kind, made with eggs and oil), and butter until the mixture has a smooth, creamy texture. Store the cream in a tightly closed glass jar in your refrigerator and be sure to label it so no one uses it in their sandwich! Use it as you would any facial cleanser, and rinse with cold water for refreshing results.

Powerful Pore Reducer

■ To lessen the appearance of large facial pores, reach for this potent (but gentle) fixer: Beat one egg, and mix it with about 1 tablespoon of honey. Spread the mixture onto your face, and leave it on for 20 minutes or so. You'll feel it working as it tightens up your skin. Then rinse it off to reveal skin that's softer, firmer, and smoother than before.

Almond Scrubber

■ For a super-simple cleanser, you can't beat this simple trick: Grind shelled almonds to a fine powder in an old blender or coffee grinder. Wet your face, rub the almond powder into your skin, and rinse it off with cold water.

EUREKA!

WHEN IT COMES to moisturizing dry skin, this mask can't be beet, er, beat. Just whirl 1 grated beet and 1 cup of sour cream in a blender, and smooth the mixture over your face and neck. Wait 10 minutes or so, and rinse it off with warm water.

Cucumber and Honey Cleanser

Your face takes a lot of punishment during the day—wind, dirt, sun, and pollutants are all bombarding it, which leads to problems. And there's nowhere to hide. So when you want to soothe and revitalize your skin at the same time, whip up this simple cleansing solution.

¼ of a small cucumber, peeled and seeded
2 tbsp. of honey
1 tbsp. of whole milk

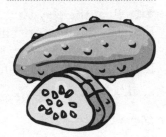

➡ Puree the cucumber, strain it, and pour its juice into a bowl. Mix in the honey, add the milk, and stir. Using cotton pads, apply the mixture to your face and neck. Wait 20 minutes, then rinse it away for a nice refreshing feeling.

Baking Soda Scrub

■ Take a tip from my Grandma Putt: Keep a jar of baking soda by your bathroom sink, and use it to gently deep-clean your face. It'll lift out the traces of oil, dirt, and makeup that even the best cleansers leave behind. Here's how to use it: Start by washing your face with your regular soap. Then mix 3 parts baking soda with 1 part water, and gently massage the mixture into your damp skin, being sure to avoid the delicate eye area. Rinse thoroughly with clear, cool water, and pat your face dry.

EUREKA!

YOU COULD WAIT 'til the cows come home and not find a better facial cleanser than this one: Mix ¼ cup of buttermilk with ¼ cup of whole dry milk (not nonfat) to form a paste. Spread it evenly over your face and neck, using a clean new paintbrush or pastry brush. Let it dry for 15 to 20 minutes, and then rinse it off with cool water. Store any leftovers in a covered container in the refrigerator until next time.

Egg It On Skin Softener

It's no secret that you can spend a fortune on fancy skin-softening and toning concoctions—and plenty of women do. But why follow the crowd when this oh-so-easy routine will do the job as well as any of 'em?

1 large egg white
Juice of ½ lemon
Bottled water
Witch hazel

➤ Beat the egg white, then fold in the lemon juice. Smooth the mixture onto your face and neck. Wait 20 minutes, and rinse it off with bottled water. Pat dry, then use a cotton ball to dab on a little witch hazel to tighten up your pores.

Mop Up the Oil

■ Here's a facial mask that Bugs Bunny would love. And it really works wonders on oily skin. Boil three large carrots until they're soft, then mash them and add 5 tablespoons of honey. Using a circular motion, massage the mixture gently onto your face, then leave it there for 20 minutes. Rinse with warm water and pat dry. Before you use this on your face, test it on an inconspicuous spot, such as inside the crook of your arm, to make sure it doesn't turn your skin slightly—but temporarily—orange.

Q: *I need a quick and easy way to take care of my face every day. It just needs a little perking up, but never so much to warrant using one of those heavy-duty cleansers. Do you have anything I can use?*

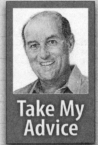

Take My Advice

A: Here's a simple skin treatment: Just mash a banana and add 1 tablespoon of honey to it. Cover your face with the mixture, let it sit for 15 minutes, and rinse with warm water. Away you go!

Fabulous Face Freshener

Dab this fixer onto your face after exercising, or any time you feel like you need a quick pick-me-up. It also makes a great after-cleansing astringent to remove all traces of soap or cleansing cream.

½ tsp. of borax
¾ cup of distilled water
2 tbsp. of vodka

➡ Mix the borax in the water until the powder is thoroughly dissolved. Add the vodka and stir well. Store the mixer in a glass bottle with a tight-fitting cap to prevent the alcohol from evaporating. When you feel the need for facial refreshment, apply the solution to your skin with a cotton ball or pad. If you prefer a scented lotion, use 6 tablespoons of distilled water and 6 tablespoons of your favorite flower water, such as orange, rose, or lavender.

Blackhead Eliminator

■ For a quick and easy facial cleanser, mix 2 tablespoons of whole milk with 2 tablespoons of warm (not hot) honey. Rinse your face with water and massage the cleanser in for a couple of minutes, then rinse it off and pat your face dry. This mixture doesn't keep well, so only make it as you need it.

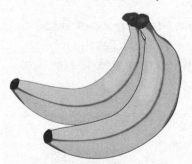

Banana Skin Refresher

■ Here's a facial you'll go bananas for: Puree one banana and one avocado in a blender. Apply the mixture to your skin and leave it on for at least 20 minutes, then rinse with warm water and pat your face dry. If you have dry skin, follow up with a good moisturizer.

EUREKA!

YOU CAN USE EVAPORATED MILK straight from the can to remove eye makeup. Just dip a cotton ball into the milk, and gently rub your eyelids. Then rinse with cool water.

Facial Power Mask

Like the saying goes, if you don't look good, you don't feel good. So when your skin is looking shabby and making you feel just plain crabby, give it what it's hungry for. This marvelous mask will make you look and feel your very best by cleaning your face and making it shiny smooth. Trust me—you'll feel like your beautiful self again!

½ cup of dry oatmeal
1 tbsp. of cider vinegar
1 tbsp. of honey
1 tsp. of ground almonds

➡ Mix all of the ingredients together in a bowl. Moisten your face with a warm washcloth. With your hands, smooth the mixture onto your skin, being careful to avoid your eyes. When the mask is dry, remove it with a warm, damp washcloth.

Nicely Natural

■ Rub peanut, avocado, or sesame oil on your face for a nice natural moisturizer. Leave it on for about 10 minutes, rinse with warm water, and pat dry.

Remove Makeup the Milky Way

■ To take off full-face makeup quickly and gently, put 1 tablespoon of evaporated milk into a small bowl and add a few drops of almond oil. Pat the mixer onto your face with a cotton pad, remove it by wiping with a clean pad (or two), and rinse with lukewarm water.

Snappy Solutions

When you're in the mood for a quick, soothing facial, just use your head—of lettuce, that is! Here's how to do it: Separate the leaves from a small head of lettuce. Wash them, and cook the leaves in boiling water for five minutes. Remove them from the water, let them cool, and apply the leaves to your face. Leave them on for 5 to 10 minutes (they'll be slippery!). Pat your face dry without rinsing and you're done.

Homemade Cold Cream

You *could* go out and pay a lot of money for a fancy cold cream. After all, if they're on the market, then they must work to a certain degree. Or, you could save yourself a whole lot of money by making your own version at home with this easy recipe.

1 egg yolk
2 tbsp. of lemon juice
½ cup of olive oil
½ cup of vegetable oil

➥ Combine the egg yolk and lemon juice, and stir with a wire whisk. Gradually add the oils, continuing to stir, until the mixture thickens. If it's too thick, add more lemon juice; if it's too thin, add a little more egg yolk. Store in a covered container in the refrigerator for up to three days.

Clogged-Pore Cleanser

■ Here's an easy-to-make peel-off facial mask. Mix 1½ tablespoons of unflavored gelatin with ½ cup of raspberry fruit juice in a microwave-safe container, then nuke it until the gelatin is completely dissolved. Put the mixture in the refrigerator until it's almost set (about 25 minutes). Then spread it on your face, let it dry, and peel it off.

E-zee Off

■ You're going to love this quick and gentle way to get off eye makeup: Simply use vitamin E oil to get the job done. It won't sting your eyes, and it's a super moisturizer for delicate eye area skin.

What Would Grandma Do?

🦋 MY GRANDMA PUTT never fussed with fancy astringents. After she washed her face, she filled the bathroom sink about halfway with water, added a few tablespoons of apple cider vinegar, and splashed the solution onto her face. Try this trick at home for 30 days. It will close your pores, restore the acid balance to your skin, and leave your face feeling clean, soft, and refreshed!

Honey of a Facial

It's truly amazing that all you have to do is reach into your fridge for a few ordinary items that can keep you looking your best. Whip up this mixer that'll look good enough to eat—but use it to soften your face instead!

2 egg whites
2 tbsp. of mashed avocado
2 tbsp. of honey

➤ Thoroughly combine all of the ingredients in a small bowl, and using your fingers, apply the mixture to your face. Leave it on for 30 minutes or so, rinse with warm water, and pat dry. That's all there is to it!

Marigolds for Me

■ If your skin is oily and/or sensitive, try this refreshing herbal tonic. Put 6 tablespoons of fresh (3 tablespoons of dried) marigold petals in a bowl and pour 8 ounces of boiling water over them. Stir, and let cool, stirring occasionally. Strain out the petals, add 4 tablespoons of witch hazel and 3 drops of your favorite essential oil to the infusion, and mix well. To use, pat the tonic over your freshly washed face once or twice a day with a cotton ball. Store the tonic in a glass jar or bottle with a tight-fitting lid.

Peachy Skin

■ Winter can be rough on your skin, both indoors and out. Hot, dry indoor air can leave your face feeling sore and irritated. And on sunny days, bone-chilling outdoor breezes can deliver a nasty windburn before you know it. To ease both kinds of discomfort, cut a fresh peach in two, and rub the juicy surface over your ailin' skin. You'll feel peachy keen in no time at all!

Nifty, Thrifty Tips

Stop paying an arm and a leg for fancy facial exfoliators! Instead, use this old-time technique: Add 1 teaspoon of Epsom salts to either your normal cleansing cream or warm water. Then massage the mixture into your face, followed by a quick rinse with cold water.

In from the Outdoors Refreshing Facial

If you love spending time outside, you've got to be extra careful when it comes to your skin. Too much of a good thing can really do a number on your face. This natural mixer is vitamin-enriched to soothe even the most delicate areas for refreshing results!

5 vitamin E capsules
2 tsp. of plain yogurt
½ tsp. of honey
½ tsp. of lemon juice

➡ Prick the vitamin E capsules and drain the contents into a bowl. Add the yogurt, honey, and lemon juice, and combine well. Apply the mixture to your face with a cotton ball, wait about 10 minutes or so, and rinse with warm water. Your face will feel rejuvenated and rarin' to go.

Make Mine Mayo

■ Believe it or not, you can use mayonnaise to clean your face. Simply apply a layer of the creamy condiment as you would any deep-cleansing facial soap. After 15 or 20 minutes, wipe it off and rinse your face thoroughly. The oils and salt in the mayo will remove any impurities and restore moisture to your skin.

Pamper with Papaya

■ If your skin is dry and patchy with uneven tone, try a papaya. Slice a fresh one and lay the slivers on your face—avoiding your eyes—for about five minutes. The papaya will dissolve dead skin cells at the surface and leave you looking fresh.

What Would Grandma Do?

🦋 GRANDMA PUTT OFTEN USED CLAY *on her face to soak up excess oil and slough off dead skin cells without irritation. So pick up some green clay at your local health-food store. Add a little water to 1 teaspoon of clay, and mix a few drops of lavender oil into the paste. The oil's antibacterial and anti-inflammatory properties will help heal any blemishes you may have, and its lovely aroma will help you relax. Leave the mask on for 15 minutes, rinse it off, and say good-bye to oily skin!*

Lemon Face Cream

If you don't always have time to give your body the pampering it deserves, then here's a fast fixer that delivers speedy tender loving care to your skin. Use it every night to keep your face satiny soft.

1 lemon
¼ cup or so of heavy cream (whipping cream)
Piece of muslin or other light cloth

➤ From the center of the lemon, cut a slice that's about ¼ inch thick. Lay it flat in a clean glass jar with a lid. Pour in enough cream to cover the lemon slice, cover the container with the cloth, and let it sit at room temperature for 24 hours, or until the contents are about the thickness of face cream. Replace the cloth with the regular jar lid, and put the mixture in your refrigerator. Rub the cream into your skin every night at bedtime. The mixture will eventually spoil, so you'll have to make a new batch every week or so.

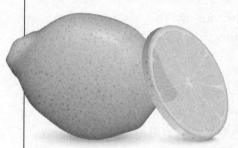

Lemon Blackhead Eraser

■ You can clear up blackheads and blemishes by rubbing them with lemon juice several times a day. Just juice half a lemon, dip a cotton swab into the juice, and gently apply it to your blemishes. Soon your face will feel refreshed and look a whole lot healthier.

Nifty, Thrifty Tips

Nowadays, you hear a lot about exfoliating creams and lotions, and you can pay big bucks for them. But you don't have to. Just mix cold-pressed vegetable oil (like sunflower or safflower) with enough salt to make a gritty paste. Then add a few drops of your favorite essential oil. Rub this mixture over your wet skin—face, hands, elbows, and knees—and rinse well. Those rough-skinned areas will be clean and moisturized at the same time. **Caution:** Don't use this treatment on raw, irritated, or broken skin.

Molasses Face Mask

You need to keep your face looking happy and healthy because of all the damaging things (like pollutants) it's confronted with each and every day. There are plenty of products that you could try, but why waste your money? Instead, rummage through your fridge and pantry and you'll be able to soften and deep-clean your skin with this fantastic facial fixer.

½ of an avocado
2 tbsp. of orange juice
1 tsp. of honey
1 tsp. of molasses

➡ Puree the ingredients in a blender. Smooth the mixture onto your skin, wait 30 to 40 minutes, and remove the mask, using a warm, damp washcloth. Store any extra mixture in a covered container in the refrigerator; it will keep for two or three days.

Tomato on Your Face

■ If you have oily—but not sensitive—skin, this from-the-kitchen cleanser is just for you. Puree a very ripe medium-size tomato in a blender or food processor, strain out the solids, and mix the juice with an equal amount of fresh whole milk. Apply the solution to your face and neck with cotton pads, wait 10 minutes or so, and then rinse with lukewarm water. Be sure to discard any remaining cleanser. Make and use a fresh batch two to three times a week to keep the oil under control.

What Would Grandma Do?

🦋 WHEN GRANDMA Putt and her friends wanted to pamper their faces, they didn't run off to a fancy spa, or even the local beauty parlor. Instead, they made their own skin cleansers and softeners using ingredients fresh from their gardens and kitchens. This was one of the simplest—and it still works as well as it did decades ago. Mix ¼ cup of grated carrots with 1½ teaspoons of mayonnaise. Spread the softener on your face and neck, wait 15 minutes, and rinse it off with lukewarm water.

Nutty Facial Scrub

Soft skin is something that all women want and deserve. It just plain feels good to be able to touch cheeks that feel like they're made of porcelain. So if your skin could stand for a little smoothing, this facial fixer will also keep it soft and squeaky clean.

2 tbsp. of almond slivers
2 tsp. of milk
½ tsp. of flour
Honey

➡ Grind the almond slivers in an old blender or coffee grinder, and mix the resulting powder with the milk, flour, and enough honey to make a thick paste. Rub the scrub into your skin, and rinse with warm water. Your face will go from dull and dirty to healthy and glowing in no time at all!

Rosemary Facial Cleanser

■ Make this soothing facial cleanser by mixing 1 tablespoon of dried rosemary in ½ cup of safflower oil. Let the oil sit in a covered container in your refrigerator for three days. Then take it out and use it once or twice a day for best results. Just smooth the mixture onto your face, rinse with lukewarm water, and pat dry.

Yeast Away Oil

■ Here's a terrific way to cleanse oily skin: Mix a tablespoon or so of brewer's yeast with just enough warm water to make a paste. Rub it onto your face, let it dry, and rinse with warm water. You can find brewer's yeast at health-food stores or in the natural-foods section of a drugstore or supermarket.

Nifty, Thrifty Tips

Here's a mild, all-natural astringent that you can make from ingredients right out of your garden. Boil a few sprigs of fresh thyme in 2 cups of water. Remove the pot from the heat, and let the thyme steep for five to seven minutes, or until the water cools to room temperature. Take out the thyme, and add 2 teaspoons of fresh lemon juice. Pour this concoction into a glass bottle with a cap and store it in your refrigerator. To use, simply apply it with a cotton ball or pad after washing your face.

Say "Aah!" Mask

Want a soothing facial fixer that'll both soften and invigorate your skin? Of course you do! Just say "Aah!" (as in *a*vocado, *a*lmonds, and *h*oney).

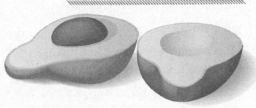

2 tbsp. of mashed avocado
1 tbsp. of crushed almonds
½ tsp. of honey

➡ Stir all of the ingredients together until the mixture is creamy. Smooth it onto your face with your hands, and leave it on for 30 minutes or so. Rinse with warm water and pat dry.

Watermelon Facial

■ When it's summertime and the livin' is not so easy, take a little time away from the daily grind and treat yourself to a wonderful watermelon facial. Simply peel a slice of the fruit, and mash it in a glass or ceramic bowl until it's about the consistency of thin applesauce. First, wash your face so that it's really clean. Then spread the melon over your skin, making sure to avoid your eyes. Lie down and put a piece of gauze or cheesecloth over the fruit (otherwise, it will probably slide off). Relax and think lovely thoughts for 20 to 30 minutes, then rinse the mash off and pat your face dry.

Honey of a Remedy

■ Here's a tasty way to get rid of blackheads. Just heat about ⅛ cup of honey, and dab it onto the blemishes. Let it sit in place for a couple of minutes, wash it off with warm water, and rinse with cool water. Then gently dry your skin with a nice soft towel.

EUREKA!

YOU'LL NEVER FIND a simpler—or more effective—moisturizer than this: Just rub some olive oil onto your face, wait about 10 minutes, rinse it off with warm water, and pat dry.

Sea Salt Shower Scrub

Take a trip to a seaside spa without ever leaving home. This DIY bath mixture will leave your skin feeling as soft and satiny smooth as the most expensive exfoliating cream.

¼ cup of sea salt
1 tablespoon of baking soda
Almond oil

➥ Mix the salt and soda and add enough oil to make a thick paste. In the bath or shower, rub the mixture on your face and all over your body, then rinse well. **Caution:** Don't use this treatment on broken skin.

Time for Tea Toner

■ Make a skin toner by mixing ½ cup of strong green tea with ¼ cup of witch hazel. Dab it onto your face with a cotton pad—there's no need to rinse. Pour the leftover toner into a jar or bottle with a lid and store in the refrigerator for up to three weeks.

Wonderful Wine Pick-Me-Up

■ Here's a simple skin freshener that your face will love: Put 1 cup of white wine and 1 sliced lemon in a glass or enamel pot, and bring the liquid to a boil over medium heat. Boil it for another full minute, remove the pan from the heat, and stir in 1 tablespoon of sugar. Let the mixer cool, strain it, and store it in a tightly capped bottle. Whenever you feel the need for some fast facial refreshment, just dab the lotion onto your skin with a cotton ball.

Snappy Solutions

Save yourself the expense of day spa treatments with this simple, yet effective moisturizer. Combine 1 egg yolk with ¾ cup of milk. Apply it to your face with your fingertips, using a gentle circular motion. Leave it on for about five minutes, then rinse. Store any unused portion in the refrigerator, covered, and use it within a week.

Strawberry Facial

Skip the fancy spas—the pampering is not worth the price. And if you've got oily skin, this herbal fixer will leave your face looking fresh, clean, and healthy for a fraction of the cost.

1 tbsp. of facial clay (available at health-food stores)
1 large ripe strawberry, mashed
1 tbsp. of witch hazel
1 drop of lavender oil

➤ Combine all of the ingredients in a small bowl to form a paste. Apply it to your face (being careful to steer clear of your eyes), leaving it on for 15 minutes or so. Despite how beautiful you look with the mask on (ugh!), the best is yet to come. Head for the bathroom sink and rinse off the mask with warm water. Your skin will glow, but not from the oil produced by your overactive oil glands!

Banish Blackheads

■ You can banish blackheads the same way your grandma did, by making a paste of roughly 3 parts oatmeal to 1 part water, and rubbing it into the affected areas. Leave it on for about 10 minutes, then rinse it away with warm water, and pat dry. It's that easy!

Yogurt Cleaner

■ To cleanse and tone your skin at the same time, nothing beats plain old unflavored yogurt. Just smooth it onto your face and throat, wait a couple of minutes, and then rinse it off with warm water.

What Would Grandma Do?

🦋 GRANDMA PUTT *rarely wore eye makeup (or any other kind). But when she did brush on mascara for a very special occasion, like a wedding or christening, she took it off by dabbing a little vegetable shortening onto her eyelids, then gently wiping it away with a soft cotton pad.*

Super Skin Smoothie

You can blend up a super "smoothie" of sugar, fruit, and milk to discourage blemishes as well as delight your taste buds. The ingredients are packed with plenty of alpha hydroxy acids, which help unclog pores by dissolving the "glue" that holds dead skin cells together. So mix it up, slather it on, and then bottoms up to any leftovers!

3 tbsp. of milk
1 tsp. of sugar
5 grapes
1 kiwi, sliced
1 apple, sliced

➡ Combine the milk (for lactic acid), sugar, grapes (for tartaric acid), kiwi (for citric acid), and apple (for malic acid) in a blender. Apply the puree to each blemish, leave it on for 10 minutes, and rinse with warm water. These acids will help your pores loosen up and release the gunk.

Facial Bleach

■ If you're troubled by dark hair on your upper lip, this old-time tip is just for you. Mix 1 teaspoon of ammonia with ¼ cup of 6% hydrogen peroxide, and dab the solution onto the offending hair with a cotton ball. Let it sit for 30 minutes, then rinse it off with cool water. If you have sensitive skin, do a patch test on your inner arm before trying this on your face.

A Gentle Exfoliator

■ You can keep your complexion glowing by sloughing off dead skin. Just mix a bit of cornmeal in with your normal face cleanser, or wash with a paste made from steel-cut oats (which are rougher than rolled oats) and warm water. Then pat dry.

EUREKA!

HONEY HAS BEEN used as a beauty aid since ancient Egyptian times because it retains moisture and can be applied to the face for smoother skin. Make a refreshing mask by smoothing a thin layer of honey on your face and leaving it on for 20 minutes. Then rinse it off with first cold, then warm water. You'll feel tingly, fresh, and smooth immediately.

Sweet-and-Sour Scrub

You just can't beat a good facial scrub. There's nothing like that feeling when your face has been rubbed free of dirt, dead skin, and other grime. This simple energizing rub will leave you rarin' to go—and make your skin squeaky clean and satiny soft all over.

½ cup of brown sugar
Juice of ½ small lemon
1 tsp. of honey

➡ Mix the ingredients together in a bowl. In your bath or shower, gently massage the mixture into your skin, and rinse it off. When you step out, your face will feel like a million bucks. And what a deal—it only cost you a few pennies!

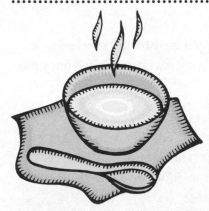

Breakfast Food for Your Face

■ Here's a terrific cleanser for all skin types: Grind about ¼ cup of old-fashioned oatmeal in a coffee grinder or food processor until it's the consistency of coarse flour. In a bowl, mix it with heavy cream to form a paste. (If you have oily skin, substitute skim milk.) Let the cleanser thicken for a minute or two, then massage it into your face and throat. Rinse with cool water.

Q: *I have a scar on my face that's more prominent than I'd like. Is there any way (short of plastic surgery) that I can get rid of it or at least make it less noticeable?*

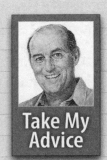

Take My Advice

A: Just massage a little olive oil into the scar once a day. How quickly you'll see results will depend on the size and depth of the scar. But over time, it will lighten the mark and reduce the raised "proud" flesh.

Tutti-Frutti Facial

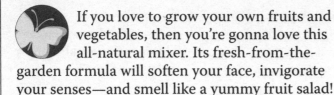

If you love to grow your own fruits and vegetables, then you're gonna love this all-natural mixer. Its fresh-from-the-garden formula will soften your face, invigorate your senses—and smell like a yummy fruit salad!

6 strawberries
½ of an apple
½ of a pear
4 tbsp. of orange juice
Honey

➡ Puree the fruits with the orange juice in a blender or food processor. Apply a thin layer of honey to your face, then smooth on the fruit mixer. Leave it in place for 30 to 40 minutes, rinse with warm water, and pat dry. Your complexion will have a nice healthy glow.

Epsom Salts Booster

■ Give your face an extra-thorough cleaning at night by mixing ½ teaspoon of Epsom salts with your regular cleansing cream. Gently massage it into your skin, and rinse it off with cold water.

(Don't) Hold the Mayo!

■ It's not just for sandwiches—mayonnaise makes a great skin moisturizer, too! Just scoop some out of the jar and apply it to your clean face at bedtime. Leave it on for 10 minutes or so, then wipe it off with a tissue. And be sure to store any leftover mayo in the fridge.

Nifty, Thrifty Tips

When you decide it's time for a professional facial, do your bank account a favor and head to one of your local cosmetology schools. They offer hands-on experience to their students, and they welcome customers with open arms—at a fraction of the price you'd pay at a commercial salon. The students who are permitted to work on customers usually have completed most of their course work and are close to graduation. And you needn't worry about a true cosmetic catastrophe because a competent instructor is always standing by to make things right.

Violet Cleansing Milk

There was nothing Grandma Putt loved more than the sweet scent of violets. She had them in the house all year round. And there wasn't a day when the smell wasn't in her home. That's also why she washed her face every night with this oh-so-fragrant soothing cleanser.

2 tbsp. of sweet violets
1¼ cups of evaporated milk
¼ cup of whole milk

➡ Put the sweet violets in the top half of a double boiler with both milks. Simmer for about 30 minutes, but don't let the milk boil! Turn off the heat, let the mixture sit for two hours or so, and strain it into a bottle that's got a tight stopper. Store it in the refrigerator for up to one week. To use, pat it onto your face with a cotton ball, massage it gently in with your fingers, and rinse with cool water.

Once and Done

■ Many dermatologists recommend a simpler skin regimen for the "mature" woman. If you're 50 or older, limit your face cleansing to once a day, at bedtime. Take off your makeup and the day's grime, moisturize, and hit the hay. Come morning, just splash your face with cool water, and apply moisturizer.

A Sweet Facial Treat

■ You can make an instant granular cleanser by adding a teaspoon of sugar to the cleanser you normally use to clean your face. Simply scrub with this mixture when you wash your face, then rinse it off with cold water.

What Would Grandma Do?

🦋 GRANDMA USED TO MAKE her own herbal vinegar to add pizzazz to recipes and to use as a beauty treatment. Just mash some dried herbs (choose ones with aromas you enjoy), and mix ½ cup of the herbs with 2 cups of white vinegar. Let the mixture sit in a cool, dark place for one to three weeks. Then use it as a skin cleanser, toner, and astringent.

Fruity Fix-Up

Some folks condition their hair periodically with mayonnaise by smooshing the gloppy stuff on, covering it with a shower cap, and letting it sit for half an hour. Then they follow up with a shampoo and rinse. If your hair is dry, frizzy, or damaged, this all-natural mixer will whip it back into shape—and it's a lot less messy than mayonnaise!

½ of a ripe avocado
½ of a ripe banana
1 tbsp. of extra-virgin olive oil
3 drops of lemon oil

➡️ Mash the avocado and banana together in a bowl, then mix in the olive oil and lemon oil. Work the mixture into your dry hair, and cover it with a shower cap. Wait about one hour, and then shampoo as usual. For badly damaged hair, repeat this treatment up to three times a week until the bounce and shine return.

Count on Bunny Food

▪ Carrots can help absorb excess hair oil without drying out your scalp. To put them to work for you, chop up three raw carrots, and puree them in a blender or food processor. Apply this mixer to your scalp, leave it on for 15 minutes, then hop along to rinse it off with some nice cool water.

Q: *I've noticed that my hair gets really dry and looks terrible after I use my favorite shampoo. What's causing it?*

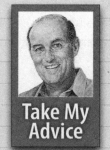

Take My Advice

A: Check your shampoo first. The products that claim they clean and condition in one application really can't do a great job of either. It's better to use a gentle shampoo that's designed for dry hair and follow it up with a conditioner that's intended for the same thing. You'll find plenty to choose from in the hair-care aisle. Good luck!

Hair's to Bananas Hair Cream

 Make no mistake, no one holds on to their luxurious locks forever. Every day, we shed about 100 of our 100,000 scalp hairs. Whether this loss is replaced with new strands depends on several factors, including hormones, genetics, and age. To give yourself a fighting chance, revive dry or damaged hair with this fantastic fixer.

1 banana
1 tbsp. of mayonnaise
1 tbsp. of olive oil

➡ Puree the banana in a blender until it's smooth and lump-free. Add the mayonnaise and olive oil, and blend until the mixture is creamy. Massage it into your hair, wait 15 to 30 minutes, rinse with warm water, and then shampoo as usual. Your hair will look (and smell) terrific!

Be a Hothead

■ Here's a mixer that may help you keep a full head of hair. Add 1 or 2 drops of red pepper (cayenne) oil to 1 ounce of rosemary oil in a small clean bottle, then massage your entire scalp with the mixture for at least 20 minutes every day. Afterward, add 5 drops of rosemary oil per ounce of shampoo you'll use, and wash your hair with it.

Break an Egg

■ Old-timers used to swear by this treatment for hair loss: Once or twice a week, beat a raw egg into about 1 tablespoon of olive oil, and massage the mixture into your hair and scalp. Leave it on for a few minutes, then rinse with warm water.

EUREKA!

WHAT'S THE CURE FOR DRY HAIR? How about a ripe (overripe is even better) avocado that's been skinned and mashed? Simply apply the puree, leave it on for 15 minutes, and then rinse it out with cool water. Your locks will be luscious—guaranteed!

Hair-Taming Treatment

 When your hair is so dry that split ends are appearing, bring those unruly tresses under control with this sweet and pungent tamer. This is one fast fix that is guaranteed to help, and the best part is, it only costs pennies to make!

2 tbsp. of garlic oil
1 tsp. of honey
1 egg yolk

➡ Combine the oil and honey, then beat in the egg yolk. Rub the mixture into your hair one small section at a time. Cover it with a shower cap or plastic bag, and wait at least 30 minutes. Then rinse thoroughly, and shampoo as usual.

Soften More Than Fabric

■ Fresh out of hair conditioner? No problem! Just mosey on into the laundry room, and pick up the liquid fabric softener. Use it as you would your normal conditioner, pouring a similar-size dollop of the liquid into your hand and working it in thoroughly. Wait two to three minutes, and rinse. (Be sure you use a quality product for the job. The lower-priced brands don't seem to work as well—or so I'm told by my lady friends, who have a lot more on top than I do!)

Fix Flat Hair

■ There's no need for pricey mousses and gels! Just rub some good old-fashioned shaving cream into the roots of your locks. It'll give lifeless hair plenty of texture, lift, and bounce.

Nifty, Thrifty Tips

Here's a cheap and easy way to revitalize dry hair with an intensive conditioning treatment. Simply massage 1 cup of olive oil into your hair, and cover it with a plastic bag or shower cap. Cover that with a towel, secure it well with safety pins, and leave it on overnight. In the morning, wash your tresses with your regular shampoo, and rinse with a half-and-half solution of white vinegar and water. Your hair will feel like a million bucks!

Healthy Hair Herbals

Just like your fingernails, hair health is a reflection of your internal health. So make it a regular habit to drink nutritive teas that are rich in minerals to optimize your skin and hair health. These helpful herbs will do just fine.

Horsetail
Nettles
Oat straw
Red clover
1 cup of hot water

➥ Combine equal parts of all the herbs, and add 1 heaping teaspoon of the mixture to the water. Steep the tea for 10 to 15 minutes, and strain out the solids. Drink 1 to 2 cups daily. **Caution:** Be sure to wear gloves when handling fresh nettles so you don't get stung.

Natural Old-Time Conditioner

■ Grandma Putt conditioned her hair with this old-time kitchen formula, and it still works as well as any product on the market—maybe even better. Beat the white of one egg until it's foamy, then stir it into 5 tablespoons of plain yogurt. Apply the mixture to one small section of your hair at a time. Leave it on for 15 minutes, then rinse and you'll have a beautiful shine.

Herbal Hair Saver

■ Comb the hair-care aisles of your local supermarket or drugstore for herbal hair products that contain camphor and eucalyptus. They dilate the blood vessels in your scalp, which will discourage hair loss and help you hang on to what you've got longer.

Snappy Solutions

Because hair is made up of protein, it's especially important to beef up the protein content of your diet. The best way is to drink plenty of milk and eat lots of other protein-rich foods, such as poultry, lean meat, and fish. It'll save you from having to waste your day on different and expensive hair treatments.

Heirloom Hair Lightener

 Make your hair a few shades lighter without spending a small fortune at the beauty parlor. Just whip up this old-time concoction to brighten up your day.

Juice of 2 limes
Juice of 1 lemon
2 tbsp. of mild shampoo

➤ Mix the ingredients in a container, pour the solution onto your hair, and massage it in well. Then sit in the sun for 15 to 20 minutes. Rinse thoroughly, and apply a good conditioner. Repeat the process until you think you're blonde enough to have more fun!

Epsom Salts Wash

■ You can wash excess oil right out of your hair with good old Epsom salts. Simply mix 1 cup of the salts and 1 cup of lemon juice in 1 gallon of water, and let the mixture sit for 24 hours. Pour the solution onto dry hair, wait 20 minutes or so, then shampoo as usual.

Home Hair Coloring

■ If you color your tresses yourself at home, here's a helpful hint: Before you begin, put on a stretchy, terry-cloth headband, and tuck cotton balls or pads inside. It's a more efficient way to catch drips than the usual method of "pasting" cotton to your head with petroleum jelly. (This headband trick also works to keep home-permanent solution out of your eyes.)

What Would Grandma Do?

GRANDMA PUTT *could never be bothered with coloring her hair, but she certainly knew how to go about it. If you ever told her you wanted to put red highlights in your curly locks, she'd have given you this advice: After shampooing in your usual way, rinse your hair with strong black coffee that's been cooled to room temperature. Give it 15 minutes or so to work its magic, then rinse thoroughly with cool water.*

Lemon-Fresh Hair Spray

There are plenty of different products you can use to hold your hair temporarily in place, but a lot of them can do your tresses more damage than good. So, if you're tired of forking over your hard-earned dough for store-bought sprays, try this super-simple DIY alternative.

2 cups of water
2 lemons
1 tbsp. of vodka

➡ Boil the water in a saucepan. While the water is boiling, peel and finely chop the lemons. Add them to the boiling water, and simmer the mixture over low heat until the lemons are soft. Cool, strain, and pour the solution into a spray bottle. Add the vodka, and shake well. If the solution is too sticky, dilute it with a little water and you're good to go.

Flee, Flakes!

■ Residue from shampoos and conditioners can leave your scalp flaky and irritated. Fortunately, I know a fast and easy fixer for that nasty feeling: Just rinse your hair with a solution of 3 tablespoons of white vinegar in a cup of warm water. Work it in well, and follow with a clear water rinse until the vinegar is gone.

Color Me Full

■ If your hair color is close to your skin color, your scalp will be less noticeable. So if you're thinning out, use hair coloring to reduce the see-through scalp look. And if you decide to color your hair at home, use only semi-permanent dyes. They are not harsh, and they will plump up your hair shafts so they look thicker. Avoid permanent dyes that don't wash out and create a color line between natural and dyed hair that seems to make thinning hair more obvious.

EUREKA!

ONE HANDY WAY to disguise thinning hair is to get a perm for fullness. Curls cover a lot more real estate than straight hair does, and by gently mussing your curls, you can camouflage any thinning areas.

Longer Locks Shampoo

You say your hairdresser got carried away and trimmed your tresses too short for your liking? Believe it or not, this herbal fixer will hasten the growth of your hair, so it'll be back to a more pleasing length sooner than you might expect—and will also give it a healthy sheen. **Note:** The herbs in this formula work best for dry hair. See "Accept Substitutions" below for the oily-hair alternatives.

1 part calendula flowers
1 part fresh or dried
    marshmallow root
1 part fresh or dried
    nettle leaf
1 cup of distilled water
3 oz. of liquid castile soap
¼ tsp. of jojoba oil
25 drops of peppermint oil
    (not extract!)

➤ Mix the calendula, marshmallow, and nettle leaf together, and measure out 2 tablespoons of the combo. In a pan, bring the water to a boil, and add the herbs. Cover, reduce the heat, and let the formula simmer for 15 to 20 minutes. Strain, and let the brew cool. Slowly add the castile soap, then stir in the jojoba and peppermint oils. Pour the mixture into a plastic bottle with a flip-top lid, and use it as you would any other shampoo. **Caution:** Be sure to wear gloves when handling fresh nettles to avoid their stinging hairs.

Accept Substitutions

■ To make Longer Locks Shampoo (above) for oily hair, keep the distilled water and liquid castile soap, and follow the instructions above, but replace the herbal ingredients with these winners: 1 part rosemary leaf, 1 part witch hazel bark (not extract), 1 part yarrow leaf and flower, ¼ teaspoon of rosemary essential oil, and 25 drops of basil essential oil.

EUREKA!

HAS SWIMMING IN A CHLORINATED POOL turned your blonde curls bright green? Not to worry! Just grab a bottle of club soda, and wash those chemicals right out of your hair.

More Color for More Fun

Herbal rinses add sheen to hair shafts while relieving any scalp irritations. You can choose which herbs to use based on your hair color. Try rosemary and sage for dark hair, chamomile and marigold for blonde, and cloves for auburn or red hair.

4 tsp. of herb (your choice)
1 qt. of boiling water
¼ cup of apple cider vinegar

➡ Make a strong tea by adding your herb of choice to the boiling water. Steep for 15 minutes, and add the apple cider vinegar to restore the scalp's proper pH. Use this mixer as a final rinse after shampooing your hair.

Let Natural Oils Out

■ Before you color your hair, avoid shampooing it for three or four days to build up the natural oils on your scalp. They will protect your hair from becoming too dry from the processing. Also, because the wrong dye can harm your hair, always experiment with a patch test before you color, especially if you have not used that particular product before.

Potato Highlights

■ To add glistening highlights to brown hair, try this neat trick: Dip a pastry brush in potato water (water that you've previously boiled potatoes in), and saturate your hair, being careful not to get any water in your eyes. Wait 30 minutes, and then rinse thoroughly with cool water. Repeat this treatment every few weeks to retain the highlights.

What Would Grandma Do?

🦋 *When Grandma Putt didn't have time to wash her hair, she gave herself a dry shampoo with oatmeal. She'd put a handful on her head, work it through her hair with her fingers, and brush it out. That cereal removed all the oil, leaving Grandma's hair clean and shiny.*

Noggin Massage

Barbers have long known that massaging the scalp stimulates circulation, feeding both oxygen and nutrients to hair follicles and perhaps stimulating hair growth. Now that *you* know that, you should treat yourself to regular scalp massages. This fast fixer really gives your scalp a workout.

6 drops of lavender oil
½ cup of warm almond, soy, or sesame oil
Bay oil (also called bay laurel)

➡ Add the lavender oil (which stimulates blood flow) to the almond, soy, or sesame oil (all of which easily penetrate the skin), and massage the mixture into your scalp for 20 minutes. Then wash it out with shampoo, adding 3 drops of bay oil per ounce of shampoo.

Rhubarb Lightener

■ When Grandma's women friends wanted to lighten their hair, they'd go about it this way—and you can, too. Start by stirring 3 tablespoons of chopped rhubarb stems into 3 cups of hot water. Simmer for 10 minutes, strain out the rhubarb, and cool the remaining liquid. Then use the solution as a rinse after each shampoo until you get the desired color.

Don't Let Your Hair Get Thirsty

■ If your hair is overprocessed, it's crucial to add lots of moisture to it—the more, the better. Moisture makes follicles stronger and more resilient. An easy way to get the job done is to deep-condition your hair several times a week.

EUREKA!

WHEN DRY, HEATED AIR leaves your locks full of static, head to your laundry room and grab a dryer sheet. Rub it all over your tresses, from the roots toward the ends. Your hair will lose the electricity and stop standing on end every time you wave a hand near it.

Thickening Conditioner

Shampoo is great for cleaning your hair, but the wrong shampoo can leave it drier than it should be. That's where a good conditioner comes in to give your hair back the life it's lost. This rich blend will leave your locks looking thicker, shinier, and healthier, too!

1 egg yolk
½ tsp. of olive oil
¾ cup of lukewarm water

➡ Beat the egg yolk until it's thick and light colored. As you continue beating, slowly drizzle the oil into the egg. Still beating, slowly add the water. When you're done, pour the mixture into a plastic container. After shampooing, massage all of the conditioner into your hair. Leave it on for three or four minutes, then rinse thoroughly.

Keep Those Tresses Sparkling

■ Grandma Putt never dyed her hair, but when the gold had turned to silver (as the old song goes), she had a little trick for keeping her tresses sparkling white: After she washed her hair, she added a few drops of bluing (found in the supermarket laundry aisle) to a quart of water, and used this as a final rinse. Some folks use this treatment after every shampoo, but Grandma only did it when she felt she needed a nice whitening boost.

Nifty, Thrifty Tips

Tired of paying beauty-shop prices just to have your bangs trimmed? Then close up your wallet, and cut 'em yourself like the old-timers did. Here's how: When your hair is wet, run transparent tape across your forehead, with the top edge where you want the bottom of your bangs to be. Looking in a mirror, cut just above the tape. You'll have a professional salon look that cost you nothing— and you can't beat that at twice the price!

Chocolate Lip Balm

When harsh winter air leaves your lips cracked and dry, reach for this mixer. While you're at it, make a few extras so you'll have gifts to give to all the chocoholics in your life!

2 tbsp. of petroleum jelly
1 vitamin E capsule
1 tbsp. of powdered chocolate milk mix (or to taste)

➡ Put the petroleum jelly in a micro-wave-safe container, and nuke it at 30-second intervals until the jelly is melted. (Be patient—it might take several minutes.) Snip open the vitamin E capsule and squeeze the oil into the melted petroleum jelly, and then stir well. Mix in the chocolate milk powder (you can use vanilla or strawberry if you'd prefer), return it to the microwave for another 30 seconds, and mix again until smooth. Let the mixture cool a bit, and pour it into small, clean, airtight containers.

Stop the Smoke

■ Smoking dries out your lips and makes them more prone to chapping. Since it also robs you of your B vitamins, the skin tissues in the corner of your mouth get weak, causing unsightly cracks or splits to appear. If you cut out the smoking, your lips should be back in good smacking order in no time at all. So add this item to the long list of good reasons to kick the habit.

Snappy Solutions

What's that—you woke up in the middle of the night with dry, chapped lips, and you're fresh out of lip balm? Don't run out to the all-night convenience store—if you have a store-bought cucumber handy in your kitchen. Just wash the cuke, dry it with a clean towel, and run your lips back and forth over the waxy peel several times. This veggie stand-in will never replace real lip balm, but it will let you sleep in comfort until you can get to the store the next day.

Flavored Lip Gloss

There are plenty of glosses on the market to give your lips a healthier-than-healthy shine. But those pricey products can really put a pinch on your wallet. So don't waste your money—make your own tinted, flavored fixer with this recipe.

1 tbsp. of petroleum jelly
¼ tsp. of lipstick
2 to 4 drops of your favorite extract

➤ In a bowl, mix the petroleum jelly, lipstick, and your favorite extract—like orange, rum, or peppermint. Then scrape the gloss into a small lidded container—that's all there is to it! Take out a glob and rub it on your lips whenever they're feeling a little too dry for your liking.

Lip Gloss Holders

■ When you whip up homemade gloss, you may decide to make a day of it by preparing as many different flavors as you can think of. But all those little containers can create quite a mess to try and keep cleaned up. So after you bottle your homemade gloss, pack it in clean movie-film canisters. You can fit a lot of jars in one canister, keeping your gloss right where you want it for right when you need it most.

Make Cold Sores Scram

■ If your lips are prone to cold sores, don't despair. The virus-fighting compounds in lemon balm have been found to be effective on these ugly nuisances. Just steep 2 to 3 teaspoons of the dried herb in hot water, let it cool a bit, then dab the liquid onto each cold sore with a cotton ball.

What Would Grandma Do?

🦋 FOLKS IN GRANDMA PUTT'S DAY knew how to cope with emergencies—even minor ones, like running out of lipstick. They'd make a stand-in supply by putting a teaspoon or so of petroleum jelly in a small dish, and mixing in some red food coloring. How much food coloring they used depended on how dark they wanted their lips to be.

Luscious Lip Gloss

Hey, candle makers! The next time you practice your craft, save some of the beeswax and use it to whip up a batch of this smooth, tasty, and great-smelling lip gloss.

1 tbsp. of grated beeswax
4½ tsp. of coconut oil
1 vitamin E capsule
⅛ tsp. of pure vanilla
    extract (not artificial)

➡ Put the beeswax and coconut oil in an ovenproof container, and add the contents of the vitamin E capsule. Place the dish in the oven, and heat it at 250°F until the wax is melted. Pour in the vanilla extract, stir well, and let the mixture cool completely. Then store it in a container that's got a tight lid. To apply the gloss to your lips, use a lip brush or your little finger. Coconut oil is available in health-food stores and the cooking-oil section of many supermarkets. You can also substitute almond extract for the vanilla extract, depending on your personal taste.

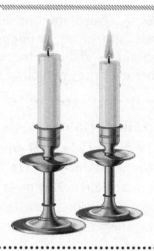

Baby Your Lips

■ When your lips are cracked and dry, there's one surefire way to give them back a great sheen and make them at least *look* healthy again. What is it? Baby oil! Just rub a small amount on and watch your lips glow. As an alternative, you can use olive oil for the same effect.

EUREKA!

IF YOUR LIPS are lacking the vibrant color you envy in everyone else's, try eating more green vegetables. They're rich in zinc, essential fatty acids, and riboflavin—everything your lips need to retain moisture and stay healthy all year long. It's a great way to keep your lips in the pink!

A Dilly of a Deal for Your Nails

If you're sick and tired of living with dull, brittle nails, then you need to hit the herbal gym. This mixture is just what your personal trainer ordered. The dill in this mixer contains nail-strengthening calcium and other minerals, while the horsetail provides silica, which gives nails (and also hair and skin) flexibility and strength.

**1 cup of water
½ tsp. of dill extract
½ tsp. of horsetail
    extract**

➡ Heat the water until it's almost boiling, then add the dill and horsetail extracts (available at health-food stores and herb shops). Wait until the brew cools, then soak your fingertips in the solution. Do this three times a week for stronger, healthier nails.

Straight from Your Lips

■ Are dry cuticles driving you crazy? Then reach into your pocket, purse, or medicine chest, and pull out a tube of lip balm. Rub it onto the base of your nails, and bingo—instant moisturizing!

Hold the Knox

■ Thanks to the Knox family, which in the 1890s began making powdered gelatin from the ground-up hooves and bones of cows that died on their farm in upstate New York, most of us think that gulping thick, protein-rich gelatin will strengthen our nails. Wrong! Gelatin does provide protein—but in an incomplete form that your body can't use. So skip the gelatin and instead apply a clear polish to halt moisture loss and fortify your nails.

Snappy Solutions

If you use a professional manicurist, keeping long fingernails in tip-top shape is time-consuming, and an expensive process to boot. To make your life simpler and your bank account plumper, wear your nails on the short side and take care of them yourself.

Mineral Magic

While your eyes may be the mirror of your soul, your fingernails can be a portal to your basic health. Calcium and magnesium are essential to nail health, and this elixir is loaded with both of these minerals.

Horsetail
Nettles
Oat straw
1 cup of hot water

➡ Combine equal parts of the horsetail, nettles, and oat straw and steep 1 heaping teaspoon of the mixture in the water for 10 minutes. Drink 1 to 2 cups daily to strengthen your nails. **Caution:** Be sure to wear gloves when handling fresh nettles to avoid their stinging hairs.

Lemon Scrub

■ Clean up your dingy, tired-looking nails with a quick lemon scrub. Just cut a fresh lemon in half, and dig your fingers into the juicy flesh. Make sure your fingers don't have cuts or scrapes on them, or you'll be in for a stinging surprise!

Don't Cover the Moon

■ When you polish your nails, be sure you don't cover the white half-moon at the base with polish. Why? Because it's live tissue that needs air. As I learned on that long-ago day before surgery, the color of those half-moons provides a quick way to tell if oxygen is circulating to the tips of your fingers.

Nifty, Thrifty Tips

Wearing nail polish all the time can make your nails brittle, and buying all those little bottles of polish can put a pinch on your wallet. So give both some breathing room by periodically laying off the polish. And don't paste on false nails either, because some of the adhesives can cause severe allergic reactions. Speaking of allergies, both nail polish and polish remover contain harsh chemicals that can cause an allergic reaction on your eyelids and the sides of your neck, even though the chemicals are on your nails.

Nail Strengthener

Nails are made of keratin, which is the same protein that is found in your hair and outer skin. Your nail growth slows down as you age, but during their peak period, they grow about ⅛ inch a month. So until your nails slow down, keep them looking their best with this mixer that will both strengthen and add shine to them.

2 tsp. of castor oil
2 tsp. of salt
1 tsp. of wheat germ oil

➡ Combine the ingredients in a small bowl, mixing them well. Pour the mixture into a bottle. Shake it vigorously before using, and apply the oil to your nails with a cotton ball. You'll be amazed at the results!

Start a Glove Collection

■ Buy some latex or rubber gloves to protect your hands and nails when you do dishes or clean house. Constant immersion in water makes your nails brittle; plus, they swell when they're wet and shrink when they're dry. As expected, this repeated change makes them vulnerable to chipping, cracking, and other damage.

Grapefruit Nail Paint

■ Fungal infections on or beneath nails can be difficult to get rid of. Before resorting to more toxic therapies, try a regimen of nail painting with grapefruit-seed extract (available at most health-food stores). Paint only the affected nail one to two times a day, taking care not to get the extract on the surrounding skin, which may become irritated. Continue the treatment for about six weeks for best results.

✚ If you are diabetic or have poor circulation, you need to be very vigilant in caring for your toenails because nail infections can spread to surrounding areas. It's best to make friends with a podiatrist, and have your toenails trimmed by him or her so you don't risk serious problems.

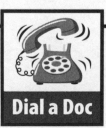

Dial a Doc

Natural Nail-Fungus Fighter

Foul fungi that attack your toe- or finger-nails can be major menaces to your health and well-being as well as your good looks. But before you resort to prescription drugs, which can damage your kidneys, give Mother Nature a chance to work her magic with this simple fixer.

1 tsp. of olive oil
2 drops of oregano oil

➡ Combine the oils and apply the mixer to the affected area three times a day. The key ingredient, oregano, has potent antifungal properties that should clear up the problem within a few weeks. If you do not see any relief within three weeks, call your doctor.

Castor Oil to the Rescue

■ Not only are cracked cuticles unattractive, but they can also hurt like the dickens. To repair the cracks and ease the pain, rub castor oil into the skin around your nails every night at bedtime. Before you know it, you'll see—and feel—an amazing difference.

Farewell, Fungus!

■ When you're battling a fungus, whether it's in your finger- or toenails, or both, you can get relief from this unexpected source—namely, the same mentholated rub that clears up chest colds. Just massage the aromatic rub into the skin around your afflicted nail(s) twice a day until the trouble disappears. And if you're prone to nail fungi, you should apply the mentholated rub daily to prevent repeated outbreaks.

What Would Grandma Do?

🦋 WHEN YOU'VE GOT A HANGNAIL *that's driving you crazy, relieve the pain with this favorite Putt family remedy: Add 4 capfuls of bath oil (any kind will do) to 1 pint of warm water and soak your ailing fingertip in the solution for about 15 minutes.*

Terrific Toenail Tea

This fabulous fungus-fighting fixer owes its success to two of the most powerful healers in nature's medicine chest: garlic and echinacea. Just one word of warning: You may need to use this, um, fragrant tonic for a period of weeks or even months before your fungus infection goes away, so do your family and friends a favor and stock up on mouthwash and breath mints before you start your treatment!

1 cup of water
2 tsp. of dried
    echinacea root
15 garlic cloves, minced
Honey and/or lemon

➡ Pour the water into a pan and bring it to a boil. Add the echinacea and garlic and simmer for 15 minutes. Remove the pan from the heat, and steep for 10 to 20 minutes. Strain out the solids, and stir in the honey and/or lemon to taste. Then drink the brew, either cool or reheated. Drink 1 cup a day until your foul fungus is history. If you find the flavor too strong, dilute the potion with 1 cup of water, and drink two milder doses daily. **Caution:** Don't take echinacea if you have an autoimmune disease, such as rheumatoid arthritis, lupus, or multiple sclerosis.

Crack an Egg for Cracked Nails

■ The fruit of the hen is jam-packed with protein and sulfur (both of which speed nail growth) along with biotin, the B vitamin that helps your body make and use amino acids, the building blocks of protein. So unless your doctor advises against it, eat eggs several times a week.

EUREKA!

DO YOU BREAK A NAIL every time you open an aspirin bottle? Then save your nails (and your good humor) by keeping a bottle opener next to the aspirin—or any other bottle that has a hard-to-pop top.

Aaahhh Aftershave

Okay, guys—this one's for you. Here's an easy mixer that will make the women in your life go "Aaahhh" and leave your freshly shaven face feeling like it was just treated at a spa.

2 cups of rubbing alcohol
1 tbsp. of glycerin
1 tbsp. of dried lavender
1 tsp. of ground cloves
1 tsp. of dried rosemary

➥ Thoroughly mix all of the ingredients, pour the solution into a bottle with a tight-fitting cap, and refrigerate. Shake well before using, and strain the solids out as you use the liquid. This oh-so-soothing aftershave will keep, refrigerated, for up to two months. Enjoy!

Replace Your Razor

■ During a folliculitis outbreak (hair follicle inflammation), it's easy for your razor's edge to be contaminated with bacteria. If that happens, then every time you shave, you can push hordes of bacteria under your skin. To prevent this from happening, buy disposable razors and use each one only once during an outbreak.

Forget the Antibiotics

■ A lot of people insist on using antibiotic soaps and creams to treat or prevent ingrown hairs. Don't do it. These products tend to irritate your skin, including areas where hairs may be growing inward. Instead, if you frequently get ingrown hairs or irritated bumps, try using a soothing skin cleanser that contains alpha hydroxy acids or benzoyl peroxide to keep them at bay.

EUREKA!

ONE OF THE EASIEST WAYS to prevent ingrown hairs and allow for smoother, faster shaving is to wash your face or legs with soap and water before, as well as after, shaving. Thorough cleansing reduces the risk that bacteria will survive long enough to colonize tiny shaving nicks or ingrown hair follicles and multiply.

Bay-Rum Aftershave

Let's face it: Too many men are just too hard to shop for around holiday time. If you're looking for a homemade gift idea for the men in your life, look no further. This classic potion is the perfect answer—especially for those guys who have everything!

½ cup of vodka
2 tbsp. of dark rum
2 dried bay leaves
¼ tsp. of allspice
1 cinnamon stick
Rind from 1 small
   orange, shredded

➡ Combine all of the ingredients. Pour the mixture into a clean jar with a tight lid, and set it in a cool, dark place for two weeks. Strain out the solids, and pour the liquid into a nice-looking bottle. Add a label, if you'd like. That's all there is to it, and the men will love it!

Turn Off the Juice

■ Electric shavers may allow you to shave without using lather or water, but they're more likely to irritate your skin than non-electric razors are. So if you're having skin problems, go back to the blades at least until the irritation has subsided.

Lose the Razor

■ For some men with extremely curly facial hair, not shaving may be the only solution to persistent ingrown hairs. Give it a try and see how well the bearded look suits you—or at least go a few days between shaves to give your skin a much-needed break to recuperate.

Snappy Solutions

Save yourself some time in the morning by shaving in the shower. It'll keep your skin clean and your pores open. This practice also reduces the chances that your skin will be irritated, and it allows for a closer shave, which can keep hairs from growing inward.

Extra-Gentle Aftershave

Hey, fellows! Is your skin too sensitive for regular aftershave lotions? If so, then you've come to the right place—this elixir has your name written all over it!

½ cup of witch hazel
2 tbsp. of dried
      chamomile flowers
2 tbsp. of vodka

➡ Combine the ingredients in a clean glass jar with a tight-fitting lid. Let the mixture steep in a cool, dark place for two weeks, strain out the solids, and splash it on.

Help from the Orange Box
◼ No matter how sensitive your skin is, a simple ingredient in your kitchen can end your razor burn problems once and for all. Simply add 1 tablespoon of baking soda per cup of water, and splash the solution onto your face or legs either before or after you shave (or both, if you like).

Baby Your Legs
◼ Before you shave your legs with an electric razor, dust them with baby powder. That way, you'll prevent painful (and unattractive) friction burns.

Soothe the Burn
◼ Razor burn is no fun, especially if it's in the sensitive bikini line area. Ladies, here's a way to ease the irritation and get rid of those unsightly bumps. Snip the ends off several vitamin E capsules and gently apply the oil directly to the inflamed area. Vitamin E works quickly to speed healing, so your skin will be silky smooth in no time at all.

Nifty, Thrifty Tips

If you've checked the price of razor blades lately, this tip will be music to your ears: To make a blade last up to five times longer, dry it well after each use, coat it with a thin layer of petroleum jelly, and wipe off any excess using a washcloth or several layers of tissues—but do it *very* carefully, please!

Shave and Soothe Solution

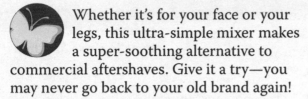

Whether it's for your face or your legs, this ultra-simple mixer makes a super-soothing alternative to commercial aftershaves. Give it a try—you may never go back to your old brand again!

1 part apple cider vinegar
1 part witch hazel

➡ Mix the vinegar and witch hazel in a bowl, and slap the bracing solution on after shaving. That's all there is to it!

Help for Wayward Hairs

■ It's not necessary to pull an ingrown hair out of your skin; your body will eventually expel it. But you should gently clean the affected area twice a day with soap and water, and keep an eagle eye out for infection. Warning signs include increasing heat, redness, swelling, pain, or pus. If an infection doesn't clear up on its own in a day or two, see your doctor.

Hit It with Heat and Cold

■ To ease painful or infected ingrown hairs, alternate hot and cold compresses. Soak a washcloth in hot water, wring it out, and drape it over the sore area. Keep it there for three minutes, then replace it with a cold cloth for one minute. Repeat the cycle two more times, ending with the cold compress. This fixer, called contrast hydrotherapy, improves skin circulation and speeds healing.

A Dream of a Shaving "Cream"

■ All out of shaving cream? No worries—simply grab some baby oil to get the job done. It'll lubricate your razor, keep the hairs standing up for a clean shave, and won't dry out your skin.

✚ If an ingrown hair bump becomes large and very painful and/or if the infection spreads and causes fever, dizziness, or other symptoms, see your doctor ASAP.

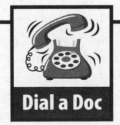

Dial a Doc

Get-Lost Garlic Mash

Here's how to take advantage of garlic's anti-viral superpowers to get rid of a bothersome wart. This powerful fixer will work like nobody's business!

1 vitamin E capsule
1 garlic clove, mashed

Prick the vitamin E capsule with a pin, and apply the oil to the skin surrounding the wart to protect it from the volatile oils in the garlic. Place the mashed garlic on the wart, and cover the area with a bandage. After 24 hours, remove the bandage and wipe the area clean. A blister will soon form, and before you know it, you'll be wart-free!

Vim and Vinegar

■ Annoying and unsightly warts will vanish when you use this simple, old-time fixer. At bedtime, cover the bump with apple cider vinegar. Simply soak a gauze pad in apple cider vinegar, put it over the wart, and cover it with a bandage to hold in the moisture. Leave it on overnight. In the morning, remove the bandage, but don't rinse off the vinegar. Repeat each night until the bump is gone.

Watch Your Step

■ The virus that causes warts is everywhere, and you can easily pick it up by following in someone's footsteps in a shower, locker room, or public pool. Always wear flip-flops or sandals when you're walking around, and don't shower in the same stall or tub of someone who has warts. It takes about three months for a wart to appear once you've been infected, but the virus can also lie dormant for years, so you probably won't remember where you got it.

What Would Grandma Do?

ANYTIME I GOT A WART, Grandma Putt would tell me firmly, "Whatever you do, don't pick it!" She knew that would be asking for more trouble, because even if you picked the whole thing off, you'd just spread the virus that caused it—and the original wart would grow back bigger and nastier to boot!

Oil's Well Wart Remover

Like many effective solutions to life's minor woes, this one may seem too simple to be true. But I've tried it, and it works—trust me!

1 pinch of baking soda
2 drops of castor oil

➡ At bedtime, mix the baking soda and the castor oil, dab the paste onto the wart, and leave it on overnight. Repeat the procedure until the nasty blemish is history, which should happen within a few days.

Bark Up the Right Tree

■ Folklore from Michigan holds that all you need to cure a wart is a strip of bark from a birch tree. (If you don't have a birch tree handy, you can find birch bark in many health-food stores.) Soak the bark in water until it softens, then tape it directly to your wart. Nobody knows exactly why it works, but birch bark contains salicylates, the main ingredient in some FDA-approved wart treatments.

An A-Peeling Idea

■ When a wart is on the sole of your foot, it's known as a plantar wart. The pressure of walking on it makes it grow inward and press on nerves in your foot—so it hurts like all get-out. Often these growths need to be removed by a doctor, but before you pick up the phone, try this old-time fixer: At bedtime, tape a piece of banana peel, inner side down, over the wart. Cover the peel with a large bandage or tight sock, and leave it on overnight. Repeat the procedure each night until the wart is gone.

✚ If your warts won't go away, if they are tender, or if they are a cosmetic nuisance, ask your doctor about having them removed. There are many treatments available—from freezing them with liquid nitrogen to zapping them with lasers and injecting them with virus-killing drugs. The resulting wound can be cauterized with chemicals or an electric needle.

Dial a Doc

Yellow Cedar Oil

Everyone's immune system responds differently to the virus that causes warts, so some people's warts clear up faster than others'. Jump-start your war on warts with this potent cedar salve. **Caution:** If a wart changes color or size, or if it morphs into a new shape or begins to bleed, see your doctor.

Yellow cedar (thuja) leaves
Vegetable oil
1 vitamin E capsule

➡ Fill a small jar with thuja leaves, and cover them with vegetable oil. Open the vitamin E capsule and squeeze out the oil. Let the mixture sit in a sunny window for 10 days, shaking well each day. Strain, and keep the oil in a cool, dark place. Stored in the refrigerator, the mixer will last four to six months. Apply two to three times daily to the surface of the wart.

Separate Your Grooming Gear

■ If you have a wart on the finger of one hand, don't use the same nail clipper or nail file on your unaffected hand. Likewise, if the bump is on your nose, don't powder it with the same puff you use for the rest of your face. In fact, you should segregate all your personal-care tools to keep the virus from spreading.

Miracle Wart Weeds

■ If you have dandelions growing in your lawn, go pick yourself a wart cure. Herbalists say you should apply the sap from the flower stem to the unsightly bump three times a day for as long as it takes for the wart to disappear.

Nifty, Thrifty Tips

Basil, say folk healers, can banish a wart. Basil contains several anti-viral compounds that make warts disappear faster than you can say, "Watch me pull a rabbit out of a hat!" Just crush a few basil leaves, place them on the bump, and cover the area with a bandage. Change the dressing every day, and the wart should disappear within a week.

Fantastic Face Food

You'd be hard-pressed to find a more emollient fruit than an avocado. Its high fat content makes it an ideal base for an anti-aging and anti-wrinkle mask.

½ of an avocado
½ tsp. of vitamin E oil
1 tbsp. of plain yogurt

Mash the avocado, then blend in the vitamin E oil and yogurt. Apply the mixer to your face, paying close attention to any crow's-feet, laugh lines, or wrinkles around your eyes and mouth. Leave it on for 20 minutes, then rinse it away with warm water.

Oil Your Insides

■ Essential fatty acids are vital to skin health, and a deficiency can leave you looking dried out and wrinkled. So make sure you eat at least one serving of omega-3 oils every day (salmon, almonds, and sesame seeds are good sources), or take them in capsule form. You can find flaxseed oil, black currant oil, borage oil, and evening primrose oil at health-food stores or in the natural-foods section of a supermarket. The recommended dose is 1,000 milligrams once or twice daily.

Q: *Ever since I started smoking, I've noticed that I've been getting little lines around my eyes and cheeks. What's causing it?*

Take My Advice

A: The culprit could be right there with you. In addition to bringing on death, disease, and other forms of disaster, cigarette smoke is a major culprit in prematurely wrinkled skin! Not only does it damage skin cells, but smoking also causes you to spend countless hours every day squinting. That's why smokers usually have much more pronounced crow's-feet (not to mention more wrinkles of all sorts) than other folks do.

Pure and Simple Wrinkle Remover

 As we all know, life has its little ups and downs. And after a while, the accompanying smiles and frowns begin to leave their mark. But you don't have to spend a small fortune on fancy cosmetics or painful Botox® treatments to eliminate the signs of aging. Instead, erase those lines with this old-time fantastic fixer.

Mild soap
Warm water
Milk of magnesia
¼ cup of virgin olive oil
Witch hazel (refrigerated)

➡ Wash your face with the soap and water, dry it, and wait 10 minutes. Using a cotton pad, spread a thin layer of milk of magnesia all over (making sure to keep it away from your eyes!), and let it dry completely. Apply a second layer of milk of magnesia, which will dissolve the first one. Wipe it all off with a warm, damp washcloth. Next, heat the olive oil in a small pan over low heat until it's just lukewarm. Apply it to your face with a cotton pad, leave it on for five minutes, and wipe it off with the witch hazel. Repeat this procedure twice a week, and within a couple of weeks, you'll be looking considerably less, um, experienced.

Grape-tastic Wrinkle Eraser

■ Here's a grape way to minimize those tiny lines around your eyes and mouth. Just cut seedless green grapes in half, and squeeze the juice right into the little creases. That's it!

EUREKA!

ONE OF THE EASIEST wrinkle-prevention maneuvers of all is to simply get in the habit of wearing sunglasses every time you go outdoors—even when the sun's not shining brightly. This way, your eyes will stay relaxed. (Along with radiation damage, which can occur even on cloudy days, it's those constant muscle contractions that form wrinkles.) Choose shades that block UV light, and opt for a wraparound style, or glasses with wide sidepieces.

INDEX

Caffeine *(continued)*
  for headaches, 148
  postnasal drip and, 210
  for sciatica, 214
Calamine lotion, 219
Calcium, 177, 248
Calendula
  for burns, 46
  Calendula Cream, 270
  for canker sores, 50
  for facial care, 305, 307
  for foot care, 139
  for sore throat, 228
  for sunburn, 246
  for vaginal dryness, 103
Calendula Cream, 270
Calf-Pain Reliever, 185
Canker Sore Counterattack, 49
Canker sores, 49–51
Cantaloupe, 106
Capsaicin, 21, 220
Capsule Cure, 242
Caraway Cramping Cure, 175
Caraway seed, 119, 122
Carbohydrates, 113, 114
Carbonated beverages, 121
Carminative herbs and seeds, 119
Carrot-Combo Cure, 105
Carrots
  carrot neck wrap, 58, 229
  for eye health, 106
  for facial care, 310, 317
  for hair care, 326
Cast-iron cookware, 7
Castor oil, 120, 194, 298, 342
Catnip, 82, 222
Cauliflower, 115
Cayenne pepper
  for cellulite, 283
  for colds, 61, 69

  for hair care, 327
  Red Pepper Mouthwash, 264
Cedar Soother, 47
Cellulite, 281–283
Cent-Sible Stomach Settler, 120
Cereals, high-fiber, 100
Cereal Scrubber, 297
Chamomile
  caution, 10
  Chamomile Cure, 208
  for foot care, 139
  Gratitude Tea, 10
  for stress, 232, 235
Chamomile Cure, 208
Chapped lips, 336
Chard, 106
Cherries, 18
Chest pain, 150
Chewing gum, 41, 96, 142, 164
Chicken soup, 45, 68
Chickweed Salve, 168
Chicory, 203
Child care, 284–288
Chilling Spray, 109
Chlorophyll, 264, 271, 276
Chlorophyll Cleansing Tonic, 271
Chocolate, 128, 233
Chocolate Lip Balm, 336
Cholesterol levels, 54
Cholesterol medication, 181
Cinnamon, 61, 124
Cinnamon Stick Tea, 22
Cinnamon Tea, 95
Circulation, 52–55, 341
Circulation-Boosting Solution, 52
Circulation Enhancer, 53
Citrate magnesia, 71
Citrus fruit, 23, 96. *See also specific fruits*

Citrusy Smooth Face Cream, 308
Classic Anti-Corn-and-Callus Concoction, 289
Clean and Soft Facial Scrub, 256
Clothing, as remedy, 160, 165, 173, 275
Clover Tea, Anti-Arthritis, 14
Cloves, 77, 247
Club soda, 332
Clutter, in bedroom, 222
Coffee. *See also* Caffeine
  arthritis and, 16
  for bloating, 34
  body odor and, 273
  for cellulite, 281
  for hair care, 330
  indigestion and, 159
Cognitive therapy, 10
Cola, 159, 197
Cold Cream, Homemade, 313
Cold (and Vampire!) Repellent, 57
Colds, 56–69
  vs. allergies, 5
  Appalachian remedies for, 69
  avoiding, 59, 66
  chicken soup for, 68
  Cold (and Vampire!) Repellent for, 57
  Crooner's Delight for, 58
  dairy products and, 64
  doctor needed for, 56
  Echinacea Tincture for, 59
  Essential Oil Solution for, 60
  foot rub for, 63
  garlic for, 58, 59, 61
  Ginger-Cinnamon Tea for, 61
  ginger for, 63
  Herbal-Oil Rub for, 63

Neck wraps and compresses, 58, 62
Neem, 216
Nettles, 204
No, No Nosebleed Tonic, 201
Noggin Massage, 334
Nonsteroidal anti-inflamma- tory drugs (NSAIDs), 14
Nosebleeds, 201–202
Nose blowing, 67, 201
NSAIDs, 14
Nutrition. *See* Diet and eating habits
Nutty Facial Scrub, 318
Nutty Sipper, 71

O

Oatmeal baths, 169, 219, 245
Oatmeal Scrub, 301
Oats
  for dry skin, 301
  for facial care, 321, 323
  for hair care, 333
  Oatmeal Scrub, 301
Oat straw, 117
Odor-Killing Herbal Swipe, 276
Oil Away Aches, 194
Oil's Well Wart Remover, 349
Old-Time Cough Stopper, 81
Old-Time Mustard Plaster, 68
Old-Time Tummy Tamer, 199
Olive oil
  for brain function, 43
  caution, 71
  for constipation, 71
  for facial care, 319, 323
  for hair care, 328
Olives, 197
Omega-3 fatty acids
  for acne, 255
  for anxiety, 10
  for brain function, 43

for depression, 86, 93
for dry skin, 294
for itches, 169, 170
for wrinkles, 351
Onion Poultice, 44
Onions, 36, 52, 63, 257
On-the-Spot Bleach, 260
Oral hygiene
  for bad breath, 262–266
  denture care, 247
  for gingivitis, 142–144
  tooth care, 247–250
Oranges, 232
Oregano, 46, 119, 131, 139
Osteoporosis, 203–204
Overweight, 17, 31, 33, 141

P

Pain-Away Spray, 227
Pain Be Gone Paste, 218
Painful intercourse, 205–206
Pain relievers
  for arthritis, 14, 20
  music and, 185
  Power-Packed Pain Reliever, 19
  for sunburn, 244
Pantothenic acid, 239
Papaya, 123, 151, 315
Papaya Acid Reflux Reducer, 3
Parsley, 162, 174, 263, 271
Passionflower, 9, 235
Peaches, 314
Peanut butter, 44
Peanut oil, 298, 312
Pennyroyal, 120
Pens, gripping, 17
Peppermint
  Aching-Muscle Magic, 179
  caution, 163
  for diarrhea, 98
  for fatigue, 118
  for headaches, 145

Make Mine Minty Bath Powder, 236
Mint Magic, 252
Minty Syrup Sweetener, 11
Minty Tea, 66
  for nausea, 200
Perfect Peppermint Toothpaste, 249
Perfumes, as allergen, 24
Peripheral vascular disease, 137
Petroleum jelly, 267, 337, 346
Pets, 225, 235, 286
Phone calls, fatigue and, 111
Photolyase, 244
Pica, 129
Pickles, 264
Pillows
  for acid reflux, 3
  back pain and, 29
  for coughs, 79
  headaches and, 145
  for hemorrhoids, 156
Pineapple, 123, 196
Pinkeye, 207–208
Plantar warts, 349
Pleasing Poppy Potion, 12
Plums, 50
Pneumonia, 44, 82
Podiatrists, 341
Pollen, as allergen, 5. *See also* Bee pollen
Pomegranate, 53
Poppy Potion, Pleasing, 12
Poppy Seed Paste, 158
Postnasal drip, 209–210
Potassium
  Back-in-Balance Bath, 182
  dandelion cautions and, 35, 70
  for fatigue, 109
  for heart health, 152
  sources of, 152
  for stroke prevention, 240